DEPRESSION AND PERSONALITY

Conceptual and Clinical Challenges

DEPRESSION AND PERSONALITY

Conceptual and Clinical Challenges

Edited by

Michael Rosenbluth, M.D.
Sidney H. Kennedy, M.D.
R. Michael Bagby, Ph.D.

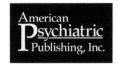

American Psychiatric Publishing, Inc.

Washington, DC
London, England

Manufactured in the United States of America on acid-free paper
09   08   07   06   05   5   4   3   2   1
First Edition

Typeset in Adobe's Palatino and Formata

American Psychiatric Publishing, Inc.
1000 Wilson Boulevard
Arlington, VA 22209-3901
www.appi.org

Library of Congress Cataloging-in-Publication Data
Rosenbluth, Michael.
    Depression and personality : conceptual and clinical challenges / edited by Michael Rosenbluth, Sidney H. Kennedy, R. Michael Bagby. -- 1st ed.
        p. ; cm.
    Includes bibliographical references and index.
    ISBN 1-58562-154-4 (pbk. : alk. paper)
    1. Depression, Mental. 2. Personality. 3. Personality disorders.
    I. Rosenbluth, Michael. II. Kennedy, Sidney H. III. Bagby, R. Michael. IV. Title.
    [DNLM: 1. Depressive Disorder. 2. Personality Disorder. 3. Personality.
WM 171 R8135d 2005]
RC537.R6383 2005
616.85'27--dc22   2005002351

British Library Cataloguing in Publication Data
A CIP record is available from the British Library.

CONTENTS

CONTRIBUTORS ix

PREFACE. xiii

Hagop S. Akiskal, M.D.

INTRODUCTION................................. xvii

Michael Rosenbluth, M.D.
Sidney H. Kennedy, M.D.
R. Michael Bagby, Ph.D.

PART   I

CONCEPTUAL ISSUES

1 PERSONALITY AND TEMPERAMENT:
HISTORICAL PERSPECTIVES 3

Jerome Kagan, Ph.D.

2 THE PSYCHOBIOLOGY OF PERSONALITY DISORDERS... 19

Kurtis L. Noblett, Ph.D.
Emil F. Coccaro, M.D.

3 PERSONALITY TRAITS/DISORDERS AND
DEPRESSION: A SUMMARY OF CONCEPTUAL
AND EMPIRICAL FINDINGS 43

M. Tracie Shea, Ph.D.
Shirley Yen, Ph.D.

4 THE DEPRESSIVE PERSONALITY:
PSYCHOPATHOLOGY, ASSESSMENT,
AND TREATMENT 65

Andrew G. Ryder, Ph.D.
R. Michael Bagby, Ph.D.
Margarita B. Marshall, B.Sc.
Paul T. Costa Jr., Ph.D.

P A R T   I I

TREATMENT IMPLICATIONS

5 THE IMPACT OF PERSONALITY ON THE
PHARMACOLOGICAL TREATMENT OF DEPRESSION 97

Sidney H. Kennedy, M.D.
Peter Farvolden, Ph.D.
Nicole L. Cohen, M.A.
R. Michael Bagby, Ph.D.
Paul T. Costa Jr., Ph.D.

6 CLINICAL STRATEGIES FOR EFFICIENT
TREATMENT OF MAJOR DEPRESSIVE DISORDER
COMPLICATED BY PERSONALITY DISORDER. 121

Ari Zaretsky, M.D.
Michael Rosenbluth, M.D.
Daniel Silver, M.D.

7 REFRACTORY AND CHRONIC DEPRESSION:
THE ROLE OF AXIS II DISORDERS IN
ASSESSMENT AND TREATMENT 157

Robert H. Howland, M.D.
Michael E. Thase, M.D.

8 BIPOLAR DISORDER AND PERSONALITY:
CONSTRUCTS, FINDINGS, AND CHALLENGES 187

Peter Bieling, Ph.D.
Glenda MacQueen, M.D., Ph.D.

9 EVALUATING THE CONTRIBUTION OF PERSONALITY
FACTORS TO DEPRESSED MOOD IN ADOLESCENTS:
CONCEPTUAL AND CLINICAL ISSUES 229

Darcy A. Santor, Ph.D.
Michael Rosenbluth, M.D.

10 THE IMPACT OF PERSONALITY DISORDERS
ON LATE-LIFE DEPRESSION 267

J.P. Cooper, M.D.
Alastair Flint, M.D.

INDEX 293

CONTRIBUTORS

Hagop S. Akiskal, M.D.
Professor of Psychiatry and Director, International Mood Center, University of California at San Diego and Veterans Affairs Hospital, San Diego, California

R. Michael Bagby, Ph.D.
Professor of Psychiatry, University of Toronto, and Director, Clinical Research, Centre for Addiction and Mental Health, Toronto, Ontario, Canada

Peter Bieling, Ph.D.
Mood Disorders Program, St. Joseph's Healthcare; Associate Professor, McMaster University, Hamilton, Ontario, Canada

Emil F. Coccaro, M.D.
Ellen C. Manning Professor and Chairman, Department of Psychiatry, Clinical Neuroscience and Psychopharmacology Research Unit, The University of Chicago, Chicago, Illinois

Nicole L. Cohen, M.A.
Ph.D. candidate, Department of Psychology, York University, Toronto, Ontario, Canada

J.P. Cooper, M.D.
Assistant Professor of Psychiatry, University of Toronto; Staff Psychiatrist, Geriatric Psychiatry Program, University Health Network; Toronto, Ontario, Canada

Paul T. Costa Jr., Ph.D.
Professor of Behavioral Biology and Psychiatry, The Johns Hopkins University Medical School, Baltimore, Maryland; Senior Investigator, Chief, Laboratory of Personality and Cognition, National Institutes of Health, Bethesda, Maryland

Peter Farvolden, Ph.D.
Assistant Professor of Psychiatry, University of Toronto; Research Scientist, Centre for Addiction and Mental Health, Toronto, Ontario, Canada

Alastair Flint, M.D.
Professor of Psychiatry, University of Toronto; Program Head, Geriatric Psychiatry, University Health Network, Toronto, Ontario, Canada

Robert H. Howland, M.D.
Associate Professor of Psychiatry, University of Pittsburgh Medical Center, Pittsburgh, Pennsylvania

Jerome Kagan, Ph.D.
Starch Professor of Psychology, Harvard University, Department of Psychology, Cambridge, Massachusetts

Sidney H. Kennedy, M.D.
Professor of Psychiatry, University of Toronto; Psychiatrist-in-Chief, University Health Network, Toronto, Ontario, Canada

Glenda MacQueen, M.D., Ph.D.
Mood Disorders Program, St. Joseph's Healthcare; Associate Professor, McMaster University, Hamilton, Ontario, Canada

Margarita B. Marshall, B.Sc.
Department of Psychology, McGill University, Montréal, Québec, Canada

Kurtis L. Noblett, Ph.D.
Research Fellow, Department of Psychiatry, Clinical Neuroscience and Psychopharmacology Research Unit, The University of Chicago, Chicago, Illinois

Michael Rosenbluth, M.D.
Assistant Professor of Psychiatry, University of Toronto; Director, Psychiatric Rehabilitation Treatment Program, Toronto East General Hospital, Toronto, Ontario, Canada

Andrew G. Ryder, Ph.D.
Assistant Professor, Department of Psychology, Concordia University, Montréal, Quebec, Canada

Darcy A. Santor, Ph.D.
Associate Professor of Psychology, Dalhousie University, Halifax, Nova Scotia, Canada

M. Tracie Shea, Ph.D.
Associate Professor of Psychiatry, Department of Psychiatry and Human Behavior, Brown University Medical School, Veterans Affairs Medical Center, Providence, Rhode Island

Daniel Silver, M.D.
Associate Professor of Psychiatry, University of Toronto, Toronto, Ontario, Canada; Staff Psychiatrist, Mount Sinai Hospital, Toronto, Ontario, Canada

Michael E. Thase, M.D.
Professor of Psychiatry, University of Pittsburgh Medical Center, Pittsburgh, Pennsylvania

Shirley Yen, Ph.D.
Assistant Professor of Psychiatry, Department of Psychiatry and Human Behavior, Brown University Medical School, Providence, Rhode Island

Ari Zaretsky, M.D.
Assistant Professor of Psychiatry, University of Toronto, Toronto, Ontario, Canada; Head, Cognitive Behavior Therapy Clinic, Sunnybrook and Women's College Health Sciences Centre, Toronto, Ontario, Canada

PREFACE

The boundaries among temperament, character, personality, and personality disorder are not clearly demarcated. If one adheres to the DSM-IV-TR definition of Axis II, it is obvious that *personality disorder* refers to abnormal behavior in the interpersonal domain and hence pathology that should be in a manual for mental disorders. This book then is about how Axis II pathologies relate to mood disorders.

Whereas it is customary to say in erudite scientific articles that personality can precede, modify, or complicate mood disorders, it is difficult to say the same with any certainty about personality disorders. This is so because nearly always the diagnosis of a personality disorder is given when the clinician meets the patient in an affective episode. On paper, according to DSM-IV-TR rules, one must not diagnose a personality disorder before giving the Axis I disorder a chance to resolve. Unfortunately, many clinicians are tempted to diagnose a personality disorder during symptomatic phases of affective illness. This diagnosis may be made in the spirit of using all relevant axes of DSM-IV-TR to provide an understanding of the patient in a multidimensional model, or often it reflects a premature opinion about the presence of a personality malfunction underlying the persistence of the affective illness.

As a clinician, I am well aware of the complexities posed by the foregoing clinical scenarios. I appreciate the invitation to write this Preface, especially because the distinguished editors know quite well from our numerous past encounters, both in Canada and the United States, that I write on this topic not just from a position of research but from that of having seen a considerable number of such patients followed prospectively in mood clinics. Although personality disorders do not always recede when one clinically manages the affective illness, in my clinical experience, *the patient is generally better served if characterological manifestations are viewed as an integral part of the affective illness.*

Two main lines of observations have led me to the foregoing conclusion. The first is that the most common characterological diagnoses given to the affectively ill (e.g., dependent, masochistic, obsessive, narcissistic, and borderline) were shown by me, my colleagues, and others to have the same *sleep neurophysiological abnormalities* (e.g., shortened REM latency) that one observes in affective illness in its neurotic, atypical, and endogenous forms. More important, through applying the art of *psychopharmacotherapy*, it has been possible to attenuate or even reverse characterological ills. Obviously, such results can be enhanced with practical psychosocial interventions. I also note that social interventions, which are relatively neglected in the current therapy scene, in my experience are far more important than psychological issues per se.

Is this model simplistic? Exaggerated? Biased? What I have outlined is what I teach in practice. It works more often than it fails. The success of the professed clinical approach depends on whether one believes in it—and is not discouraged and derailed by theoretical distractions. The first task is to get the patient well in regard to the mood disorder. Associated personality problems will gradually come under control, and one has to take a long-term perspective on this. As we understand them today, depressive and bipolar disorders are chronically relapsing diseases. The application of this long-term view is insufficiently emphasized in the relatively short curriculum of our trainees.

I also wish to emphasize that DSM-IV-TR Axis II focuses on what is wrong with the patient's character. Thus, it is very important to obtain information from significant others about the patient's antecedent temperament with all its liabilities and assets. It is far easier to help affectively ill patients by enhancing their past assets and achievements than by focusing on current interpersonal pathology. I am particularly critical of the notion that patients who do not get well are somehow "resisting" because they benefit from being ill, or that it is "easier" to be ill than to be well, or that they want to frustrate their doctors. True, affectively ill patients often harbor self-defeating thoughts, but in practice these are best regarded as being an integral part of the illness. As a field, we need to graduate to a new era in which we *help patients maximize their personal assets to overcome their illness instead of blaming their character.*

What I think as a clinical scientist about the relationships between temperament, character, personality, and personality disorder is far more complex than what I have outlined in this Preface. But intricacies of scientific methodology and the various conceptual frameworks bearing on them are not immediately relevant to patient care. For this reason, I have avoided boring readers with these intricacies and, instead, have provided what I as a physician and a clinician believe works best.

The reader of this book will find expressions of this as well as alternative positions. It is ultimately the clinician who will choose what approach is best for his or her patients.

Temperamental issues are far more complex when it comes to bipolar disorder. This is a fascinating area that more eloquently highlights the importance of capitalizing on patients' assets. This is not to say that their liabilities are minor. The therapeutic challenges involving their characterological peculiarities are often formidable. Although much ingenuity has gone into recent publications on this subject by research psychiatrists and psychologists, in the end it is the clinician's art and human qualities that will be decisive in obtaining favorable outcomes. But such art cannot bypass the increasingly complex science of mood stabilizers. My point is that, as in the case of depressive illness, pharmacotherapy of bipolar disorder can often achieve good functional outcomes in both the *trait* and the *episode* domains. The most dramatic example of this outcome is that we have recently obtained long-term and full remission of severe borderline personality disorder among several bipolar II, or "soft," bipolar patients treated with lamotrigine. The bottom line is that the clinician must refrain from condemning affectively ill patients to Axis II diagnoses.

The invoking of biological processes for affective illness and of psychological constructs for personality and personality disorder is not founded in fact. Etiology is multifactorial for each. It may therefore be useful to think of pathological personality traits as subthreshold protracted states or episodes that permit only short remissions and eventually coalesce into chronicity. The genetics of traits and affective episodes has provided data in support of such a model. The best example perhaps is the shared familial-genetic factors between neuroticism and depressive illness. Concerning a point that I made earlier on the basis of clinical experience, such science strongly concurs in favoring the view that in many instances characterological manifestations are very much part of affective illness and that it is heuristic to conceptualize them as intimately interwoven in both pathogenesis and the recovery process.

Hagop S. Akiskal, M.D.
Professor of Psychiatry and Director of the International
Mood Center, University of California at San Diego and
Veterans Affairs Hospital, San Diego, California

INTRODUCTION

In the Preface, Dr. Akiskal notes that the patient with presumed personality disorder is better served if characterological manifestations are viewed as an integral part of the affective illness. He finds it clinically useful to think of pathological personality traits as "subthreshold protracted states or episodes that permit only short remissions and eventually coalesce into chronicity."

We agree that clearly there is value in emphasizing the robust treatment of affective illness. However, we also believe that a careful and detailed review of where we are with regard to understanding the relationship between personality dimensions, disorders, and affective disorder is important for clinicians working with these patients.

This book brings together contributors who can help clinicians and researchers in the field understand this issue by their review of the historical antecedents, neurobiological dimensions, and conceptual models regarding the relationship between personality and depression.

Subsequent chapters discuss the impact of personality on pharmacotherapy and review assessment and therapy issues in working with the personality disorder patient with comorbid depression, chronic depression, bipolar disorder, and issues particular to this topic in the adolescent and geriatric populations. This book also attempts to clarify issues regarding depressive personality from a dimensional and categorical perspective.

In Chapter 1, Dr. Kagan provides a valuable historical perspective on the evolution of personality from "humors" to body constitution and temperament. Dr. Kagan defines *temperament* as "stable sets of behavioral and emotional reactions that appear early in life and are influenced in part by the child's genome." He contrasts the temperamental dimensions of Thomas and Chess's descriptions of "easy," "slow-to-warm-up," and "difficult" children that reflect interviews with parents with the "Big Five" personality dimensions described by McCrae and Costa. He challenges the validity of the five-factor model on the basis of self-report and lack of objective validation, an issue that is addressed by Dr. Ryder and colleagues in Chapter 4.

Dr. Kagan describes the role of cultural setting in the salience of a trait; the critical interaction between temperamental bias and subsequent social experience; and the recognition of the indeterminate relations among brain states, conscious feelings, beliefs, and behaviors. He looks forward to further integration of biology, behavioral observations, phenomenological report, and social context to provide new conceptual schemata to understand human behavior and illness. His observations invite clinicians to assess and factor into treatment considerations regarding the patient's temperament.

In Chapter 2, Drs. Noblett and Coccaro present evidence to support neurobiological dimensions of personality. Focusing on affect-related traits, they review the evidence for serotonin (5-HT) and norepinephrine disturbance based on challenge paradigms. They also point out links between hypercortisolism and sustained childhood abuse in patients with borderline personality disorder. This is an area of increasing importance in understanding potential differences among subpopulations of depressed patients. These neurotransmitter disturbances have been used to provide evidence to support the use of antidepressant and mood-stabilizing anticonvulsant medications in populations with personality disorder.

The authors also highlight the impulsivity/aggression dimension and its neurobiological links to 5-HT. This issue has received further support from neuroimaging studies, leading the authors to suggest that different serotonergically linked anatomical pathways may be involved in depression and personality disorders such as antisocial personality disorder. They conclude that promising etiological findings, although helping to define dimensions of affective instability, impulsivity, and anxiety, have not yet had a substantial impact on pharmacotherapy selection.

The authors encourage clinicians to appreciate the complex interplay of state-versus-trait variables in formulating diagnoses and treatment plans. They also encourage clinicians to appreciate the nuances and limitations of conventional pharmacotherapy within the context of personality comorbidity.

In Chapter 3, Drs. Shea and Yen describe the range of models used to understand the interrelationship between personality and depression. These include independence, pathoplasty, common cause, predisposition or vulnerability, and complication or scar hypotheses. The authors explore the stress-diathesis model, based on "sociotropy/dependency" and "autonomy/self-criticism," which borrows from both cognitive and psychoanalytic literatures. They also explore the "positive-and-negative-affect" model, which is closely allied to extraversion and neuroticism dimensions and forms the basis for the tripartite model of Clark and Watson.

Drs. Shea and Yen also review the literature on how these models apply to clinical populations and conclude that the neuroticism/negative affect construct has the strongest association with depression as a vulnerability but not as a complicating or scar factor. They briefly consider the neurobiological model of Cloninger, who has defined *harm avoidance, reward dependence,* and *novelty seeking* in terms of their postulated relationship to neurotransmitter systems. The authors bring this theoretical discussion to a practical level as they explore the historical recognition by clinicians of personality contributions to depression under terms such as *neurotic depression, depression spectrum disease,* and *subaffective dysthymic disorder.* They also point out the ubiquitous nature of neuroticism and its lack of specificity as a risk factor for depression, and that neuroticism may also predispose patients to anxiety and substance abuse disorders. The authors also view Axis II disorders as vulnerabilities to some Axis I disorders.

In Chapter 4, Dr. Ryder and colleagues discuss the justification for depressive personality in categorical and dimensional terms as an addition to the diagnostic armamentarium of DSM-IV-TR, tracing the debate from Kraepelin's depressive temperament to the contributions of Schneider and Akiskal.

The perceived gap in our current diagnostic system relates to the inclusion of dysthymic disorder as an Axis I diagnosis that requires somatic symptoms, meaning that there is no current diagnostic category for an individual who displays depressive traits in the absence of somatic symptoms. The authors caution, however, that overlap between depressive personality disorder and Cluster C personality disorders is approximately 50%, limiting support for including depressive personality disorder (DPD) as an additional Axis II disorder.

With regard to a dimensional approach, the authors focus on the five-factor model to provide a link between several facets of neuroticism and DPD. They cite evidence to show that harm avoidance is higher in DPD compared with major depressive disorder (MDD) or dysthymic disorder. They also offer some clinically useful ways to distinguish between DPD and avoidant, dependent, or obsessive-compulsive personality disorders or dysthymic disorder. The growth of research in this field has been hindered by the limited availability of valid, easily administered measures. The authors recommend several DSM-IV-TR Axis II instruments that have been modified to detect DPD as well as two instruments developed by Gunderson and by Huprich specifically to detect DPD.

In the absence of research findings on treatment, Dr. Ryder and colleagues can only speculate on the choice of psychotherapies. They suggest that cognitive-behavioral analysis system psychotherapy might help, as might cognitive-behavioral approaches tailored to specific DPD traits. However, they point out that any therapeutic approach should also consider the strengths and overall context in which DPD traits occur within the individual. The authors note that although there have been no pharmacotherapy studies, DPD traits are predictive of a negative outcome to pharmacotherapy when they coexist with MDD. This may imply that the patient with chronic low-grade depression who meets criteria for dysthymic disorder is more likely to respond to pharmacotherapy than the patient with DPD.

In Chapter 5, Dr. Kennedy and colleagues explore the impact of personality on various aspects of treatment. Their main thesis is that individual differences have tended to be neglected during the evaluation of treatment outcomes for depression, particularly in the pharmacotherapy literature. The authors examine six aspects of treatment, beginning with help seeking, in which they cite evidence that men with low neuroticism and an external attributional style are less likely to seek treatment. They note that individual personality differences may also influence symptom presentation. On the basis of Cloninger's temperament and character model of personality, individuals with high levels of harm avoidance are likely to display greater symptom severity; those with high levels of novelty seeking have greater likelihood of suicide attempts and alcohol use; and those with a combination of high harm avoidance and high novelty seeking are associated with admission to a hospital. The authors briefly explore the relevance of personality measures in treatment selection between pharmacotherapy and psychotherapy when individuals had an option to choose. The data are limited, but no evidence was found to support personality variables influencing treatment selection. With respect to compliance, there is evidence to suggest that high levels of neuroticism increase side-effect reporting, irrespective of treatment, whereas high levels of extraversion or novelty seeking may be associated with early improvement and subsequent medication discontinuation.

Treatment outcome is examined from both dimensional and categorical perspectives. Conventional wisdom has tended to suggest that patients who have been diagnosed with comorbid personality disorder and MDD are likely to have a worse outcome than those with MDD in the absence of an Axis II diagnosis. However, this is not always the case. For example, Fava and colleagues showed that Cluster B diagnoses were associated with a more favorable antidepressant response. At the dimensional level, most emphasis has been on examining neuroticism and extraversion as predictors of outcome. The conclusion from Mulder and colleagues in New Zealand is particularly pertinent here: In the best-designed studies, personality pathology had the least impact on outcome. This group has also examined a related question: Do personality variables influence specific pharmacotherapy responses? The group initially reported differences between response to clomipramine and desipramine on the basis of personality measures. For example, women with high levels of reward dependence were more likely to respond to the serotonergic tricyclic antidepressant clomipramine than to the noradrenergic tricyclic antidepressant desipramine. Subsequently, Mulder and his group explored predictors of response to fluoxetine compared with nortriptyline and showed that patients with a Cluster B personality disorder who received nortriptyline demonstrated significantly less improvement. This did not apply to fluoxetine. It is also noted that dimensional influences on response to specific antidepressants have not been replicated.

The authors conclude that personality pathology, whether assessed in terms of dimension or disorders, can affect the patient's capacity to seek, be engaged in, or be compliant with treatment. They emphasize that clarifying maladaptive attributional styles, helping patients overcome denial of their depression, and avoiding an overemphasis on side effects may all have a beneficial effect on treatment.

In Chapter 6, Dr. Zaretsky and colleagues outline key assessment and treatment issues that are expanded on in Chapters 7–10 with more reference to refractory depression, bipolar disorder, and the adolescent and the elderly patient.

The authors indicate that although mood disorders with comorbid personality disorders have been traditionally associated with a poor prognosis, recent research suggests that such therapeutic nihilism is not warranted. They advocate a multimodal-phased treatment approach that involves targeted pharmacotherapy and integrative individual psychotherapy.

The authors note that optimal treatment of depressed patients with Axis II comorbidity requires different modalities that extend beyond pharmacotherapy and individual psychotherapy, including group therapy, family psychoeducation therapy, and occupational therapy. A thorough assessment that includes the use of rating scales is advocated.

They note that patients with Axis II conditions are different from patients with Axis I conditions in that even when they are not severely depressed, they still experience high activation of negative cognitive schemas that constantly filter and distort information processing such that positive experiences are ignored or minimized and negative experiences are magnified and attended to.

With regard to pharmacotherapy, the authors note that it is important for the clinician and patient to have a mutual understanding regarding the role of medication when working with patients with borderline or other personality disorders who have Axis I issues. The authors also note that exploring the patient's experience and perception of medication is critical and that reviewing ambivalence and maladaptive attitudes about medication will improve adherence to a medication plan. They note the importance of reviewing the past history of medication trials as well as clarifying which medications have been used, their mechanism of action, and the degree of response and the reason medication was stopped (i.e., side effects or nonresponse).

The authors note that patients with both Axis I and Axis II disorders may require not only a maximum dose of medication but also a longer trial before switching medications. They emphasize that once a patient has responded to medication, it is important to empower the patient by ensuring that he or she, not the medications, gets the credit for the changes that have occurred. They note that it is important to emphasize that the pills allowed the patient to handle specific stressful situations and function in spite of the difficulties that were encountered.

The psychotherapeutic emphasis is on skill acquisition, structured treatment, and helping patients handle affect dysregulation and multiple crises. The treatment approach emphasizes understanding vulnerability and nurturing strengths. The important role of the therapist is to help the patient see the positive changes that are occurring as treatment unfolds and to be explicit about the nature of the change. The authors note that optimizing the pharmacotherapy of the Axis I disorder allows further attention to be paid to treating the comorbid personality disorder. Restructuring the concomitant core beliefs associated with the personality problems may facilitate relapse prevention.

In Chapter 7, Drs. Howland and Thase consider the role of personality disorder in the assessment and treatment of chronic depression. They note the mixed literature regarding whether personality disorders diminish outcome in depressive disorders and note that there is no consistent finding regarding specific dimension variables predicting the response to antidepressants. They call for research into whether personality disorder traits modify the response to cognitive therapy or to interpersonal psychotherapy and whether modifications of these therapies tailored to comorbid personality psychopathology are more effective.

Although noting that personality disorders appear more prevalent in patients with various forms of chronic depression, they advise that personality disorder diagnoses may be less valid when people have been depressed for many years. They present an interesting overview of biopsychosocial factors regarding how personality may alter antidepressant effects, including decreasing social supports, contributing to stressful life events, and medication nonadherence.

With regard to assessment and treatment, they emphasize a comprehensive assessment of Axis I comorbid disorders. A longitudinal history from patient and collateral sources regarding premorbid psychosocial functioning and traits and review of prior response to medication and psychotherapy is called for. They caution that the collateral history may be colored by assortative mating issues. Also, the negative effects of the patient's depression on the quality of life of the collateral source can color the perception and description of premorbid personality. Practical, individually tailored therapy strategies are called for. The importance of the therapist and patient reaching agreement on goals and strategies is noted. The authors provide a concise and practical overview of medication and psychotherapy issues regarding the role of Axis II disorders in the treatment of chronic depression.

In Chapter 8, Drs. Bieling and MacQueen address the complex relationships between bipolar disorder and personality factors by reviewing clinical and conceptual issues related to the comorbidity of bipolar and Axis II factors, the personality-bipolar continuum, the bipolar/borderline personality disorder spectrum, temperament and trait markers of bipolar disorder, and treatment implications of personality factors and bipolar disorder.

The authors outline methodological problems and suggest that clinicians be vigilant regarding the presence of comorbid personality disorder in patients with bipolar disorder, especially in the presence of refractory symptoms. They explain that comorbid personality disorder is common in patients with bipolar disorder (up to 45%) and note that patients with multiple episodes appear to have increased personality disorder as a reaction to the multiple episodes. The controversies in the area of bipolar spectrum disorder are outlined. Concerns are expressed regarding denying a clear distinction between temperament and illness as well as regarding the possibility of misidentifying a group of individuals whose temperamental characteristics did not warrant aggressive intervention with pharmacological agents whose safety has not been established for each developmental period. (This refers to the controversy about using antidepressants in the adolescent patient, which is discussed in Chapter 9.)

While reviewing the relationship between bipolar disorder and borderline personality disorder, the authors conclude that it is still necessary to use different sets of terms for bipolar and borderline personality disorder. They note that those who view patients with borderline personality disorder as having a form of mood disorder are concerned that such patients may be undertreated with medication and stigmatized if labeled as having a character disorder. Those who believe that borderline personality disorder is a valid clinical entity believe that considering this disorder as a mood disorder will lead to undertreatment with psychosocial interventions.

The authors call for research involving a more longitudinal approach, either in a large population or in a sample of high-risk participants, to clarify the predictive value of personality traits in bipolar disorder and to explore the extent that temperament variables of all kinds (not only "bipolar" temperament) are associated with bipolar disorder. They note the importance of the issue of personality disorders and traits on outcome in bipolar disorder but note that there are very few studies that have systematically examined the issue.

They conclude that clinicians must be comfortable assessing and managing personality disorders because these occur frequently in patients with mood disorders. They note that maladaptive personality features may significantly influence treatment outcome through the development of therapeutic alliance, adherence to treatment, and the type and efficacy of psychotherapy and pharmacotherapy.

In Chapter 9, Drs. Santor and Rosenbluth review the complexity involved in adolescent depression with personality disorder. They provide a conceptual framework for understanding what factors of personality contribute to vulnerability for depression in adolescents. Issues related to tendencies versus characteristics, exogenous risk factors, and endogenous factors are discussed. Biopsychosocial factors including biology and temperament, familial environment, and childhood adverse events and their interplay are noted. Cognitive vulnerabilities including attribution style and schema containing predisposing attitudes and dysfunctional beliefs are described, with an emphasis on how individuals explain the occurrence of bad events and the vulnerability for depressive symptoms.

The authors clarify key concepts in understanding the complexity and the interaction of personality, developmental stage, and depressive symptoms. Clinically, agreeing with the assessment guidelines described in Chapters 6 and 7, they emphasize the importance of deferring personality assessment until after the patient has recovered from his or her depression, of asking the patient to describe his or her personality before the onset of the depressive illness, and of obtaining collateral history. Because obtaining a longitudinal history is relatively limited in adolescents (vs. in adults and the elderly), the authors emphasize careful review of family and school functioning. They provide an overview of key assessment and treatment issues, emphasizing robust treatment of all Axis I disorders, practical approaches to psychotherapy, and consideration of the use of antidepressants in depressed adolescents in the post-FDA warning era.

In Chapter 10, Drs. Cooper and Flint outline difficulties conceptually and clinically in considering the impact of personality disorder on depression in late life. Agreeing with the emphasis in previous chapters, they emphasize the importance of a longitudinal view. However, in the elderly, they advocate a decade-by-decade review of behavior to determine whether current behavior is of long-standing origin (Axis II) or is related to Axis I disorders such as chronic depression, organic brain changes, or age-related life events. Dramatic behaviors may decrease with age and be replaced with somatic complaints, depressive withdrawal, and/or aberrant family interactions. They raise questions about the effects of chronic or recurrent depression on personality, referring to the scar hypothesis noted by Drs. Shea and Yen in Chapter 3.

The authors emphasize the importance of obtaining relevant history and current mental status; assessing physical health; and providing feedback to the patient, family, and caregivers to assist in management. They advocate vigorous treatment, noting that the combination of personality disorder and depression, especially in late life, may diminish the chances of patients receiving adequate treatment trials—an observation that agrees with comments expressed in earlier chapters.

They note that age per se is not a contraindication to psychotherapy and emphasize the fit between the patient's needs and capacities and the mode of therapy. They conclude that more studies are required to clarify treatment issues because of the complexity of biopsychosocial factors in the depressed elderly with a personality disorder. They conclude that unless there is evidence to the contrary, the presence of a personality disorder in the depressed elderly should not affect therapeutic optimism. Issues more particular to the elderly include the role of physical illness and organic factors in the clinical presentation of personality and affective disorders.

This book emphasizes the importance of understanding the relationship between personality dimensions, personality disorders, and mood disorder. A clear view of the conceptual issues allows for careful consideration of assessment and treatment issues. Considering the impact of personality on mood disorders allows for more robust and strategic use of both psychotherapy and pharmacotherapy to optimize treatment outcomes.

Michael Rosenbluth, M.D.
Sidney H. Kennedy, M.D.
R. Michael Bagby, Ph.D.
Toronto, Ontario, Canada

PART I

CONCEPTUAL ISSUES

PERSONALITY AND TEMPERAMENT

Historical Perspectives

Jerome Kagan, Ph.D.

Definitional Issues

An essay charting the history of the concepts *personality* and *temperament* must first attend to definitions because meanings change over time. No nineteenth-century scholar would have predicted that the primary referent for the word *inhibition* would change from a desirable brain state that mediated adaptive behavior to children who were consistently shy and timid (Kagan 1994).

Personality has had three different definitions in Western writings over the last 2,000 years. The earliest conception referred to distinct types of psychological profiles that were caused, in part, by a particular balance among the biological substances blood, phlegm, and yellow and black bile. The balance among these "four humors," which was always monitored by diet and climate, created a set of distinct personality types. Galen called four of these types *sanguine, melancholic, phlegmatic, and choleric* (Siegel 1968).

The ancient Chinese, by contrast, assumed a balance among types of energy rather than bodily humors. Because energy was always changing, a person's moods and behaviors could not be permanent; therefore, the Chinese were less interested than the Greeks in positing personality types (Yosida 1973).

The Arabs, who dominated North Africa and the Middle East in the seventh century, translated Galen's writings and adopted his ideas with minimal alteration. An eleventh-century Islamic physician, Ibn Ridwan, attributed the impulsivity and timidity of Egyptians to an unhealthy balance among the humors that was traceable to the humid, hot climate of the Nile (Dols 1984). Even Kant accepted Galen's four types, although he distinguished between emotion and behavior because he recognized the imperfect relation between private processes and overt action. Kant was certain humans possessed a will that could control behaviors urged on by strong desire or emotion. Nineteenth-century commentators saw the wisdom in Kant's ideas and contrasted temperament with character. The former was the result of inherited emotional biases; the latter referred to behaviors that were a function of both temperament and experience.

Nineteenth-century commentators also moved the material cause of a personality type from blood, phlegm, and bile to the brain. Franz Gall (1835) incurred the anger of segments of his community when he suggested that a personality type was caused by a profile of brain tissue that could be measured by examining the skull. Spurzheim (1834), impressed with Gall's ideas, suggested that there was a location in the brain for each primary human trait and, reflecting the prejudices of his time, assigned more space in the cranium to emotional than to intellectual processes. For reasons that seem bizarre to modern readers, Spurzheim located love in the cerebellum, aggression in the temporal lobe, and timidity in the parietal cortex.

As the nineteenth century ended, there was an expansion in the number of physical features that revealed personality. The shape of the body and face and the color of eyes, hair, and skin were believed to be associated with particular personal qualities. George Draper (1924), a physician at Columbia University, noting that some body types were especially vulnerable to contracting polio during an epidemic, suggested that there was an association between certain body constitutions and particular diseases. He observed that people with brown eyes seemed more likely to have ulcers and gallbladder problems, whereas those with blue eyes seemed to be more at risk for tuberculosis. It is of interest that Hippocrates also believed that tall, thin adults were especially vulnerable to diseases of the lungs. Both Lombroso (1911) and Kretschmer (1925) suggested associations between body type and crime or mental illness. Kretschmer believed that people who suffered from schizophrenia were often tall, thin, narrow-faced asthenic individuals, whereas those who were diagnosed as manic depressive were likely to be chubby, broad-faced individuals with short, stout body types.

The Influence of Freud and Psychoanalytic Theory

These materialistic views, which ignored the role of social experiences, persisted in Europe and North America until the end of the nineteenth century when Freud made theoretically significant changes in the meaning of personality. The most important was his insistence that childhood experiences, rather than body chemistry or body type, were the bases for personality categories, and he invented terms like *hysterical, obsessive,* and *narcissistic* to name some basic personality types that were defined primarily by different socialization regimens (Freud 1933[1932]/1964). Like Galen, Freud assumed that his personality types were universally applicable. That is, he expected that the same personality profiles would emerge from a particular set of childhood experiences independent of cultural setting or historical era.

Freud substituted one substance, the energy of the libido, for the four Galenic humors and assumed a balance among the psychological processes he named *id, ego,* and *superego.* Freud located the libidinal energy in sexuality and accepted the view, popular at the time, that heredity influenced the amount of libido each person possessed. Psychological energy was not a completely novel notion. Nineteenth-century physicians had elaborated the ancient belief that energy level—called *vis nervosa*—was an inherited property and was less abundant in those who developed fears, depression, and *neurasthenia* (a term coined in 1869 by the neurologist Charles Beard, who theorized that individuals who experienced tension, depression, and insomnia were doing so because their brains had run out of energy [Gosling 1987)]). Even V.I. Lenin, one of the leaders of the Bolshevik revolution, received this diagnosis. Pavlov (1928) exploited these hypotheses to explain why some of the dogs in his laboratory conditioned easily, whereas others were resistant. Pavlov conjectured that the former group had a stronger nervous system with more energy than the latter.

The hypothesis that humans vary in psychological energy and therefore in strength of brain activity may seem odd to modern readers. However, norepinephrine, an important neurotransmitter in the sympathetic nervous system, maintains body temperature by producing energy through metabolism, and some contemporary theorists believe that depressive patients have lower levels of brain norepinephrine than nondepressive subjects.

Freud's views were popular in the United States for half a century, from 1910 to about 1960, but were celebrated with less enthusiasm in Europe because Freud implied that the proper arrangement of childhood experiences could create a maximally adaptive personality. This optimistic belief was more consonant with the egalitarian premises of most American psychiatrists and psychologists than with their European counterparts. Freud's conviction that acquiring insight into one's unconscious wishes would free a compromised ego appealed to Americans because it implied that psychic freedom was a seminal component of psychological health. The Freudian metaphor equated political liberty with the psychological state gained from releasing one's desires from the prison of repression.

Another reason for the receptivity of Freud's writings was that the presumed mechanisms of personality development applied to everyone, not just to those with psychiatric disability. Freud, and his supporters, persuaded many that because every individual is capable of feeling shame, guilt, or anxiety over sex or hostility, anyone could develop a phobia or obsession. Thus, a terror of leaving home and worry about a child's health could be derivatives of the same conflict. Psychoanalytic theory slowly turned minds away from a category of person who was especially vulnerable to acquiring a phobia to the idea of environmental experiences that produced anxiety. The adjective "anxious" or "fearful" became a continuous dimension on which any person could be placed. As a result, the earlier conception of a vulnerable individual was replaced with the notion of unusually stressful life experiences.

A metaphor of a bridge that collapses under a load captures the contrast. The traditional assumption had been that all bridges must carry loads of varying weight; hence, a bridge that collapsed under a load in the normal range must have been structurally weak in the first place. Freud argued that most of the time the collapse was caused by an unusually heavy load. For Freud, the psychological loads were childhood seduction, harsh socialization of hostility and sexuality, loss of a love object, and fear of parental anger.

The broadly based acceptance of the Freudian edifice by psychiatrists, psychologists, and educated citizens began to dissipate after World War II. One reason for this diminished acceptance was that historical events had led to a palpable decrease in the intensity of guilt and anxiety linked to sexual behaviors and intentions. Psychoanalytic theory would have predicted a significant decrease in anxious symptoms and a change in the distribution of personality types because repression of libidinal impulses was supposed to be the primary cause of the personality categories. The failure to validate that prediction led to a more critical attitude toward Freud's assertions.

A second reason can be traced to research with animals. The discovery that closely related strains of animals raised under identical laboratory conditions behaved differently to the same intrusions implied the operation of biological differences among strains. Scott and Fuller (1965) observed puppies from five different breeds at the secluded Jackson Laboratories in Bar Harbor, Maine. The five breeds differed dramatically in the degree of timidity displayed to unfamiliar events or people. Subsequent work revealed that mice, rats, wolves, cows, foxes, monkeys, birds, and even paradise fish differ within species in the tendency to approach or to avoid unfamiliarity (Wilson et al. 1994).

A final reason for the growing disenchantment with psychoanalytic theory was the increase, after 1950, in the number of younger psychologists joining university faculties. These younger scholars, trained in a positivistic tradition, were unfriendly to case studies and intuition as the bases for theoretical progress and filled the niche that Freudians had occupied. These scientists wished to use the objective tools and approaches of the natural sciences to infer personality types. This cohort of investigators decided that factor analyses of the questionnaire answers provided by large numbers of young adults—often middle-class, white college students—would reveal the fundamental dimensions, or categories, of personality.

The Emergence of Dimensional Perspectives

The personality dimensions inferred from this evidence, popularly called the Big Five, are *neuroticism* (a calm vs. a worried manner), *extraversion* (a socially avoidant vs. a sociable persona), *openness* (a conservative vs. a liberal ideology), *agreeableness* (an irritable vs. a good-natured manner), and *conscientiousness* (a careless vs. a reliable character) (McCrae and Costa 1987). Unfortunately, these bold psychologists failed to realize that the source of data influences the meaning of a scientific concept. The Big Five advocates assumed, without detailed argument, that a person's consciously given judgments about behaviors, beliefs, and moods were the most valid bases for inferring fundamental personality types. This claim is surprising.

It is surprising because no biologist would use the reports of informants to decide on the basic human diseases; no economist would rely only on interviews with consumers to discover the fundamental economic concepts; and no cognitive psychologist would analyze adults' descriptions of their perceptions, memories, and problem solutions to infer the basic cognitive competences. A different set of personality types would emerge if the subjects who had filled out the questionnaires had been observed directly in varied contexts and those observations had been factor analyzed. Also, a factor analysis of a dozen biological measurements gathered under varied conditions would reveal a third set of personality types. Further, there is usually a weak relation between a personality trait based on questionnaire data and theoretically related behavior or physiology. The most important critique of questionnaire evidence is that it reveals only a select set of properties available to conscious report and does not provide information on traits that are very private, unavailable to consciousness, or linked to physiological states. Thus, the Big Five personality dimensions represent a specific, and limited, answer to the question "What are the basic personality types?" even though this view dominates contemporary discussions of personality in American journals.

The Rise and Fall of Temperament

The term *temperament* refers to stable sets of behavioral and emotional reactions that appear early in life and are influenced, in part, by the child's genome (Kagan 1994). This meaning differs from that proposed by Galen, for whom personality and temperament were almost synonymous. A temperamental bias, like a genetically programmed motor circuit, can lead to a variety of behavioral outcomes. A child's culture selects the behaviors and moods that are desired and adaptive for that setting. Thus, a temperamental bias is only a potentiality because the child's experiences determine the personality profile that will be actualized. The journals of the writer John Cheever (1993), who died in the second half of the twentieth century, and the biography of William James's sister, Alice James (Strouse 1980), who died 100 years earlier, suggest that both inherited a very similar, if not identical, diathesis for a chronically dysthymic, melancholic mood. But Cheever, whose ideas about human nature were formed when Freudian theories were ascendant, assumed that his emotional life was caused by childhood experiences, and he tried to overcome the distress he believed that his family had created with drugs and psychotherapy. By contrast, Alice James believed, as did most of her contemporaries, that she inherited her dour mood, and she concluded, after trying baths and galvanic stimulation, that because she could not alter her heredity, she wished to die. The historical era in which these writers lived had a profound influence on their coping strategies and the quality of their emotional lives and, therefore, on their personality.

An infant born with a particular temperamental bias—for example, a high activity level—is embedded in a family context, and this combination creates the child's personality. The infant temperament is an intimate part of the school-age child's personality, but it cannot be observed as a separate component, even though scientists write about a temperamental bias as if it were an independent entity. A physical metaphor is helpful. A drop of black ink placed in a rotating cylinder of glycerin disappears into the clear liquid. The drop of black ink cannot be detected as an entity separate from the glycerin in which it is embodied.

Furthermore, *temperament* is defined currently in psychological terms, and therefore a description of a temperamental category or dimension is not equivalent to a description of the biological features that comprise its foundation. A description of the transparent property of a pane of glass is not equivalent to a description of the chemical structure of silica. This position is neither a defense of traditional mind-brain duality nor an attack on biological reduction. It simply states that all psychological phenomena, including personality and temperament, are emergent with respect to their underlying biological conditions.

Although temperamental concepts were popular in the nineteenth century and the first two decades of the twentieth century, they vanished suddenly in the 1930s as behaviorism came to dominate psychology departments and psychoanalysis found favor in departments of psychiatry. Two important reasons for the rejection of temperamental influences were Hitler's announcement that "Aryan" people were superior to others and America's need to assimilate large numbers of illiterate European immigrants living in urban slums. Both historical conditions motivated American scientists to minimize the contribution of biology to personality development.

An American psychiatrist or psychologist who would have suggested in the 1930s that inherited temperamental biases contributed to personality would be regarded as affirming a fascist philosophy. Ernst Hooton (1939), a Harvard anthropologist, wrote that some bodily constitutions were naturally inferior. This 1939 essay had a defensive tone because Hooton was aware that his views were unpopular among Americans.

The Reemergence of Temperament

A renascence of interest in temperament emerged in the 1960s following the creative work of Alexander Thomas and Stella Chess (1977, 1990). These New York psychiatrists used interviews with well-educated, professional parents to infer nine infant temperamental dimensions that they collapsed later into three abstract categories called the "easy," the "slow-to-warm-up," and the "difficult" child. It is probably not a coincidence that the two most extensively studied temperamental categories over the past two decades refer, on the one hand, to the shy, timid, inhibited child and, on the other, to the sociable, bold, uninhibited child (Kagan 1994). These two categories are analogous to Thomas and Chess's "slow-to-warm-up" versus "easy" child and to Galen's "melancholic" and "sanguine" types.

Thomas and Chess insisted on an interaction between the child's temperament and the environment and declared, wisely, that the personality that developed from the temperamental bias was dependent on the match between the infant's behaviors and the ideal the parent held for the child. Thomas and Chess affirmed that a temperamental bias represented a potential for an envelope of personality types that, although varied, was nonetheless limited. Some temperamental types could not develop particular personalities. Thomas and Chess acknowledged that the temperamental dimensions they inferred were a function of their evidence, namely, interviews with parents. It is not surprising that middle-class mothers describing their infants to an interviewer emphasized characteristics that made caregiving easy or difficult and that either conformed to or were inconsistent with the traits they hoped their children would acquire.

The ideas of Mary Rothbart (1989) have dominated the study of temperament over the last two decades. Rothbart, who relies on both parental reports and behavioral observations, suggested that *reactivity* and *regulation* are two significant temperamental biases in infants. *Reactivity* refers to the ease of arousal of motor, emotional, autonomic, and endocrine reactions. *Regulation* refers to processes that modulate reactivity, especially distribution of attention; approaching, withdrawing, or attacking an object or person; restraint; and self-soothing. One problem with this parsimonious solution is that an infant's level of reactivity depends on the nature of the arousing event and the response chosen to index it. Rothbart implies that infants who cry in response to the recording of a woman speaking sentences have the same level of reactivity as those who cry in response to a moving mobile because both were distressed by an external stimulus. However, the evidence reveals that infants who cry in response to a recording of a woman's voice without the visual support of a face are different behaviorally in the second and third years from infants who cry in response to a moving mobile but not to the taped voice (Kagan 1994). Thus, one serious problem with the concept of reactivity is an indifference to the nature of the incentive that produces the arousal.

The idea of self-regulation shares similar problems. First, if an infant does not cry or react behaviorally to a stranger, it is not possible to decide if the infant regulated his or her arousal well or was simply not aroused. Rothbart also fails to differentiate among the different forms of self-regulation. A 1-year-old child who shows a wary face to a stranger and then retreats may be different from one who also displays a wary face but does not retreat and subsequently vocalizes to the intruder. Most infants do something when aroused by an event; therefore, most regulate to varying degrees. It is important to accommodate to the specific incentive producing the reactivity and the specific regulatory behaviors that follow.

Neurochemistry and Temperament

It is likely that the biological bases for many, but certainly not all, temperamental categories rest with neurochemical profiles. There is heritable variation in the concentration of, and density and location of receptors for, the more than 100 different neurotransmitters that can affect brain function. This fact implies that there will be a large number of neurochemical profiles. Even if a majority of these profiles have little relevance for mood and behavior, given the extraordinarily large number, it is likely that human populations contain many temperaments, many more than the nine suggested by Thomas and Chess. Each temperament will rest on a neurochemistry that influences the child's usual psychological reaction to particular classes of events.

These transmitters and their receptors could affect the activity of neuronal ensembles in at least four different ways. A neuronal ensemble could secrete a greater amount of a neurotransmitter or modulator; it might have more receptors for a particular molecule; a second ensemble that projects to the one of interest might secrete more of a particular transmitter; or a second ensemble that modulates the one of interest could be inhibited by a third ensemble. Given the massive interconnectedness of the brain, it is reasonable to expect that there will be a large number of ways in which a particular neurochemistry could influence the emotional and behavioral patterns that define a temperament.

Temperamental Constraint

Longitudinal research on infants who possess temperamental categories distinguished by high and low reactivity to unfamiliar events reveals that an infant's temperament is more likely to constrain certain outcomes in adolescents rather than determine a particular personality trait. In one study (Kagan 1994), 4-month-old infants were classified as high reactive if they showed high levels of vigorous motor activity and distress to unfamiliar visual, auditory, or olfactory stimuli. In contrast, 4-month-old infants were classified as low reactive if they showed minimal motor activity and little distress to the same battery of events. It is presumed that these behavioral differences are the result of variations in the excitability of the amygdala and its projections. About one-third of the high-reactive infants preserved a timid, cautious personality and an expected biology through preadolescence, but very few of the high-reactive infants preserved a bold, sociable persona combined with low cortical and autonomic arousal through age 11 years. Similarly, about one-third of low-reactive infants preserved sociable, affectively spontaneous traits combined with low autonomic and cortical arousal, and very few developed the timid features of the high-reactive infant (Kagan 2002; Kagan and Snidman 2004). Thus, each temperamental bias eliminated many more psychological possibilities than it determined. A temperamental bias, therefore, resembles the basic form of a song that characterizes a particular bird species. The animal's genome constrains the song's architecture but does not determine all of its features, because the adult song depends on exposure to songs of conspecifics and the opportunity to hear its own sounds.

The same principle applies to environmental conditions. If all one knows about a sample of children is that they were born to economically secure, well-educated, nurturing parents, and if one must predict their adult psychological profile, the most accurate guesses will refer to the characteristics that will *not* be actualized, for example, criminality, homelessness, drug addiction, and poverty. However, predictions of the specific characteristics that *will* be part of the adult personality are less likely to be correct.

Combining Temperament and Personality

A personality type is a stable profile of behaviors, beliefs, and moods that differentiates one group of individuals from others in the same society. The assignment of an animal to a species shares features with the mission of the personality psychologist. The biologist takes into account the species' phylogenetic history, distinctive anatomical and physiological features, reproductive isolation from genetically related animals, and chance events. Analogously, a personality category is defined by the person's inherited and temperamental biases, past history, contemporaneous social contexts, and chance. Certain problems must be solved before scientists can create a more valid set of personality concepts. First, investigators must find fruitful ways to measure in adolescents and adults the psychological products of childhood histories and temperamental biases and, in addition, discover the historical factors that maintain, or alter, the profiles acquired during earlier development.

With the completion of the Human Genome Project, it is hoped that scientists will have something to say about the genetic contribution to temperament. These discoveries will be delayed, however, if the personality categories remain as heterogeneous as they are at the present time. It is not possible to discover the genetic contribution to a personality type if the category consists of genetically diverse individuals. Had medical investigators insisted on the unity of a disease category called "stomach aches," they would not have discovered the genetic contribution to bowel cancer. It is unlikely that a deeper understanding of adult personality will be gained if investigators continue to rely only on the evidence supplied by interviews and questionnaires.

How General Are Personality Types?

The influence of culture has been lost in the excitement over the elegant discoveries in molecular biology and neuroscience. The mood among scientists in these disciplines, as well as among the public, resembles the belief held 100 years earlier that genes were the only important influence on evolution and that local ecology and natural selection played a negligible role. Fortunately, biologists came to their senses by the late 1940s, and evolutionists such as Ernst Mayr argued, persuasively, that biologists had to combine mutations with selection to explain the distribution of animal forms. It is reasonable, therefore, to question the assumption held by both Galen and Freud that there is a basic set of personality types present in all cultures throughout history. It is unlikely, for example, that the major personality types present in nineteenth-century Swedish villages would be found in ancient Alexandria.

One reason for this claim is that human groups that have been reproductively isolated for long periods of time probably possess different genomes and therefore have different distributions of temperaments. Asians and Europeans represent two such isolated groups, and there are temperamental differences between infants born to parents from these two populations. For example, healthy infants born to Asian parents are less easily aroused by stimulation than those born to Caucasian parents (Freedman and Freedman 1969; Kagan et al. 1994).

Second, each society's geographical isolation from others, economic structure, and ethics can restrict or expand the range of variation in the behaviors and moods that define personality. Villages in rural Tibet, for example, limit seriously the opportunity for extreme levels of autonomy, achievement, and power. Therefore, there will be less variation in these traits in Tibet than in Europe and North America, and they will not be salient personality categories in the former location. If there is little variation in a quality within a society, it will not emerge as a personality type because the purpose of the type is to differentiate among individuals in a cultural setting.

In addition, individuals who are temperamentally vulnerable to high levels of anxiety but fortunate enough to live in a place with minimal threat and supportive groups will be less anxious than those individuals living in most urban settings. That is why patients with social phobia living in small towns are more likely to recover than those living in large cities. Criminality is overrepresented among adults who grew up in poor, less well educated families because of the effects of disadvantaged class status on beliefs and values. Analogously, a child with a low-reactive temperament is more likely to become a class leader if raised in a middle-class home in a neighborhood with well-socialized children and good schools than if raised in an urban slum by uneducated parents who do not socialize asocial behavior. The latter child is at higher risk for a criminal career. These facts imply that theories of personality should accommodate to the individual's historical and current social setting.

A comparison of European and Asian cultures in the eighteenth century, especially before Western influence, is illustrative. The individual is the primary social entity in European society of that era, and each person feels a moral imperative to attain salvation, accomplishment, wealth, or happiness on his or her own. By contrast, the imperative for Asian adults of that era is to seek harmony with, and become part of, a group. Each person's pride or shame rests on the success or failure of the groups of which he or she is, or was, a member and not only on his or her talent or perseverance. Both profiles are equipotential in the human genome.

This principle is supported by observations of animals. Young male elephants occasionally experience surges in male hormone that are accompanied by increased aggression and sexual behavior. This state, called *musth*, usually lasts for a few weeks. However, musth can last for 5 months if no adult males are present. When older males are introduced into such a group, the duration of the episode of musth is decreased dramatically (Slotow et al. 2000).

Theoretical and Referential Meanings

Contemporary scholarship on personality and temperament is divided into distinct research camps that rely on different methodologies. The largest group uses questionnaires or interviews as the sole source of evidence. The Big Five personality types are a product of this strategy. A smaller group adds behavioral observations and, on occasion, biological variables to the self-report information. The personality concepts derived from distinctly different sources of data may be incommensurable. That is, the meaning of the term *introvert* based on questionnaire data may be different from the meaning based on behavioral observations in diverse settings. Consider the Big Five personality construct called *neuroticism*. Individuals are classified as high in neuroticism if they admit on a questionnaire to chronic feelings of worry, concern, or anxiety, often combined with sadness or depression. However, investigators who remain loyal to Freudian ideas use the term *neurotic* as a hypothetical construct to explain compulsions or obsessions in individuals who might not report chronic feelings of worry, anxiety, or depression. Further, an unemployed high school dropout living in poverty who feels angry because of his current circumstances and poor life prospects would not be classified as high in neuroticism, even though some theorists might argue that the anger is a reaction to an unconscious feeling of vulnerability caused by a compromised sense of potency in the society. Moreover, a high or a low score on the personality dimension *neuroticism* is heterogeneous with respect to the individual's prior history, temperament, and context of action. If investigators possessed this information, they would have a deeper insight into the varied profiles of those classified as high in neuroticism from questionnaire evidence.

Current psychiatric categories for mental disorders are vulnerable to a similar critique because these categories are usually based on the patient's (or an informant's) descriptions of their behaviors and moods. Self-report evidence guarantees that patients in North America and Europe will emphasize their conscious feelings first because they are phenomenologically salient and second because many Western adults assume that their emotions are likely to be a primary cause of their symptoms. By contrast, many adults in India and China believe that the state of their body is the primary cause of symptoms and, as a result, report somatic disturbances such as tachycardia, headache, and muscle tension rather than their emotions. Both the judgment that one is anxious and somatic sensations are present in most patients with an anxiety disorder. Cultural beliefs determine which features are awarded salience and reported to therapists. An unpleasant feeling of distress is present in most human diseases, but it is usually epiphenomenal and not the primary cause for the illness—headache is an example.

A similar argument can be applied to depressive disorder. The central features leading to a diagnosis of depression are reports of feelings of sadness, apathy, sleeplessness, and poor appetite. If these symptoms occurred in a person who failed to meet an important personal standard for fidelity to a partner, the profile is more accurately classified as a guilt reaction. The same features reported by an adolescent who is pessimistic about his future because he lives in poverty with an alcoholic parent in rural Manitoba are more accurately classified as a state of hopelessness. Deep pessimism about one's future should be differentiated from guilt over failing a moral imperative. A third category of patient might report the same symptoms because of an inherited diathesis caused by neurochemical abnormalities. These three individuals should be placed in different personality categories even though their reports of depressive feelings seem similar. The important suggestion is that psychiatric classifications should be based on a complete profile of evidence that includes phenomenology, behavior, and biology, rather than only verbal reports of conscious feelings. If verbal reports were the only source of data for the classification of physical illnesses, the primary categories in modern internal medicine would be abdominal pain, headache, chest pain, itching, and fatigue.

Students of personality and temperament may be moving toward a fruitful change in research strategy—Thomas Kuhn would call it a "paradigm shift"—as they combine biology, behavioral observations, and phenomenological report to arrive at a new set of categories. These categories will be defined by a stable profile of behavior, mood, and usual emotional reaction to novelty, threat, or uncertainty that acknowledges the individual's temperamental biases, experiential history, and the demands imposed by contexts of action. In this new scheme, individuals with different temperaments and life histories will be placed in different personality categories even though they might report similar levels of worry, depression, or loneliness. This suggestion is not radical. Contemporary physicians place individuals with complaints of chronic headache in different diagnostic groups as a function of their physiology and lifestyle. A restless American child who has difficulty paying attention in school and a neurochemistry characterized by dopamine deficiency in the frontal lobes will be placed in the category called attention-deficit/hyperactivity disorder. A child with exactly the same biological and cognitive features would not belong to this category if he lived with a family who raised goats in an isolated village in Indonesia without a school. Galen might approve of these suggestions because he acknowledged that aspects of the local context, especially diet and climate, affected the balance of humors and therefore the personality type that would be actualized.

Conclusions

History has changed the meanings of *personality* and *temperament*, as it has for many other words. The most obvious alterations include acknowledging the effect of cultural setting on the salience of a trait; the profound interaction between a temperamental bias and subsequent social experience; and recognition of the indeterminate relations among brain states, conscious feelings, beliefs, and behaviors. The next set of personality constructs, based on a rich set of empirical data, will blend these phenomena into new clusters that will dominate theory until the next fresh perspective emerges.

References

Cheever J: The Journals of John Cheever. New York, Ballantine Books, 1993

Chess S, Thomas A: The New York Longitudinal Study. Can J Psychiatry 35:557–561, 1990

Dols MW: Medieval Islamic Medicine. Berkeley, CA, University of California Press, 1984

Draper G: Human Constitution. Philadelphia, PA, WB Saunders, 1924

Freedman DG, Freedman N: Behavioral differences between Chinese-American and American newborns. Nature 224:12–27, 1969

Freud S: New introductory lectures on psycho-analysis (1933[1932]) (Lectures XXIX–XXXV), in Standard Edition of the Complete Psychological Works of Sigmund Freud, Vol 22. Translated and edited by Strachey J. London, Hogarth Press, 1964, pp 1–182

Gall FJ: On the Organ of the Moral Qualities and Intellectual Faculties in the Plurality of the Cerebral Organs. Boston, MA, Marsh, Copen, & Lyon, 1835

Gosling FG: Before Freud. Urbana, IL, University of Illinois Press, 1987

Hooton EA: Crime and the Man. Cambridge, MA, Harvard University Press, 1939

Kagan J: Galen's Prophecy. New York, Basic Books, 1994

Kagan J: Childhood predictors of states of anxiety. Dialogues in Clinical Neuroscience 4:287–292, 2002

Kagan J, Snidman N: The Long Shadow of Temperament. Cambridge, MA, Harvard University Press, 2004

Kagan J, Arcus D, Snidman N, et al: Reactivity in infants. Dev Psychol 30:342–345, 1994

Kretschmer E: Physique and Character. New York, Harcourt Brace, 1925

Lombroso C: Crime and Its Causes. Boston, MA, Little Brown, 1911

McCrae RR, Costa PT Jr: Validation of the five-factor model of personality across instruments and observers. J Pers Soc Psychol 52:81–90, 1987

Pavlov IP: Lectures on Conditioned Reflexes, Vol 1. New York, International Universities Press, 1928

Rothbart MK: Temperament in childhood, in Temperament in Childhood. Edited by Kohnstamm GA, Bates JE, Rothbart MK. New York, Wiley, 1989, pp 59–73

Scott JP, Fuller J: Genetics and the Social Behavior of the Dog. Chicago, IL, University of Chicago Press, 1965

Siegel RE: Galen's System of Physiology and Medicine. Basel, Switzerland, Karger, 1968

Slotow R, van Dyk G, Poole J, et al: Older bull elephants control young males. Nature 408:425–426, 2000

Spurzheim JG: Phrenology. Boston, MA, Marsh, Copen, & Lyon, 1834

Strouse J: Alice James. Boston, MA, Houghton Mifflin, 1980

Thomas A, Chess S: Temperament and Development. New York, Brunner/Mazel, 1977

Wilson DS, Clarke AB, Coleman K, et al: Shyness and boldness in humans and other animals. Trends Ecol Evol 9:442–446, 1994

Yosida M: The Chinese concept of nature, in Chinese Science. Edited by Nakayama S, Sivin N. Cambridge, MA, MIT Press, 1973, pp 71–90

CHAPTER 2

THE PSYCHOBIOLOGY OF PERSONALITY DISORDERS

Kurtis L. Noblett, Ph.D.

Emil F. Coccaro, M.D.

The growth in empirical evidence suggesting unique biological profiles of DSM-IV-TR (American Psychiatric Association 2000) personality disorders has stimulated a flurry of research activity over the past 15–20 years. A corresponding growth in research technology has also allowed investigators to begin delineating Axis II disorders along distinct neurobiological dimensions, prompting some to even suggest that biology serve as the foundation for classification. Accordingly, the DSM-IV-TR categorizes the 10 different personality disorders within discrete clusters based on their similarity of clinical presentations. Although originally developed as a heuristic device, this taxonomy has been particularly useful in directing research and developing psychopharmacological treatment strategies. Cluster A disorders, characterized by odd and eccentric presentations, all share some degree of schizotypy. Cluster B disorders are typified by impulsivity, aggression, and/or emotional dysregulation. Cluster C is characterized largely by social or interpersonal anxiety. Although schizotypy, impulsivity, aggression, emotional dysregulation, and anxiety are not unique to Axis II disorders, they all demonstrate some correlation with selected biological variables that make them particularly amenable to empirical analysis.

In this chapter, we review the existing research data concerning the biology of personality disorders. Each of the DSM-IV-TR Axis II clusters will be discussed by systematically addressing the implicated neurotransmitter systems, neurophysiological/psychological/structural function, and psychopharmacologic treatment correlates. To reflect the overarching focus of this book, discussion will begin with affective-related traits within the context of personality disorders. The remainder of the chapter will address the other core dimensions of personality disorders, including impulsivity/aggression, anxiety, and schizotypy.

Affect-Related Traits and Personality Disorders

Affect-related traits are hallmark diagnostic criteria of several of the personality disorders, particularly within Clusters B and C. Some investigators have proposed that affective instability comprises a distinct psychobiological dimension of personality disorders (Gurvits et al. 2000; Siever and Davis 1991). This proposition receives support from family studies showing that relatives of borderline personality disorder probands showed a greater risk for affective and impulsive personality disorder traits than did relatives of probands with other personality disorders or with schizophrenia (Silverman et al. 1991). There was no similarly greater risk for other disorders, including major depressive disorder, suggesting that a familial relationship between borderline personality disorder and the core dimensions of borderline personality disorder (e.g., impulsivity, affective instability) is perhaps even greater than the relationship between borderline personality disorder and major mood disorders.

Psychobiology

The psychobiology of affective instability in patients with borderline personality disorder has not been well investigated. Several studies have implicated the cholinergic system as a moderator of affect within the context of borderline personality disorder (e.g., Steinberg et al. 1994). Following administration of physostigmine, a cholinesterase inhibitor, patients with borderline personality disorder demonstrated an increased depressive response compared with healthy control subjects, a response that was highly correlated with borderline traits related to affective instability independent of impulsivity (Steinberg et al. 1997). There was no such correlation in patients diagnosed with other non-borderline personality disorders. Procaine, an agent with widespread cholinergic properties, has been shown to induce dysphoria and dissociative symptoms in patients with borderline personality disorder, a response likely mediated by paralimbic regions (Kellner et al. 1987). These regions are largely involved in the evaluation of, and responsiveness to, emotionally charged stimuli. Procaine ostensibly increases regional cerebral blood flow in paralimbic regions, a response that seems to be blunted in mood disorder patients as compared with control subjects (Ketter et al. 1996), although such a comparison with patients with borderline personality disorder has yet to be assessed.

The noradrenergic and serotonergic systems are both potential candidates for the modulation of affective response and stimulus reactivity. Growth hormone responses to clonidine, an index of central α_2-noradrenergic receptor sensitivity, in both subjects with personality disorder and healthy volunteers were found to correlate with irritability but not with depression (Coccaro et al. 1991). Similarly, correlations between prolactin responses to fenfluramine challenge have been found with irritability and assaultiveness but not with depression (Coccaro et al. 1989). The possibility exists of multiple neurotransmitter system involvement in mood dysregulation, including both norepinephrine and serotonin (5-HT) (Siever and Davis 1991). Amphetamine challenges in healthy volunteers correspond with affective lability (Kavoussi and Coccaro 1993), whereas such stimulation in patients with borderline personality disorder was associated with an improvement in global function, including mood (Schulz et al. 1988). The more global neurotransmitter effects of amphetamines versus selective neurotransmitter agents may partly explain the lack of treatment efficacy with tricyclic antidepressants (TCAs) on mood disorders in patients with personality disorders (Coccaro and Siever 1995).

Some investigators have argued that the depression often associated with borderline personality disorder has a distinct neurobiological substrate as compared with nonpersonality disorder–related depression (Siever et al. 1986). De La Fuente et al. (2002) found less dexamethasone nonsuppression and less thyroid-releasing hormone blunting following stimulation tests than in major depressives. A possible biological substrate for such effects is disturbance of the hypothalamic-pituitary-adrenal (HPA) axis. Attempts to evaluate HPA axis function in patients with borderline personality disorder have been largely inconclusive because of the confounding effects of major depression and/or posttraumatic stress disorder. Elucidation of these confounding effects has identified history of child abuse as a possible mediator of subsequent HPA axis dysfunction. Higher concentrations of adrenocorticotropic hormone (ACTH) and cortisol were found following dexamethasone/

corticotropin-releasing hormone challenge in borderline patients with a history of sustained childhood abuse as compared with nonabused or mildly abused borderline patients (Rinne et al. 2002). Correspondingly, the selective serotonin reuptake inhibitor (SSRI) fluvoxamine significantly reduced the hyperresponsiveness of the HPA axis in borderline patients with a history of sustained childhood abuse (Rinne et al. 2003), implicating the HPA axis as an important target of SSRI function. This area of research promises to provide important information on the etiology and treatment of the complex interplay between patients with borderline personality disorder and comorbid Axis I features, including mood disorders.

Psychopharmacology

Following a symptom-specific algorithm for the treatment of affect-related symptoms, Soloff (1998) has proposed a multi-tiered approach beginning with SSRIs and related antidepressants. First-line treatment with antidepressants has been found to be effective when major depressive disorder is the primary focus of treatment (Sternberg 1987). The efficacy of SSRIs in ameliorating depressive symptomatology in patients with personality disorder has been well documented (e.g., Kavoussi et al. 1994; Markowitz 1995). However, when the mood disorder is not primary or not linked with the affect-related symptoms, the results of such treatment are much more variable (Soloff 2000).

Empirical evidence for the use of TCAs in the treatment of patients with borderline personality disorder with comorbid depression has been mixed. Placebo-controlled trials have demonstrated patient improvement following amitriptyline, although effects mostly have been limited to depressive symptomatology (Soloff et al. 1989). Furthermore, Soloff and colleagues (1986) reported paradoxical effects following administration of amitriptyline among 15 borderline patients, including suicide threats, paranoid ideation, and demanding/assaultive behavior. A recent study (Joyce et al. 2003) comparing fluoxetine to nortriptyline in depressed samples of borderline personality disorder, nonborderline personality disorder, and nonpersonality disorder subjects found the nortriptyline-treated borderline group to have the poorest outcome of all treatment conditions.

Placebo-controlled studies have demonstrated some efficacy of monoamine oxidase inhibitors (MAOIs) in treating patients with borderline personality disorder. Cowdry and Gardner (1988) found significant improvement on measures of impulsivity, mood reactivity, and rejection sensitivity following 6 weeks of tranylcypromine. Cornelius and colleagues (1993) found a modest efficacy for phenelzine in the treatment of depression and irritability in borderline patients. These findings parallel those of Soloff and colleagues (1993), who found a superior efficacy of phenelzine over haloperidol and placebo on measures of depression, borderline psychopathologic symptoms, and anxiety. Despite some promise in the treatment of affect-related symptoms of borderline personality disorder, MAOIs do not receive widespread use because of concerns regarding compliance with dietary restrictions and notable side effects.

The use of anticonvulsants and mood stabilizers has also been suggested for the treatment of personality disorders, particularly as an adjunctive or alternative treatment to antidepressants (Soloff 1998, 2000). Their efficacy in the treatment of patients with borderline personality disorder with comorbid Axis I mood disorders will be discussed briefly because of the paucity of literature on the topic. A preliminary study by Hollander and colleagues (2001) suggested symptom improvement following treatment with divalproex sodium in both the amelioration of aggressive behaviors as well as depressive symptomatology. However, conclusions are somewhat limited in generalizability given the small sample size. Only one placebo-controlled study (Links et al. 1990) has been performed investigating the efficacy of lithium in the treatment of patients with borderline personality disorder. In terms of anger and irritability, therapists' and patients' ratings were discrepant, with patients reporting no significant improvement. None of the ratings demonstrated an antidepressant effect compared with placebo. The few existing studies using carbamazepine have been inconclusive with respect to depressive comorbidity, although Gardner and Cowdry (1986) found a precipitation of melancholic depression in several of their research subjects that remitted following discontinuation of treatment.

Depressive Personality Disorder

Depressive personality disorder (DPD) is a diagnostic category that has been relegated to Appendix B of the DSM-IV-TR for possible inclusion in future editions of the DSM. In spite of the controversy as to whether DPD is a valid construct (for recent reviews, see Bagby et al. 2003; Huprich 2001; Ryder et al. 2002; and Chapter 4 of this book), a dearth of literature exists regarding its biology and pharmacology. However, family history studies have shown co-aggregation of DPD with mood disorders (Klein 1990; Klein and Miller 1993; McDermut et al. 2003), indicating the possibility of shared biological substrates.

At this time, a general consensus suggests that DPD demonstrates some degree of construct validity. However, the overlap between DPD and dysthymic disorder (i.e., around 50%) calls into question the clinical utility of such a category, such that DPD may be best conceptualized as a subcategory of dysthymia (Bagby and Ryder 1999; Bagby et al. 2003) or perhaps an early-onset, traitlike variant of depressive disorders in general (Akiskal et al. 1980; Klein and Miller 1993; Wetzel et al. 1980). If the assumption is made that DPD is no more than an extension of dysthymia on the depression spectrum, then one could argue that the overlap in symptoms is tantamount to an overlap in biological substrates. On the basis mainly of its pattern of responsiveness to TCAs and SSRIs (for a review, see Kocsis 2003), dysthymia appears to have a similar neurobiological profile to major depression in terms of noradrenergic and serotonergic dysfunction. Pharmacologic challenge with the 5-HT agonists m-chlorophenylpiperazine (m-CPP) and ipsapirone in subjects with major depression or dysthymia produced similar effects on neuroendocrine responsiveness, implicating a 5-HT receptor-mediated effect in both conditions (Riedel et al. 2002). Several placebo-controlled studies (Boyer and Lecrubier 1996; Lecrubier et al. 1997) have found the atypical antidepressant amisulpride, a dopamine-receptor agonist, to be efficacious in treatment of dysthymia, implicating a mesolimbic-mediated disruption in dopamine transmission that may play a contributing role in the long-term maintenance of symptomatology.

The increased interest in the pharmacotherapy of dysthymia will continue to shed light on the biology of chronic and traitlike depression. Whether DPD is eventually included in DSM as a legitimate disorder, the ongoing investigations will certainly elucidate many of the overlapping symptom domains shared with dysthymia.

Affective Instability and Impulsivity

Cluster B disorders are defined by some degree of impulsivity. The impulsivity demonstrated by borderline patients is intimately connected with affective instability and is often triggered by feelings of abandonment or separation. Antisocial patients tend to be more self-serving, demonstrating impulsive behaviors that place immediate gratification ahead of social conformity. Impulsivity as a personality dimension appears to be partially heritable. Twin studies of borderline patients suggest that impulsivity is partially inherited, even though the diagnosis of borderline personality is not (Torgerson 1984). A recent meta-analysis of both twin and adoption studies found a moderate genetic contribution to antisocial behavior (Rhee and Waldman 2002). Given the shared association between 5-HT function and both depression and impulsive aggression, as well as shared treatment efficacy in response to SSRIs, it seems likely that depression and impulsivity are, at least in part, mediated by specific and common neurotransmitter function.

Psychobiology

One of the most consistent findings in research on the biology of personality disorders is an inverse correlation between 5-HT and impulsivity/aggression, or "impulsive aggression." Tables 2–1 and 2–2 summarize the research evidence presented in this chapter. First reported in samples of rodents (Valzelli 1980), this inverse relationship has been found across different studies using a variety of assessment measures (Coccaro and Siever 2002). Early studies of central 5-HT function demonstrated reduced activity in human subjects with impulsive aggression as evidenced by significantly lower levels of the primary 5-HT metabolite, cerebrospinal fluid (CSF) 5-hydroxyindoleacetic acid (5-HIAA), regardless of whether the aggression was self-directed (e.g., suicide attempts) or other-directed (Asberg et al. 1976; Brown et al. 1982).

TABLE 2–1. Evidence for neurotransmitter dysregulation in personality disorder

System	Sample	Result
General monoamines (norepinephrine, dopamine, serotonin)	Borderline personality disorder	Amphetamine challenge associated with improved global function in borderline subjects
Serotonin	General personality disorder	Prolactin response correlates with irritability
Norepinephrine	General personality disorder	Growth hormone response correlates with irritability
Dopamine	General personality disorder	CSF and plasma HVA correlate with positive symptoms of schizotypy
Acetylcholine	General personality disorder	Increased depressive response in borderline subjects

Note. CSF=cerebrospinal fluid; HVA= homovanillic acid.

TABLE 2–2. Biological evidence for serotonin dysregulation in impulsivity and aggression

Sample	Study type	Result
General personality disorder	CSF 5-HIAA	Inverse correlation with history of aggression ↓ CSF 5-HIAA in suicide attempters
Violent offenders	CSF 5-HIAA	↓ CSF 5-HIAA in impulsive violent offenders
Impulsive arsonists	CSF 5-HIAA	↓ CSF 5-HIAA compared with control subjects
General personality disorder	Fenfluramine challenge	Inverse correlation with assault and irritability ↓ PRL[D,L-FEN] in subjects with borderline personality disorder
Antisocial personality disorder	m-CPP challenge	↓ PRL[m-CPP] and ↑ CORT[m-CPP] compared with control subjects
General personality disorder	5-HTT binding	Inverse correlation with history of aggression
Violent offenders	TPH genotype	Violence associated with variant alleles

Note. ↑=increased; ↓=decreased; 5-HIAA=5-hydroxyindoleacetic acid; 5-HTT= serotonin transporter; CORT=cortisol; m-CPP=*m*-chlorophenylpiperazine; CSF= cerebrospinal fluid; D,L-FEN=D,L-fenfluramine; PRL=prolactin; TPH=tryptophan hydroxylase.

Later studies investigating indices of 5-HT functioning brought into question the relationship between 5-HT and impulsivity, independent of aggression. In a study of violent offenders, Linnoila and colleagues (1983) reported diminished CSF 5-HIAA concentrations in impulsive but not nonimpulsive subjects. A follow-up study (Virkkunen et al. 1987) including impulsive arsonists found a significant difference in CSF 5-HIAA between the arsonists as compared with habitual offenders and healthy volunteers, indicating that poor impulse control is an important contributing factor to the role of deficient 5-HT activity in aggressive behaviors.

A number of pharmacologic challenge studies have lent support to the 5-HT hypothesis of impulsive aggression. In the first such study in impulsive-aggressive personality disorder subjects, Coccaro and colleagues (1989) reported that the 5-HT releaser/reuptake inhibitor D,L-fenfluramine produced an attenuated prolactin (PRL) response (i.e., PRL[D,L-FEN]) in patients with borderline personality disorder and had an inverse correlation with aggression in all the patients with personality disorder. An inverse correlation between PRL[D,L-FEN] response and aggression has since been replicated in patients with antisocial (O'Keane et al. 1992) and other personality disorders (Coccaro et al. 1997; Siever and Trestman 1993). After the administration of the postsynaptic 5-HT agonist, PRL[m-CPP], patients with antisocial personality disorder showed a decreased PRL response as well as an inverse correlation between PRL[m-CPP] response and assaultive behaviors (Moss et al. 1990). Coccaro and colleagues found a similar profile using the cortisol and thermal responses to the 5-HT$_{1A}$ receptor agonist ipsapirone in a small sample of patients with personality disorder (Coccaro et al. 1995).

Other measures of central nervous system (CNS) function have supported a crucial role of 5-HT in the expression of aggressive tendencies. Blood platelet receptor markers have provided a useful model of 5-HT receptor function in the CNS. Patients with personality disorder demonstrated an inverse correlation between the number of platelet [3H]imipramine (5-HT transporter [5-HTT]) binding sites and self-mutilation and impulsive behaviors (Simeon et al. 1992). Similarly, the number of platelet binding sites for [3H]paroxetine was found to be inversely correlated with life history of aggression in patients with personality disorder (Coccaro et al. 1996).

Genetic variation in 5-HT receptor coding, as well as other regulatory components of 5-HT functioning, have shown associations with aggressive behaviors. Nielsen and colleagues (1994) found that a largely personality-disordered population of violent offenders with a variant allele (LL or UL genotypes) for the tryptophan hydroxylase (TPH; the rate-limiting enzyme in 5-HT synthesis) gene had significantly lower levels of CSF 5-HIAA than their comparison group with the UU genotype. Although the presence of personality disorders was not assessed, DNA polymorphisms in TPH (Manuck et al. 1999) and MAO-A (the enzyme that breaks down 5-HT and norepinephrine within the neuron) (Manuck et al. 2000) were found to associate positively with self-reported aggression. An earlier study of a personality-disordered population with the LL genotypic variant showed a similar association with aggression scores (New et al. 1998).

Neuroimaging and neuropsychological studies have provided a unique perspective in identifying neuroanatomical dysfunction as possible contributors to impulsivity and aggression in personality disorders. One of the more robust neuroimaging findings in the study of antisocial behavior is decreased involvement of prefrontal cortex, particularly in the lateral and medial areas (Bassarath 2001). A recent magnetic resonance imaging (MRI) study on a community sample of volunteers with antisocial personality disorder indicated a reduced volume of prefrontal gray matter as compared with control subjects (Raine et al. 2000). Positron emission tomography (PET) studies (Siever et al. 1999; Soloff et al. 2000) have found reduced responsivity to serotonergic challenge in orbitofrontal and medial frontal cortex in impulsive-aggressive and personality-disordered populations. Single photon emission computed tomography (SPECT) has largely supported the PET findings. A comparison of subjects with a history of aggression toward person or property found significantly decreased activity in prefrontal cortex as compared with psychiatric control subjects (Amen et al. 1996). Similar studies have shown prefrontal dysfunction in psychopathic men (Intrator et al. 1997) and Type II alcoholic individuals (i.e., with a history of impulsive aggression) (Tiihonen et al. 1997a).

In general, neuropsychological studies suggest a significant functional association between prefrontal integrity and antisocial and aggressive behaviors (Brower and Price 2001). Specific measures of orbitofrontal and ventromedial cortical functioning in a subpopulation of psychopathic inmates found significant deficiencies in those specific brain regions (LaPierre et al. 1995). This finding mirrors studies demonstrating that lesions of the orbital and medial prefrontal cortex and anatomically connected areas are present in patients with impulsive and aggressive behaviors, affective dysregulation, and unawareness of behavioral consequences (Anderson et al. 1999; Davidson et al. 2000). Best and colleagues (2002) compared patients with intermittent explosive disorder (IED), who were also personality disordered, with non-IED control subjects on a number of tests sensitive to impulsivity, working memory, emotional recognition, and general frontal lobe functioning. The researchers found a generalized deficit in IED-positive subjects across tasks related to orbital and ventromedial precortical function, raising the possibility of an organic etiology to the expression of impulsive-aggressive behaviors.

In terms of their biological profiles, the distinction between disorders of impulsivity and disorders of depression remains unclear. However, the frequent co-occurrence of depression in disorders of impulsivity such as antisocial and borderline personality disorders (for reviews, see Deakin 2003; Koenigsberg et al. 1999) speaks not only to shared psychosocial sequelae but also to common biological substrates. Such comorbidity has potentially serious consequences because impulsivity increases the likelihood of suicidal behaviors in individuals suffering from severe forms of depression. The biological profile of suicidality often mimics that of impulsive aggression (for a review, see Oquendo and Mann 2000), particularly in terms of diminished 5-HT activity. Individuals' possession of the short allele coding for 5-HTT, a polymorphism commonly associated with depression and anxiety disorders, has also been found to correlate with impulsivity and aggression (Reist et al. 2001; Retz et al. 2004). This finding has important treatment implications because antidepressant medications have shown efficacy in treatment of impulsivity, aggression, and Cluster B personality disorders, as will be discussed in the next section.

Psychopharmacology

SSRIs have received much scrutiny as potential pharmacological interventions for patterned aggression and Cluster B disorders (Walsh and Dinan 2001). In one of the first studies on SSRI efficacy in treatment of patients with borderline personality disorder, subjects treated with fluoxetine showed a significant reduction in anger as compared with those treated with placebo (Salzman et al. 1995). This finding was generally replicated in a sample of 17 patients with Axis I/II comorbid borderline personality disorder (Markowitz 1995). A placebo-controlled study by Coccaro and Kavoussi (1997) found significant reductions in patients' verbal aggression and aggression against objects during treatment with fluoxetine. The sample consisted of 40 nondepressed subjects with personality disorder who had a history of recurrent, impulsive-aggressive behavior. The same authors had found previously a similar treatment efficacy following administration of sertraline (Kavoussi et al. 1994). Recently, an open-label treatment with citalopram on subjects meeting diagnostic criteria for a Cluster B disorder or IED found a significant reduction in overt aggression, subjective irritability, and overt irritability as compared with placebo (Reist et al. 2003).

Another approach to pharmacological treatment of Cluster B disorders and impulsive aggression has been the use of anticonvulsants and mood stabilizers. Clinical trials with subjects with borderline personality disorder have already supported the efficacy of anticonvulsants in ameliorating aggressive tendencies (Cowdry and Gardner 1988). In addition, Kavoussi and Coccaro (1998) found divalproex sodium to be effective in reducing aggressive events in subjects with personality disorder who did not respond to SSRIs. An anti-aggressive effect for divalproex was also found in Cluster B subjects with personality disorder and IED (Hollander et al. 2003). Recent placebo-controlled clinical trials with subjects with borderline personality disorder showed significant improvement on measures of aggression and subjective anger/irritability (Frankenburg and Zanarini 2002; Hollander et al. 2001). Carbamazepine has been shown to significantly reduce the frequency and severity of behavioral dyscontrol (Cowdry and Gardner 1988). A 16-week, double-blind, placebo-controlled study of subjects meeting criteria for IED showed that administration of phenytoin reduced the frequency of aggressive behaviors by 57% as compared with baseline and by 38% as compared with placebo (Stanford et al. 2001). The presence of Axis II disorders was not assessed.

Neuroleptics traditionally used to treat patients with schizophrenia and related psychotic disorders increasingly are being used for "off-label" indications. Early placebo-controlled studies with classic antipsychotics such as haloperidol and thiothixene have shown a modest efficacy in the treatment of impulsive-aggressive behaviors in subjects with borderline personality disorder (Goldberg et al. 1986; Soloff et al. 1989). The agranulocytosis associated with clozapine has limited its off-label use, although existing studies have suggested treatment efficacy in psychotic and nonpsychotic borderline patients (Benedetti et al. 1998; Chengappa et al. 1999). The safer side-effect profiles of newer atypical antipsychotics have catalyzed a growing body of research on alternative uses. A recent 8-week, open-label trial with risperidone demonstrated significant decreases in self-rated impulsive-aggressive behaviors in a sample of 13 patients with borderline personality disorder (Rocca et al. 2002). Early indications have shown treatment efficacy in decreasing acts of self-mutilation and general impulsivity in borderline patients (Khouzam and Donnelly 1997; Szigethy and Schulz 1997) and decreasing impulsive-aggressive behavior associated with antisocial personality disorder (Hirose 2001), although controlled studies will need to support such use.

Anxiety-Related Traits and Personality Disorders

Excessive anxiety is most commonly associated with Cluster C disorders, although as a state symptom it is relatively ubiquitous among all of the personality disorder categories. Of all the personality dimensions discussed so far, probably the least systematic investigation has taken place with anxiety-related traits and Cluster C disorders, perhaps because they are often overshadowed by more problematic comorbid Axis I disorders. In fact, the comorbidity of social phobia with avoidant personality disorder may be as high as 90% (Widiger 1992). Despite the lack of specific empirical data for Cluster C disorders, family studies have indicated significant transmission of anxiety traits and anxiety disorders among family members (e.g., Mannuzza et al. 1995; Reich 1991). Such studies support the possibility of a neurobiological substrate for such symptom expression in personality disorders, a possibility that remains largely speculative.

Psychobiology

The serotonergic system has been thought to be the most likely neurotransmitter system involved in the etiology of social anxiety, a statement based solely on the efficacy of SSRIs in the treatment of anxiety disorders. Clonazepam, a benzodiazepine with notable serotonergic properties, has also shown some efficacy in the treatment of social anxiety (Davidson et al. 1993). Pharmacologic challenges have provided some evidence in support of a serotonergic etiology. Tancer and colleagues (1994), for example, found that fenfluramine challenge produced an augmented cortisol response in patients with social phobia as compared with control subjects. Noradrengeric and dopaminergic challenges using clonidine and levodopa, respectively, produced comparable results between social phobic patients and healthy control subjects.

Some limited data exist suggesting a role of dopamine in social anxiety. A neuroimaging study using SPECT analysis found lower densities of striatal dopamine receptor sites in patients with social phobia as compared with healthy control subjects (Tiihonen et al. 1997b). This finding may in part explain the higher concurrence of social anxiety disorder among patients with Parkinson's disease (Richard et al. 1996), a disease caused by degradation of the dopaminergic nigrostriatal pathway.

Psychopharmacology

The pharmacologic treatments of choice for social anxiety disorder are the SSRIs (Ballenger et al. 1998). A relatively large number of clinical trials have supported the efficacy of SSRIs, including fluvoxamine, sertraline, and paroxetine, in the treatment of patients with social phobia (e.g., Allgulander 1999; Stein et al. 1999). However, because Axis II comorbidity is not typically assessed, the efficacy in alleviating trait-related anxiety remains unclear. A recent clinical trial of sertraline and imipramine efficacy found the Cluster C (anxiety-related) personality disorders to be most prevalent (39%) among individuals with chronic depression (Russell et al. 2003). Interestingly, the presence of a comorbid Axis II disorder had no significant effect on symptom response, suggesting that symptom alleviation was caused by positive treatment response of state—as opposed to trait—anxiety, this implication being supported by the high incidence of comorbid anxiety disorders (76%) with the Cluster C disorders.

Research evidence provides some support for the use of MAOIs and benzodiazepines in the treatment of patients with social anxiety disorder. Double-blind, placebo-controlled trials have shown a positive response to phenelzine (Gelernter et al. 1991; Liebowitz et al. 1992). However, the tyramine pressor effect limits its utility. Benzodiazepines such as clonazepam, alprazolam, and bronazepam have shown promising effects (Davidson et al. 1994; Versiani et al. 1997), but the common comorbidity of alcohol abuse with social anxiety disorder, as well as the high risk of dependence, precludes its practical use. Again, the positive effects of such medications are unclear in a personality-disordered population because of the dearth of published data on the matter.

Schizotypy and Personality Disorders

Cluster A disorders, which include paranoid, schizoid, and schizotypal personality disorders, are closely related to schizophrenia. Research has demonstrated the transmission of schizotypal traits among first-degree relatives of schizophrenic patients (Asarnow et al. 2001), underscoring the likelihood of shared biological substrates. Schizotypal personality disorder is the best characterized and most severe of the schizophrenia-related personality disorders and appears to be the most closely related to schizophrenia biologically, phenomenologically, and genetically (Siever and Davis 1991).

Psychobiology

Psychotic-like symptoms in the Cluster A disorders include magical thinking, ideas of reference, and perceptual distortions, all of which distinguish the diagnostic criteria set for schizotypal personality disorder. The dopamine hypothesis of schizophrenia, which posits that excess dopamine activity contributes to the positive (psychotic) symptoms of the illness, has provided the conceptual framework for exploring the biological substrates of schizotypal personality disorder. The dopamine hypothesis is supported by studies demonstrating a high correlation between therapeutic efficacy and dopamine receptor blockade of mesolimbic neurons (e.g., Seeman and Lee 1975). Both CSF and plasma homovanillic acid (HVA; a dopamine metabolite) levels are greater in clinically selected schizotypal patients than in healthy and other personality disorder control subjects, especially those patients exhibiting more psychotic-like symptoms (Siever et al. 1991, 1993b). These preliminary data, along with evidence indicating a positive response to low-dose neuroleptics (Coccaro 1998), suggest the covariance of dopamine activity with psychotic-like symptoms in schizotypal personality-disordered subjects.

The negative, or "deficit," symptoms of schizophrenia are also characteristic of Cluster A disorders. Such symptoms include the flattened affect, anhedonia, and social detachment inherent to schizoid personality disorder. Unlike psychotic symptoms, the substrate for deficit symptoms appears to be hypodopaminergia in frontal cortical areas. An adequate dopaminergic tone, particularly involving prefrontal dopamine D_1 receptors, is likely necessary for the integrity of higher order brain functions. Evidence supporting the hypodopaminergia hypothesis of deficit symptoms comes from neuropsychologic, psychophysiological, and brain imaging studies (Siever et al. 1993a).

Neuropsychological studies have demonstrated significant impairment in executive functioning in individuals with schizophrenia, their first-degree relatives, and individuals with schizotypal personality disorder. Tests that are sensitive to the integrity of prefrontal cortical functioning are often impaired in this population. Tests of working memory, mental flexibility, and sustained attention, such as the Wisconsin Card Sorting Test (WCST), are found to be associated with symptoms of schizotypy and vulnerability to schizophrenia (e.g., Gooding et al. 1999). The positive correlation between deficit symptoms and impairment in executive function within schizotypal individuals (Dinn et al. 2002) supports an inverse correlation between prefrontal cortical integrity and negative schizotypy.

Neuroimaging studies have suggested neuroanatomical differences between subjects with schizotypal personality disorder and healthy control subjects. Increased ventricular size has been shown in patients with schizotypal personality disorder (Cazzullo et al. 1991) and schizotypal relatives of individuals with schizophrenia (Silverman et al. 1998). Although the findings have been inconsistent, studies using volumetric MRI (Raine et al. 2002) and regional cerebral blood flow (Buchsbaum et al. 1997) have suggested some degree of prefrontal impairment in conjunction with deficient performance on tests of executive functioning. Early indications of an association between enlarged ventricles and reduced concentrations of plasma HVA (Siever et al. 1993a) again implicate dopamine as a possible neurochemical substrate.

Psychopharmacology

Clinical psychopharmacologic trials have found neuroleptics to be generally efficacious in treating patients with schizotypal personality disorder (Coccaro 1998). In two relatively large placebo-controlled trials of patients with borderline and/or schizotypal personality disorder, psychotic-like symptoms were reduced following treatment with thiothixene (Goldberg et al. 1986) and haloperidol (Soloff et al. 1989). However, a more recent follow-up trial found no efficacy of haloperidol in a subject sample of patients with the same disorders (Soloff et al. 1993). The authors explain this discrepancy in findings by noting that subjects in their previous study (Soloff et al. 1989) demonstrated significantly higher ratings on measures of "psychoticism," "schizotypal symptom severity," and "global impairment." When combined with the results from the study by Goldberg and colleagues (1986), which showed that schizotypal symptom severity was a favorable predictor of response to thiothixene, the results suggest that neuroleptic treatment may be best indicated for patients with prominent psychotic features, as opposed to those with more deficit-type symptomatology.

Given the hypothesized association between prefrontal hypodopaminergia and deficit-type symptoms of schizotypy, one might expect an improvement in cognitive function following stimulation of dopamine activity in prefrontal cortical areas. Indeed, preliminary data from Siegel and colleagues (1996) suggest an enhanced performance on the WCST following administration of amphetamines to subjects with schizotypal personality disorder. The preponderance of dopamine D_1 receptors in prefrontal cortex raises the possibility that selective agonism of D_1 receptors may produce an amelioration of deficit-type symptoms. Recent preliminary data from a small clinical trial (Tsuang et al. 2002) showed that subjects meeting criteria for "schizotaxia" (a liability to schizophrenia closely related to negative schizotypy) generally showed improvement in attention, working memory, and deficit-type symptoms following a 6-week trial of risperidone. As with other atypical antipsychotics, risperidone demonstrates a high affinity for 5-HT receptors, and antagonism at these sites may very well facilitate dopamine activity within the prefrontal cortex.

Conclusions

As the empirical database grows regarding the biology of personality disorders, so, too, will our understanding of the biological interactions with comorbid Axis I disorders and their interactive effects on psychopathology. The challenge for the investigator is to identify the heritable, biological markers of Axis I/II symptomatology and the specific substrates on which pharmacologic agents exert their influence within the matrix of possible diagnostic combinations of both mood and personality disorders. The challenge for the clinician lies not only in comprehending the complex interplay of state-versus-trait variables in formulating diagnoses and treatment plans but also in appreciating the nuances and limitations of conventional pharmacotherapy within the context of psychopathological comorbidity. Both individuals are restricted by the current state of the art in taxonomy and in research technology.

Given the prevalence of depression across Axis II categories and the consequent treatment complexities, the need for continued exploration and elucidation is evident. The promise of therapeutic efficacy demonstrated by a number of preliminary clinical trials begs for more large-scale placebo-controlled studies with personality-disordered and comorbid populations. Similarly, the need exists for ongoing investigation of contributing neurotransmitters and receptor substrates of pharmacologic efficacy that will ultimately lead to "cleaner" agents targeting more specific symptom profiles. The number of studies tailored toward these objectives grows every year. Of course, every study has its limitations inherent to the diagnostic assessment measures, study duration, and sample size, to mention but a few. The primary goal for the research community is not just one of replication but one of innovation, capitalizing on the evolving research technology that will allow for the advancement of our current understanding of depression, personality disorders, and the dynamic interactions between them.

References

Akiskal HS, Rosenthal TL, Haykal RF, et al: Characterological depressions: clinical and sleep EEG findings separating "subaffective dysthymia" from "character spectrum disorders." Arch Gen Psychiatry 37:777–783, 1980

Allgulander C: Paroxetine in social anxiety disorder: a randomized placebo-controlled study. Acta Psychiatr Scand 100:193–198, 1999

Amen DG, Stubblefield M, Carmichael B, et al: Brain SPECT findings and aggressiveness. Ann Clin Psychiatry 8:129–137, 1996

American Psychiatric Association: Diagnostic and Statistical Manual of Mental Disorders, 4th Edition, Text Revision. Washington, DC, American Psychiatric Association, 2000

Anderson SW, Bechara A, Damasio H, et al: Impairment of social and moral behavior related to early damage in human prefrontal cortex. Nat Neurosci 2:1032–1037, 1999

Asarnow RF, Nuechterlein KH, Fogelson D, et al: Schizophrenia and schizophrenia-spectrum personality disorders in the first-degree relatives of children with schizophrenia: the UCLA family study. Arch Gen Psychiatry 58:581–588, 2001

Asberg M, Traskman L, Thoren P: 5-HIAA in the cerebrospinal fluid: a biochemical suicide predictor? Arch Gen Psychiatry 33:1193–1197, 1976

Bagby RM, Ryder AG: Diagnostic discriminability of dysthymia and depressive personality disorder. Depress Anxiety 10:41–49, 1999

Bagby RM, Ryder AG, Schuller DR: Depressive personality disorder: a critical review. Curr Psychiatry Rep 5:16–22, 2003

Ballenger JC, Davidson JRT, Lecrubier Y, et al: Consensus statement on social anxiety disorder from the International Consensus Group on Depression and Anxiety. J Clin Psychiatry 59 (suppl 17):54–60, 1998

Bassarath L: Neuroimaging studies of antisocial behavior. Can J Psychiatry 46:728–732, 2001

Benedetti F, Sforzini L, Colombo C, et al: Low-dose clozapine in acute and continuation treatment of severe borderline personality disorder. J Clin Psychiatry 59:103–107, 1998

Best M, Williams JM, Coccaro EF: Evidence for a dysfunctional prefrontal circuit in patients with an impulsive aggressive disorder. Proc Natl Acad Sci U S A 99:8448–8453, 2002

Boyer P, Lecrubier Y: Atypical antipsychotic drugs in dysthymia: placebo-controlled studies of amisulpride versus imipramine, versus amineptine. Eur Psychiatry 11:135–140, 1996

Brower MC, Price BH: Neuropsychiatry of frontal lobe dysfunction in violent and criminal behaviour: a critical review. J Neurol Neurosurg Psychiatry 71:720–726, 2001

Brown GL, Ebert MH, Goyer PF, et al: Aggression, suicide, and serotonin relationships to CSF metabolites. Am J Psychiatry 139:741–745, 1982

Buchsbaum MS, Trestman RL, Hazlett E, et al: Regional cerebral blood flow during the Wisconsin Card Sort Test in schizotypal personality disorder. Schizophr Res 27:21–28, 1997

Cazzullo CL, Vita A, Giobbio GM, et al: Cerebral structured abnormalities in schizophreniform disorder in schizophrenia spectrum personality disorders, in Schizophrenia Research: Advances in Neuropsychiatry and Psychopharmacology, Vol. 1. Edited by Tamminga CA, Schultz SC. New York, Raven, 1991, pp 209–217

Chengappa KN, Ebeling T, Kang JS, et al: Clozapine reduces severe self-mutilation and aggression in psychotic patients with borderline personality disorder. J Clin Psychiatry 60:477–484, 1999

Coccaro EF: Clinical outcome of psychopharmacologic treatment of borderline and schizotypal personality disordered subjects. J Clin Psychiatry 59 (suppl 1):30–35, 1998

Coccaro EF, Kavoussi RJ: Fluoxetine and impulsive aggressive behavior in personality disordered subjects. Arch Gen Psychiatry 54:1081–1088, 1997

Coccaro EF, Siever LJ: The Neuropsychopharmacology of personality disorders, in Psychopharmacology: The Fourth Generation of Progress. Edited by Bloom FE, Kupfer DJ. New York, Raven, 1995, pp 1567–1579

Coccaro EF, Siever LJ: Pathophysiology and treatment of aggression, in Psychopharmacology: The Fifth Generation of Progress. Edited by Davis KL, Charney D, Coyle JT, et al. Philadelphia, PA, Lippincott, Williams & Wilkins, 2002, pp 1709–1723

Coccaro EF, Siever LJ, Klar HM, et al: Serotonergic studies in patients with affective and personality disorders: correlates with suicidal and impulsive aggressive behavior. Arch Gen Psychiatry 46:587–599, 1989

Coccaro EF, Lawrence T, Trestman R, et al: Growth hormone responses to intravenous clonidine challenge correlates with behavioral irritability in psychiatric patients and in healthy volunteers. Psychiatry Res 39:129–139, 1991

Coccaro EF, Kavoussi RJ, Hauger RL: Physiologic responses to d-fenfluramine and ipsapirone challenge correlate with indices of aggression in males with personality disorder. Int Clin Psychopharmacol 10:177–180, 1995

Coccaro EF, Kavoussi RJ, Sheline YI, et al: Impulsive aggression in personality disorder: correlates with ^{3}H-paroxetine binding in the platelet. Arch Gen Psychiatry 53:531–536, 1996

Coccaro EF, Kavoussi RJ, Cooper TB, et al: Central serotonin and aggression: inverse relationship with prolactin response to *d*-fenfluramine but not with CSF 5-HIAA concentration in human subjects. Am J Psychiatry 154:1430–1435, 1997

Cornelius JR, Soloff PH, George A, et al: Haloperidol vs. phenelzine in continuation therapy of borderline disorder. Psychopharmacol Bull 29:333–337, 1993

Cowdry RW, Gardner DL: Pharmacotherapy of borderline personality disorder: alprazolam, carbamazepine, trifluoperazine, and tranylcypromine. Arch Gen Psychiatry 45:111–119, 1988

Davidson JR, Hughes DL, George LK, et al: The epidemiology of social phobia: findings from the Duke Epidemiological Catchment Area Study. Psychol Med 23:709–718, 1993

Davidson JR, Tupler LA, Potts NL: Treatment of social phobia with benzodiazepines. J Clin Psychiatry 55:28–32, 1994

Davidson RJ, Putnam KM, Larson CL: Dysfunction in the neural circuitry of emotion regulation: a possible prelude to violence. Science 289:591–594, 2000

Deakin JF: Depression and antisocial personality disorder: two contrasting disorders of 5-HT function. J Neural Transm Suppl 64:79–93, 2003

De La Fuente JM, Bobes J, Vizuete C, et al: Biological nature of depressive symptoms in borderline personality disorder: endocrine comparison to recurrent brief and major depression. J Psychiatr Res 36:137–145, 2002

Dinn WM, Harris CL, Ayicegi A, et al: Positive and negative schizotypy in a student sample: neurocognitive and clinical correlates. Schizophr Res 56:171–185, 2002

Frankenburg FR, Zanarini MC: Divalproex sodium treatment of women with borderline personality disorder and bipolar II disorder: a double-blind placebo-controlled pilot study. J Clin Psychiatry 63:442–446, 2002

Gardner DL, Cowdry RW: Positive effects of carbamazepine on behavioral dyscontrol in borderline personality disorder. Am J Psychiatry 143:519–522, 1986

Gelernter CS, Uhda TW, Cimbolic P, et al: Cognitive-behavioral and pharmacological treatments of social phobia: a controlled study. Arch Gen Psychiatry 48:938–945, 1991

Goldberg SC, Schulz SC, Schulz PM, et al: Borderline and schizotypal personality disorders treated with low-dose thiothixene versus placebo. Arch Gen Psychiatry 43:680–686, 1986

Gooding DC, Kwapil TR, Tallent KA: Wisconsin Card Sorting Test deficits in schizotypic individuals. Schizophr Res 40:201–209, 1999

Gurvits IG, Koenigsberg HW, Siever LJ: Neurotransmitter dysfunction in patients with borderline personality disorder. Psychiatr Clin North Am 23:27–40, 2000

Hirose S: Effective treatment of aggression and impulsivity in antisocial personality disorder with risperidone. Psychiatry Clin Neurosci 55:161–162, 2001

Hollander E, Allen A, Lopez RP, et al: A preliminary double-blind, placebo-controlled trial of divalproex sodium in borderline personality disorder. J Clin Psychiatry 62:199–203, 2001

Hollander E, Tracy KA, Swann AC, et al: Divalproex in the treatment of impulsive aggression: efficacy in Cluster B personality disorders. Neuropsychopharmacology 28:1186–1197, 2003

Huprich SK: The overlap of depressive personality disorder and dysthymia, reconsidered. Harv Rev Psychiatry 9:158–168, 2001

Intrator J, Hare R, Stritzke P, et al: A brain imaging (single photon emission computerized tomography) study of semantic and affective processing in psychopaths. Biol Psychiatry 42:96–103, 1997

Joyce PR, Mulder RT, Luty SE, et al: Borderline personality disorder in major depression: symptomatology, temperament, character, differential drug response, and 6-month outcome. Compr Psychiatry 44:35–43, 2003

Kavoussi RJ, Coccaro EF: The amphetamine challenge test correlates with affective lability in healthy volunteers. Psychiatry Res 48:219–228, 1993

Kavoussi RJ, Coccaro EF: Divalproex sodium for impulsive aggressive behavior in patients with personality disorder. J Clin Psychiatry 59:676–680, 1998

Kavoussi RJ, Liu J, Coccaro EF: An open trial of sertraline in personality disordered patients with impulsive aggression. J Clin Psychiatry 55:137–141, 1994

Kellner CH, Post RM, Putnam F, et al: Intravenous procaine as a probe of limbic system activity in psychiatric patients and normal controls. Biol Psychiatry 22:1107–1126, 1987

Ketter TA, Andreason PJ, George MS, et al: Anterior paralimbic mediation of procaine-induced emotional and psychosensory experiences. Arch Gen Psychiatry 53:59–69, 1996

Khouzam HR, Donnelly NJ: Remission of self-mutilation in a patient with borderline personality during risperidone therapy. J Nerv Ment Dis 185:348–349, 1997

Klein DN: Depressive personality: reliability, validity, and relation to dysthymia. J Abnorm Psychol 99:412–421, 1990

Klein DN, Miller GA: Depressive personality disorder in a nonclinical sample. Am J Psychiatry 150:1718–1724, 1993

Kocsis JH: Pharmacotherapy for chronic depression. J Clin Psychol 59:885–892, 2003

Koenigsberg HW, Anwunah I, New AS, et al: Relationship between depression and borderline personality disorder. Depress Anxiety 10:158–167, 1999

LaPierre D, Braun CMJ, Hodgins S: Ventral frontal deficits in psychopathy: neuropsychological findings. Neuropsychologia 33:139–151, 1995

Lecrubier Y, Boyer P, Turjanksi S, et al: Amisulpride versus imipramine and placebo in dysthymia and major depression: Amisulpride Study Group. J Affect Disord 43:95–103, 1997

Liebowitz MR, Schneier FR, Campeas R, et al: Phenelzine versus atenolol in social phobia. Arch Gen Psychiatry 49:290–300, 1992

Links PS, Steiner M, Boiago I, et al: Lithium therapy for borderline patients: preliminary findings. J Personal Disord 4:173–181, 1990

Linnoila M, Virkkunen M, Scheinin M, et al: Low cerebrospinal fluid 5-hydroxyindoleacetic acid concentration differentiates impulsive from nonimpulsive violent behavior. Life Sci 33:2609–2614, 1983

Mannuzza S, Schneier FR, Chapman TF, et al: Generalized social phobia: reliability and validity. Arch Gen Psychiatry 52:230–237, 1995

Manuck SB, Flory JD, Ferrell RE, et al: Aggression and anger-related traits associated with a polymorphism of the tryptophan hydroxylase gene. Biol Psychiatry 45:603–614, 1999

Manuck SB, Flory JD, Ferrell RE, et al: A regulatory polymorphism of the monoamine oxidase-A gene may be associated with variability in aggression, impulsivity, and central nervous system sertonergic responsivity. Psychiatry Res 95:9–23, 2000

Markowitz PJ: Pharmacotherapy of impulsivity, aggression, and related disorders, in Impulsive Aggression and Disorders of Impulse Control. Edited by Stein D, Hollander E. Sussex, UK, Wiley, 1995, pp 263–287

McDermut W, Zimmerman M, Chelminski I: The construct validity of depressive personality disorder. J Abnorm Psychol 112:49–60, 2003

Moss HB, Yao JK, Panzak GL: Serotonergic responsivity and behavioral dimensions in antisocial personality disorder with substance abuse. Biol Psychiatry 28:325–338, 1990

New AS, Gelernter J, Yovell Y, et al: Increases in irritable aggression associated with "LL" genotype at the tryptophan hydroxylase locus. Am J Med Genet 81:13–17, 1998

Nielsen DA, Goldman D, Virkkunen M, et al: Suicidality and 5-hydroxyindoleacetic acid concentration associated with a tryptophan hydroxylase polymorphism. Arch Gen Psychiatry 51:34–38, 1994

O'Keane V, Moloney E, O'Neill H: Blunted prolactin responses to d-fenfluramine in sociopathy: evidence for subsensitivity of central serotonergic function. Br J Psychiatry 160:643–646, 1992

Oquendo MA, Mann JJ: The biology of impulsivity and suicidality. Psychiatr Clin North Am 23:11–25, 2000

Raine A, Lencz T, Birhle S, et al: Reduced prefrontal gray matter volume and reduced autonomic activity in antisocial personality disorder. Arch Gen Psychiatry 57:119–127, 2000

Raine A, Lencz T, Yaralian P, et al: Prefrontal structural deficits in schizotypal personality disorder. Schizophr Bull 28:501–513, 2002

Reich J: Avoidant and dependent personality traits in relatives of patients with panic disorder, patients with dependent personality disorder, and normal controls. Psychiatry Res 39:89–98, 1991

Reist C, Mazzanti C, Vu R, et al: Serotonin transporter polymorphism is associated with attenuated prolactin response to fenfluramine. Am J Med Genet 105:363–368, 2001

Reist C, Nakamura K, Sagart E, et al: Impulsive aggressive behavior: open-label treatment with citalopram. J Clin Psychiatry 64:81–85, 2003

Retz W, Retz-Junginger P, Supprian T, et al: Association of serotonin transporter promoter gene polymorphism with violence: relation with personality disorders, impulsivity, and childhood ADHD psychopathology. Behav Sci Law 22:415–425, 2004

Rhee SH, Waldman ID: Genetic and environmental influences on antisocial behavior: a meta-analysis of twin and adoption studies. Psychol Bull 128:490–529, 2002

Richard IH, Schiffer RB, Kurlan R: Anxiety and Parkinson's disease. J Neuropsychiatry Clin Neurosci 8:383–392, 1996

Riedel WJ, Klaassen T, Griez E, et al: Dissociable hormonal, cognitive and mood responses to neuroendocrine challenge: evidence for receptor-specific serotonergic dysregulation in depressed mood. Neuropsychopharmacology 26:358–367, 2002

Rinne T, De Kloet ER, Wouters L: Hyperresponsiveness of hypothalamic-pituitary-adrenal axis to combined dexamethasone/corticotropin-releasing hormone challenge in female borderline personality disorder subjects with a history of sustained childhood abuse. Biol Psychiatry 52:1102–1112, 2002

Rinne T, De Kloet ER, Wouters L: Fluvoxamine reduces responsiveness of HPA axis in adult female BPD patients with a history of sustained childhood abuse. Neuropsychopharmacology 28:126–132, 2003

Rocca P, Marchiaro L, Cocuzza E: Treatment of borderline personality disorder with risperidone. J Clin Psychiatry 63:241–244, 2002

Russell JM, Kornstein SG, Shea MT, et al: Chronic depression and comorbid personality disorders: response to sertraline versus imipramine. J Clin Psychiatry 64:554–561, 2003

Ryder AG, Bagby RM, Schuller DR: The overlap of depressive personality disorder and dysthymia: a categorical problem with a dimensional solution. Harv Rev Psychiatry 10:337–352, 2002

Salzman C, Wolfson AN, Schatzberg A: Effect of fluoxetine on anger in symptomatic volunteers with borderline personality disorder. J Clin Psychopharmacol 15:23–29, 1995

Schulz SC, Cornelius J, Schulz PM, et al: The amphetamine challenge test in patients with borderline disorder. Am J Psychiatry 145:809–814, 1988

Seeman P, Lee T: Antipsychotic drugs: direct correlation between clinical potency and presynaptic action on dopamine neurons. Science 188:1217–1219, 1975

Siegel BV, Trestman RL, O'Flaithbheartaigh S, et al: D-amphetamine challenge effects in Wisconsin Card Sort Test: performance in schizotypal personality disorder. Schizophr Res 20:29–32, 1996

Siever LJ, Davis KL: A psychobiological perspective on the personality disorders. Am J Psychiatry 148:1647–1658, 1991

Siever LJ, Trestman RL: The serotonin system and aggressive personality disorder. Int Clin Psychopharmacol 8 (suppl 2):33–39, 1993

Siever LJ, Coccaro EF, Klar H, et al: Biological markers in borderline and related personality disorders, in Biological Psychiatry: Proceedings of the 4th World Congress of Biological Psychiatry. Edited by Shagass C, Josiassen RG, Wagner BH. New York, Elsevier, 1986, pp 566–568

Siever LJ, Amin F, Coccaro EF, et al: Plasma homovanillic acid in schizotypal personality disorder. Am J Psychiatry 148:1246–1248, 1991

Siever LJ, Kalus OF, Keefe RS: The boundaries of schizophrenia. Psychiatr Clin North Am 16:217–244, 1993a

Siever LJ, Amin F, Coccaro EF: CSF homovanillic acid in schizotypal personality disorder. Am J Psychiatry 150:149–151, 1993b

Siever LJ, Buchsbaum MS, New AS, et al: d,l-fenfluramine response in impulsive personality disorder assessed with [18F]flurodeoxyglucose positron emission tomography. Neuropsychopharmacology 20:413–423, 1999

Silverman JH, Pinkham L, Horvath TB, et al: Affective and impulsive personality disorder traits in the relatives of borderline personality disorder. Am J Psychiatry 148:1378–1385, 1991

Silverman JM, Smith CJ, Guo SL: Ventricular volume and asymmetry in schizotypal personality disorder and schizophrenia assessed with magnetic resonance imaging. Schizophr Res 27:45–53, 1998

Simeon D, Stanley B, Frances A, et al: Self-mutilation in personality disorders: psychological and biological correlates. Am J Psychiatry 149:221–226, 1992

Soloff PH: Algorithms for pharmacological treatment of personality dimensions: symptom-specific treatments for cognitive-perceptual, affective, and impulsive-behavioral dysregulation. Bull Menninger Clin 62:195–214, 1998

Soloff PH: Psychopharmacology of borderline personality disorder. Psychiatr Clin North Am 23:169–192, 2000

Soloff PH, George A, Nathan RS, et al: Paradoxical effects of amitriptyline in borderline patients. Am J Psychiatry 143:1603–1605, 1986

Soloff PH, George A, Nathan RS, et al: Amitryptiline versus haloperidol in borderlines: final outcomes and predictors of response. J Clin Psychopharmacol 9:238–246, 1989

Soloff PH, Cornelius JR, George A, et al: Efficacy of phenelzine and haloperidol in borderline personality disorder. Arch Gen Psychiatry 50:377–385, 1993

Soloff PH, Meltzer CC, Greer PJ, et al: A fenfluramine-activated FDG-PET study of borderline personality disorder. Biol Psychiatry 47:540–547, 2000

Stanford MS, Houston RJ, Mathias CW, et al: A double-blind placebo-controlled crossover study of phenytoin in individuals with impulsive aggression. Psychiatry Res 103:193–203, 2001

Stein MB, Fyer AJ, Davidson JR, et al: Fluvoxamine treatment of social phobia (social anxiety disorder): a double-blind, placebo-controlled study. Am J Psychiatry 156:756–760, 1999

Steinberg BJ, Trestman RL, Siever LJ: The cholinergic and noradrenergic neurotransmitter systems and affective instability in borderline personality disorder, in Biological and Neurobehavioral Studies of Borderline Personality Disorder. Edited by Silk KR. Washington, DC, American Psychiatric Press, 1994, pp 41–62

Steinberg BJ, Trestman RL, Mitropoulou V, et al: Depressive response to physostigmine challenge in borderline personality disorder patients. Neuropsychopharmacology 17:264–273, 1997

Sternberg DE: Pharmacotherapy and affective syndromes in borderline personality disorder. Paper presented at the 140th annual meeting of the American Psychiatric Association, Chicago, IL, May 9–15, 1987

Szigethy EM, Schulz SC: Risperidone in comorbid borderline personality disorder and dysthymia. J Clin Psychopharmacol 17:326–327, 1997

Tancer ME, Mailman RB, Stein MB, et al: Neuroendocrine responsivity to monoaminergic system probes in generalized social phobia. Anxiety 1:216–223, 1994

Tiihonen J, Kuikka J, Bergstrom K, et al: Dopamine reuptake site densities in patients with social phobia. Am J Psychiatry 154:239–242, 1997a

Tiihonen J, Kuikka JT, Bergstrom KA, et al: Single-photon emission tomography imaging of monoamine transporters in impulsive violent behavior. Eur J Nucl Med 24:1253–1260, 1997b

Torgerson S: Genetic and nosological aspects of schizotypal and borderline personality disorders. Arch Gen Psychiatry 41:546–554, 1984

Tsuang MT, Stone WS, Tarbox SI, et al: An integration of schizophrenia with schizotypy: identification of schizotaxia and implications for research on treatment and prevention. Schizophr Res 54:169–175, 2002

Valzelli L: Psychobiology of Aggression and Violence. New York, Raven, 1980

Versiani M, Nardi AE, Figueira I, et al: Double-blind placebo-controlled trial with bromazepam in social phobia. J Bras Psiquiatr 46:167–171, 1997

Virkkunen M, Nuutila A, Goodwin FK, et al: Cerebrospinal fluid monoamine metabolite levels in male arsonists. Arch Gen Psychiatry 44:241–247, 1987

Walsh M-T, Dinan TG: Selective serotonin reuptake inhibitors and violence: a review of the available evidence. Acta Psychiatr Scand 104:84–91, 2001

Wetzel RD, Cloninger CR, Hong B, et al: Personality as a subclinical expression of the affective disorders. Compr Psychiatry 21:197–205, 1980

Widiger TA: Generalized social phobia versus avoidant personality disorder: a commentary on three studies. J Abnorm Psychol 101:340–343, 1992

PERSONALITY TRAITS/DISORDERS AND DEPRESSION

A Summary of Conceptual and Empirical Findings

M. Tracie Shea, Ph.D.

Shirley Yen, Ph.D.

The relevance of personality to depression is evident in the enormous attention that their association has received over the years in the clinical and research literatures. Although the theories and conceptualizations underlying the personality-depression relationship have varied widely, the idea that personality is important to understanding the cause, manifestation, or outcome of depression has persisted. Most of the earlier work in this area focused on personality traits. With the introduction of a separate axis for personality disorders in DSM-III (American Psychiatric Association 1980), numerous studies reporting on the high rates of diagnostic co-occurrence led to a focus on the relationship between personality disorders and depressive disorders (for review, see Klein et al. 1993). Despite the large number of studies in this area, the nature of the relationship of personality traits or disorders with depression remains far from clear. This is perhaps not surprising given the complexity of the constructs and the wide variability in conceptualizations, measurement, and research designs used to investigate the association of personality and depression.

The goal of this chapter is to provide a summary of the issues and findings in this area. We first review different models of the relationship between personality traits and disorders and depression. We then review specific theories of the personality-depression relationships and some of the relevant empirical literature examining the associations.

Models of Personality-Depression Relationships

Several authors have summarized the various ways in which the personality-depression relationship has been conceptualized. One of the earlier attempts to provide clarity to the literature was an article by Akiskal and colleagues (1983). Klein and colleagues (1993) provided a detailed review of the various models proposed and how they apply to different theories and specific clinical syndromes. They emphasized the role of these models as abstract hypotheses about the ways in which personality and depression can logically be related, noting that despite the conceptual appeal of the models, it is very difficult to test them empirically (Klein et al. 1993).

Table 3–1 summarizes the models as outlined by Klein and colleagues (1993). The first, *independence,* explains associations as artifactual results of general risk or of help-seeking factors. For example, having both a personality disorder and a depressive disorder increases the likelihood of an individual's seeking treatment, resulting in increased rates of his or her co-occurrence in clinical samples. This factor is important to consider in studies of clinical samples, although studies in community (i.e., nontreatment-seeking) samples should provide an unbiased assessment of the associations. Despite the possible influence of sampling bias on some of the research findings, it is unlikely that the high rates of co-occurrence so consistently found can be explained by treatment-seeking biases.

Pathoplasty models also assume independence of conditions in terms of etiology but emphasize the influence of features of one on the presentation or course of the other. This can work both ways, in that personality style may influence the manner in which depression is experienced and expressed, and depressed mood may influence the expression of the personality style. For example, individuals with an impulsive or disinhibited personality style may respond to depressed mood with active behaviors to cope, such as substance abuse or risk-taking behaviors. A compulsive personality, in contrast, may become even more rigid, or a depressive episode might subdue a normally more

TABLE 3–1. Models of hypothesized associations between personality and depression

Model	Distinct conditions?	Shared etiology?	Nature of association
Independence	Yes	No	Chance or help-seeking factors
Pathoplasty	Yes	No	One influences the expression or course of the other
Common cause	Yes	Yes	Shared etiology
Spectrum (subclinical)	No	Yes	Manifestations of common pathological process (current and etiological)
Vulnerability (predisposition)	Yes	No	One creates risk for onset of the other
Complication (scar)	Yes	No	One is residual effect or "scar" of the other

Source. Adapted from Klein et al. 1993.

expressive personality. Although this model assumes independence of etiologies, the use of the term *pathoplasty* to describe the influence of one condition on the course of another condition does suggest the involvement of causal mechanisms in terms of course. An example of such a mechanism could be the influence of personality on the individual's response to treatment (Widiger et al. 1999). A paranoid personality style, for example, would negatively affect the likelihood of an individual's entering or maintaining a therapeutic relationship, precluding or lessening the possibility of therapeutic treatments and hence influencing the course of the depression. Personality styles could also be associated with life circumstances that increase or decrease the likelihood of an onset or recurrence of depression through such mechanisms as the "buffering" effects of social supports. The overlap of this aspect of pathoplasty with the vulnerability model, described later in this section, highlights the difficulty in clearly distinguishing among these various abstract models.

Common-cause models assume that personality and depression, although distinct and independent once developed, share a common etiology. *Spectrum,* or subclinical, models are conceptually close to common-cause models in their assumption of a shared etiology but assume that one disorder is a manifestation or variant of the other, rather than a distinct disorder. For example, one disorder may be an early stage (prodromal) or a less severe (subclinical) manifestation of the other. The "spectrum" is usually a continuum of severity or impairment. Thus, these models focus on a common pathological process, although a common-cause model would assume distinct pathological processes once the conditions have developed, despite the shared etiology. *Vulnerability*, or "predisposition," models assume that one condition precedes and increases the risk of the other condition. In contrast to the spectrum model, vulnerability models assume different pathological processes: one for the development of the condition that poses the risk, and another for the influence of the first condition (the risk factor) on the development of the second condition. Thus, the second condition develops at least in part because the first condition creates risk factors specific to the second condition. Examples of vulnerability models can be seen in various diathesis-stress models that have been articulated to describe the relationships between stress, personality, and depression. Certain kinds of environmental stressors are hypothesized to interact with the vulnerabilities (e.g., temperament, personality traits, cognitive styles) resulting in depression.

Complication, or "scar," models are similar to vulnerability models because they assume distinct conditions that are related in that one condition develops because of the presence of the other. However, complication models focus on the residual or recovery phase of an initial disorder and view the second condition or disorder as a complication, or scar, resulting from the first. It is difficult even conceptually to distinguish the complication model from the vulnerability model. The main distinction is the emphasis in the former on recovery phase of the initial disorder and the emphasis on persistence of the second condition even after recovery from the first. The complication model has typically referred to the presence of certain personality traits, such as dependency and introversion, following episodes of depression.

It is important to keep in mind that these models are abstractions that highlight certain aspects of possible associations among disorders or conditions and that they are not all mutually exclusive. Klein and colleagues (1993) note that "[e]ven from these descriptions of the models in their abstract and hypothetical forms, it is apparent that the boundaries between types of models may often be quite arbitrary or fluid" (p. 12). No single model is likely to explain the complex links among personality and depression. Nonetheless, the models provide a useful framework for approaching the large and complex literature in this area. Next, we provide an overview of theories and research on personality dimensions and depression, followed by the more recent literature on personality disorders and depression.

TABLE 3–2. Vulnerabilities to depression: sociotropy/dependence (SOC-DEP) vs. autonomy/self-criticism (AUT-SC)

Dimensions	Regulation of self-esteem	Proneness to depression
SOC-DEP	Through interpersonal relations	When relationships fail
AUT-SC	Through achievement of personal standards and goals	When goals and standards not met

Personality Traits and Dimensions

There are several different lines of research that have examined the association of personality traits and depression. These may be grouped broadly into research on the personality dimensions of sociotropy/dependency and autonomy/self-criticism (derived from psychoanalytic and cognitive theories of depression) and on the personality traits derived from factor-analytic approaches to the study of normal personality. In addition, Cloninger's (1987) model of temperament and personality has been examined in relation to types of symptoms and as a predictor of treatment response. Not surprisingly, there is overlap among the constructs derived from these diverse approaches.

Sociotropy/Dependency Versus Autonomy/Self-Criticism

Conceptual Models

The personality dimension of sociotropy/dependency (SOC-DEP) and autonomy/self-criticism (AUT-SC) has been conceptualized and studied as vulnerabilities for depression (see Table 3–2). SOC-DEP refers to a personality type that seeks to establish interpersonal relations to bolster low self-esteem and is prone to depression when relationships end or fail. AUT-SC refers to a personality type that is excessively focused on achievement of internalized standards and goals for the maintenance of self-esteem, with a tendency toward self-criticism and vulnerability to depression when these goals are not realized. These terms refer to overlapping constructs independently developed by psychoanalytic and cognitive theorists. SOC-DEP as used here incorporates the construct of *sociotropy* from Beck's cognitive theory of depression (Beck 1983) and constructs from psychoanalytic theories including *dependency* (Blatt et al. 1976), *interpersonal dependency* (Hirschfeld et al. 1977), and *anaclitic depression* (Spitz 1946). AUT-SC has reference to the overlapping constructs of *autonomy* (Hirschfeld et al. 1977), *self-criticism* (Blatt et al. 1976), *introjective depression* (Blatt 1974), and *dominant goal personalities* (Arieti and Bemporad 1980), from psychoanalytic approaches, and *autonomy,* from cognitive theory (Beck 1983). Whereas both groups of terms share conceptual similarities, there are differences between the psychoanalytically derived concepts (e.g., dependency, self-criticism) and cognitive-behavioral concepts (e.g., sociotropy, autonomy). The psychoanalytic definition presumes that these two types of personalities represent enduring stable personality traits that are fixed in early childhood experiences and are unlikely to occur simultaneously or within the same individual (Coyne and Whiffen 1995). In contrast, Beck postulated that these characteristics should not be regarded as fixed, but rather as different modes that can dominate an individual's functioning, that may be associated with different etiologies or different depressive symptoms, and that may interact with treatment. Furthermore, several empirical studies have provided evidence to suggest that the concepts are not mutually exclusive within an individual (i.e., individuals can score high on both dimensions of SOC-DEP and AUT-SC [Coyne and Whiffen 1995]).

Empirical Findings

Over the past 20 years, empirical studies have examined the association between these personality dimensions and depression. A meta-analysis of published studies from 1976 to 1989 found 21 such studies, but only four of these were prospective (Nietzel and Harris 1990). The mean effect sizes for the relationships with depression were statistically significant for both SOC-DEP and AUT-SC, but they were small (an average of 0.28 and 0.31, respectively). Effect sizes were also significantly smaller in the prospective than in the cross-sectional studies (0.25 vs. 0.29 for SOC-DEP; 0.19 vs. 0.33 for AUT-SC). Both SOC-DEP and AUT-SC scores have been found to be higher in patients who have recovered from depression compared with never-depressed control subjects, and SOC-DEP scores have been found to decrease significantly from the depressed to the remitted state (Coyne and Whiffen 1995). In their review, Coyne and Whiffen (1995) outlined a number of methodological problems with research on this topic and concluded that evidence from the few existing longitudinal studies that have examined these two personality dimensions does not support their role as risk factors for depression. One study (Hirschfeld et al. 1989) of assessments of personality before the first onset of depression did report a statistically significant association between a measure of interpersonal dependency and onset of depression within the subsequent 6 years, but only for a subgroup of 11 individuals who were 30 years or older at the time of their first episode of depression.

Research in this area has also examined hypotheses from a more complex "diathesis-stress" variant of the vulnerability model, which predict that individuals will become depressed when they experience a life event that matches their predisposing personal vulnerability (Coyne and Whiffen 1995). This congruency hypothesis predicts that individuals with high scores on SOC-DEP are more likely to become depressed when faced with interpersonal loss, whereas individuals with high scores on AUT-SC are more vulnerable to depression when faced with failure to achieve goals. A recent longitudinal investigation of this model found only partial support for the predicted relations and in general failed to support the hypothesis that SOC-DEP and AUT-SC serve as vulnerability factors for matching interpersonal and achievement-related stress (Kwon and Whisman 1998). Previous studies investigating the congruency hypothesis report mixed and ambiguous findings, and many of these studies had methodological limitations such as small sample sizes, discarding participants based on not meeting criteria for prototypes of pure dimensions, and analyzing data that obscure the temporal relationship between personality dimensions and symptom changes (Coyne and Whiffen 1995). Therefore, despite decades of research, longitudinal studies of SOC-DEP and AUT-SC have failed to substantively conclude that these dimensions, or the interaction of these dimensions with matched life stressors, serve as diatheses for depression.

Two studies (Rohde et al. 1990; Shea et al. 1996) have examined the complication model for SOC-DEP by comparing predepression scores with those following recovery. In both studies, the dependency scores did not increase from their premorbid levels following a depressive episode.

Negative Affectivity/Negative Emotionality/Neuroticism and Positive Affectivity/Positive Emotionality/Extraversion

Conceptual Models

The other predominant theme in the literature on personality traits and depression has focused on robust dimensions emerging from factor-analytic studies (see Table 3–3). In particular, the dimensions of neuroticism and introversion/extraversion from factor-analytic studies by Eysenck (1990) have been examined in relation to depression. More

TABLE 3–3. Factor-analytic studies of temperamental dimensions associated with depression

Studies	Dimensions
Eysenck (1990)	Neuroticism Introversion/extraversion
Tellegen (1985)	Negative emotionality Positive emotionality
Clark and Watson 1991)	Negative affectivity Positive affectivity

recent factor models of temperament have proposed very similar dimensions, including Tellegen's (1985) factors of negative emotionality and positive emotionality, and Watson and Clark's (Clark and Watson 1991; Watson and Clark 1992) factors of negative temperament (also called negative emotionality or affectivity), and positive temperament (also called positive emotionality or affectivity). These two dimensions also correspond to the first two dimensions, neuroticism and introversion/extraversion of the "Big Five" or five-factor model of personality, independently identified through years of research (Digman 1990; see also Chapter 4 this book).

As described by Tellegen (1985) and by Clark and colleagues (Clark and Watson 1991; Clark et al. 1994), the core of the negative affectivity/negative emotionality/neuroticism (NA/N) dimension is a stable temperamental sensitivity to negative stimuli. A broad range of negative moods are associated with this dimension, including sadness and depression but also anxiety, guilt, hostility, and self-dissatisfaction. In addition, a wide range of nonmood aspects are related to NA/N, including negative cognitions and negativistic appraisals of self and others, low self-esteem, and life dissatisfaction (Clark et al. 1994). Similar to NA/N, the dimension variously referred to as positive affectivity/positive emotionality/extraversion (PA/E) is conceptualized as a stable and heritable temperamental dimension that encompasses several lower order traits, including positive affect, energy, affiliation, and dominance. The core of this dimension is believed to be affective, reflecting a tendency to experience positive mood states (Clark et al. 1994). In the tripartite model of Clark and Watson (1991), high NA/N is viewed as a vulnerability to both anxiety and depression (or "distress" disorders more generally), whereas low PA/E is believed to be more specifically associated with depression.

These dimensions have also been conceptually linked to depression

TABLE 3–4. Negative and positive affectivity

Negative affectivity/negative emotionality/neuroticism (NA/N)	Positive affectivity/positive emotionality/extraversion (PA/E)
• Stable and heritable temperamental dimension	• Stable and heritable temperamental dimension
• Tendency to experience broad range of negative moods: sadness, dysphoria, anxiety, guilt, hostility	• Tendency to experience positive affect and mood states, energy, affiliation, dominance
• Wide range of nonmood aspects: negative cognitions, negativistic appraisals of self and others, low self-esteem, life dissatisfaction	• Low PA/E associated with low energy and activity levels, withdrawal, decreased cognitive capacity, anhedonia, depressed mood
• Vulnerability to both anxiety and depressive disorders	• Low PA/E: vulnerability to depressive disorders
• Linked with an aversive motivational system (behavioral inhibition system)	• Linked to Gray's behavioral activation system (Fowles 1993), and Depue and colleague's behavioral facilitation system (Depue and Iacono 1988)
• Increases nonspecific arousal and attention to threat-related stimuli and inhibition of behavior (Gray 1982)	

through associations with biologically based motivation systems (Clark et al. 1994; Fowles 1993). NA/N has been linked with an aversive motivational system (the behavioral inhibition system), which is believed to increase nonspecific arousal and attention to threat-related stimuli and to inhibit behavior (Gray 1982). Fowles (1993) proposed that this system is important in both anxiety and depression. Fowles also linked PA/E to Gray's behavioral activation system and to the behavioral facilitation system proposed by Depue and colleagues (1988) to underlie bipolar affective disorders (Clark et al. 1994). Poor regulation of the behavioral facilitation system would be associated, on the low end of the PA/E dimension, with low energy and activity levels, withdrawal, decreased cognitive capacity, anhedonia, and depressed mood (Clark et al. 1994) (see Table 3–4).

Empirical Findings

Measures of NA/N and PA/E similarly have been found to be elevated during episodes of depression and to decrease upon recovery from depression. Scores on these dimensions following recovery from depression also remain higher than those of healthy control subjects. In contrast to the few studies of SOC-DEP and AUT-SC, results of prospective studies with assessments before the first onset of depression have suggested that elevated scores on NA/N are predictive of developing depression (Angst and Clayton 1986; Boyce et al. 1991; Hirschfeld et al. 1989; Kendler et al. 1993; Nystrom and Lindegard 1975), consistent with the vulnerability model. Low scores on PA/E, however, have not been found to predict the first onset of depression (Hirschfeld et al. 1989; Kendler et al. 1993).

A few studies have also examined whether there are increases on these dimensions that persist following recovery from prospectively observed episodes of depression (complication model). Shea and colleagues (1996) examined whether there were increases in NA/N and PA/E following recovery from depressive episodes from premorbid levels (before the first lifetime episode of depression). There were no increases in pathology on either of these dimensions, again suggesting that the higher pathology scores found on these measures cannot be explained by persisting consequences of depressive episodes. Instead, differences in this study were found on measures of NA/N for the group of participants who became depressed, both before the first episode of depression and following full recovery from depression, which is consistent with the vulnerability model. Similarly, Duggan and colleagues (1991) did not find increases in NA/N as a result of recurrent depression. Another study (Kendler et al. 1993), however, reported moderate elevations in NA/N following recovery from prospectively observed episodes of depression compared with premorbid scores. The average length of time following recovery to the repeated assessment in this study was notably shorter than in the study by Shea and colleagues (1996), suggesting that there may be temporary increases in NA/N that subside with time. Despite the negative findings, it remains possible that longer, more severe, or repeated episodes of depression may have a persisting impact on personality because the majority of the individuals in the existing studies experienced a single episode of depression of unclear severity during the intervals studied.

With regard to the pathoplasty model, NA/N has clearly been shown to negatively affect the course of depression, predicting a more chronic course (Hirschfeld et al. 1986). The effects of NA/N have been shown in studies as long as 18 years, with higher scores associated with more chronic depression and a poorer overall outcome (Andrews et al. 1990; Duggan et al. 1990). PA/E has shown smaller effects on course, but, as noted by Clark and colleagues (1994), earlier measures of extraversion stressed different aspects of the PA/E construct, limiting conclusions about the role of PA/E as a predictor of onset and course in depression.

Thus, of all the personality traits examined, NA/N has shown the strongest associations with depression. There is consistent evidence that this broad trait predicts the first onset of depression (vulnerability) and the course of depression (pathoplasty). There is little support for NA/N as a complication of depression. Another interpretation of the vulnerability findings, however, is that rather than an independent personality trait that is a risk factor for developing a mood disorder, NA/N is a subsyndromal or prodromal manifestation of depression, consistent with a spectrum or subclinical model (Hirschfeld et al. 1989). Findings from a longitudinal twin study of personality and major depression in women (Kendler et al. 1993) have provided support for a spectrum or common-cause model for NA/N and major depression. The results from their test of a complex model led these investigators to conclude that the significant relationship between neuroticism and liability to major depression in women is "largely the result of genetic factors that predispose to both neuroticism and major depression" (p. 853).

Whatever the nature of the relationship between NA/N and depression, however, it is clearly not a specific one. NA/N has also been shown to be associated with and predictive of other psychopathology, particularly anxiety disorders. As noted previously, the tripartite model of Clark and Watson (1991) views NA/N as a vulnerability to both anxiety and depression ("distress disorders"), and studies have shown NA/N to be elevated in patients with anxiety disorders and predictive of course (Clark et al. 1994; Jorm et al. 2000). Whereas most studies have focused on single disorders, a prospective study by Krueger (1999) examined personality traits assessed in late adolescence as predictors of multiple Axis I disorders in early adulthood. NA/N in subjects at age 18 years significantly predicted affective, anxiety, substance dependence, and antisocial personality disorders at age 21 years, controlling for the presence of these disorders at age 18 years. The factor corresponding to PA/E did not show predictive associations with any of the Axis I disorders (Krueger 1999).

Temperament and Character Model

Another relevant model of personality traits, proposed by Cloninger (1986, 1987), describes a basic set of heritable traits, each associated with a different neurobiological system. The earliest version of this model included the three traits of novelty seeking, harm avoidance, and reward dependence. Different combinations of these traits are assumed to underlie anxiety, affective, and personality disorders. Reward dependence, associated with the noradrenergic system, is most closely tied to depressive symptoms ("reactive dysphoria"). A high level of reward dependence is described as including a strong need for praise and approval of others and strong sensitivity to social cues of approval or rejection, which suggests an overlap with the SOC-DEP construct. Cloninger distinguishes reactive dysphoria from a more autonomous affective disturbance, which is unresponsive to environmental stimuli and unrelated to personality features.

Personality Disorders

Given the very high frequency of depressive diagnoses in individuals with personality disorders, as well as the common presence of personality disorders in individuals with depression, a large literature on the associations between the personality disorders and Axis I disorders has developed following the introduction of Axis II disorders in DSM-III. This work has proceeded largely independent of the work on personality traits and dimensions, although more recently there have been attempts to integrate these two approaches. We first review some relevant clinical typologies that have been described that incorporate features of both personality disorders (mostly borderline) and affective disorders, followed by consideration of research on borderline personality disorder (BPD) and depression, conceptualized as distinct disorders. We then briefly summarize findings from longitudinal studies of associations between the broader group of DSM-defined personality disorders and depression.

Clinical Typologies

Neurotic Depression

Several typologies that encompass both personality and affective features, with varying assumptions regarding etiological factors, have been proposed through the years (see Table 3–5). The earlier view, encompassed in the psychodynamic notion of "neurotic depression," assumed that personality features are primary and that the depression associated with such features (which is distinguished in some cases from other forms of depression such as endogenous or melancholic depression) is secondary to the personality features. Such personality features included dependent and "anal" or obsessive character traits, similar to the constructs of SOC-DEP and AUT-SC described previously.

TABLE 3–5. Evolution of clinical typologies linking personality and depression

Clinical typology	Assumptions/features
Neurotic depression (psychodynamic)	• Assumes personality features are primary • Associated depression is secondary to personality features: "dependent," "anal," or "obsessive" character traits
Depression spectrum disease (Winokur 1972)	• Fewer melancholic features, more unstable relationship histories • More irritable, demanding, and nervous • A form of neurotic-reactive depression • Depression is viewed as secondary to personality features
Character spectrum dysphoria (Akiskal et al. 1983)	• Depression viewed as secondary to long-standing characterological features • Dependent, histrionic, antisocial, and schizoid traits • Environment developmental actors: adverse and chaotic environments
Subaffective dysthymic disorder	• Chronic depressive • Onset before age 25 years • Depressive personality temperament: quiet, passive, gloomy, self-critical, given to worry, preoccupied with failure • Melancholic features

Depression Spectrum Disease

Other typologies that view depression as secondary to personality have emerged from attempts to classify the heterogeneous domain of mood disorders. Distinctions have been made and subtypes derived on the basis of presenting features and presumed etiology, sometimes incorporating differences in family history, course, and biological variables. Winokur and colleagues (Winokur 1972; Winokur et al. 1978) described a subgroup of female depressed patients with family histories of alcoholism and/or sociopathy ("depression spectrum disease") and contrasted them with depressive individuals with family histories of depression (and no alcoholism or sociopathy). The spectrum group had somewhat fewer melancholic features; more unstable relationship histories; and was more irritable, demanding, and nervous. Winokur considered this group as a form of neurotic-reactive depression, with the depression viewed as secondary to the personality features and "stormy" lifestyle.

Character Spectrum Dysphoria

Akiskal and colleagues (1983) also described a group of patients for whom depression was viewed as secondary to long-standing character-ological features—described as a mixture of dependent, histrionic, anti-social, and schizoid traits—and was attributed to adverse and chaotic environmental developmental factors. The depressive features were also viewed as strongly influenced by the personality styles or features, without the biological markers associated with endogenous depres-sions. Despite the name "character spectrum dysphoria," the etiological assumptions of this type are more consistent with the vulnerability and pathoplasty models.

Subaffective Dysthymic Disorder

Akiskal and colleagues proposed other subtypes for whom personality characteristics were believed to represent a milder (subclinical) or alter-native (spectrum) expression of an underlying and biologically deter-mined affective disorder. One of these (subaffective dysthymic disorder) included chronic depressive subjects with an early (before age 25 years) onset of personality traits similar to Schneider's depressive personality temperament (e.g., quiet, passive, gloomy, self-critical, given to worry, preoccupied with failure) and some melancholic fea-tures of depression (Akiskal et al. 1983). The criteria for depressive per-sonality disorder, included as an appendix disorder in DSM-IV-TR (American Psychiatric Association 2000), incorporated many of these features (Phillips et al. 1995). Akiskal and colleagues (1985) also de-scribed a subgroup of BPD subjects with concurrent affective disorders (mostly dysthymia or cyclothymia), proposing a mixture of causal fac-tors. For this group with "subaffective" borderline disorders, the de-pressive symptoms were proposed to be a result of the same biological factors as in the subaffective dysthymic subjects, but the borderline traits were proposed to be the result of unstable developmental histo-ries. Despite the separate original causes, the chronic affective disorder and the borderline features are proposed to interact, influencing the course and expression of each (Klein et al. 1993).

Research Findings

Borderline Personality Disorder and Depression

Several reviews have examined the research on BPD and depressive disorders in attempts to clarify the nature of their relationship (Gunder-son and Elliott 1985; Gunderson and Phillips 1991; Koenigsberg et al.

1999). Considering findings from research on phenomenology, comorbidity patterns, biological features, family history, course, and treatment response, conclusions have differed. In the most recent review, Koenigsberg and colleagues (1999) summarize recent understandings of findings that BPD and depression share similarities but also differ from depression in biology. Briefly, shared biological dysfunction in serotonergic activity and cholinergic sensitivity may be modulated by differences in levels of adrenergic activity to explain the common vulnerability to depressed, but distinct, patterns of mood reactivity. High levels of adrenergic activity in patients with BPD are associated with increased engagement in the social environment and hence greater mood reactivity, whereas low levels characteristic of major depression may result in decreased responsivity to external stimuli, more inward focus, and a more fixed, autonomous depressed mood.

The authors note that this model is a simplistic one, but it is noteworthy in its integration of distinct dimensions of vulnerability and dysfunction to explain similarities and differences among mood disorders and BPD. In addition to some shared biological features, this review notes that the psychosocial consequences of each of the disorders may predispose each to the other. Frequent "dependent" life events, such as social and occupational failures and losses resulting from affective instability, impulsivity, and maladaptive interpersonal patterns in BPD, increase risk for depressive episodes (Perry et al. 1992). Conversely, chronic depressed mood and irritability can lead to the persistent maladaptive relationship problems characteristic of BPD. Thus, conclusions from this review of BPD and depression (Koenigsberg et al. 1999) support spectrum, vulnerability, and complication models. Another conclusion from the review is that, similar to the findings for NA/ N, the link between BPD and depression is not a specific one. BPD co-occurs with several Axis I disorders, including anxiety, substance abuse, and eating disorders, and depression co-occurs with many of the personality disorders.

Personality Disorders and Course of Depression (Pathoplasty)

Much of the empirical literature that focuses on personality disorders more broadly has examined the influence of personality disorders on the course of depression (pathoplasty model). Such studies have included treatment studies and naturalistic studies, in which treatment is uncontrolled. In a review of pharmacological and psychosocial treatment studies of depression, Shea and colleagues (1992) report that studies of depressed patients with personality disorders typically (although not always) show that patients with comorbid depression and personality disorders have a poorer response to antidepressant medication (primarily tricyclic antidepressants) and short-term psychotherapy, compared with patients without a personality disorder. However, most of the reviewed studies demonstrating a poorer response examined the broad category of personality disorders rather than specific personality disorders. Studies that have examined features of specific personality disorders, particularly those in the dramatic cluster, seem to yield more inconsistent findings. In a more recent review, Mulder (2002) reported inconsistencies across studies as well and emphasized methodological limitations that prevent conclusions regarding the influence of personality disorders on treatment response.

Several factors may contribute to the discrepancy across studies. One possible explanation is that the patients exhibiting more severe dramatic cluster personality features (e.g., suicidality, antisocial features, substance abuse disorders) were excluded from many of the treatment studies, thereby producing a less severely disturbed sample (Shea et al. 1992). Another possible explanation is that the study designs are so varied in severity of sample, nature of comparison condition, and adequacy of assessment of personality disorders that definitive conclusions regarding the impact of personality disorder on course of depression are difficult to reach. On the other hand, it is a long-standing clinical belief that patients with personality disorders are less responsive to depression treatment, and most studies support this observation. Hypothesized reasons for this lessened response include the possibility that depression comorbid with personality disorders is a different and more chronic type of depression, that personality disorders may be associated with negative behavioral patterns and life circumstances that may increase risk for depression, or that patients with personality disorders are less likely to comply with treatment.

Personality Disorders and Onset of Depression

Studies of personality disorders with prospective, naturalistic designs in community adolescent samples have addressed the vulnerability model. Such samples provide a unique opportunity to examine whether depression serves as a risk factor for personality disorder and vice versa. In a study by Lewinsohn and colleagues (1997) in which 299 individuals were assessed for Axis I disorders twice during adolescence and assessed for both Axis I and II disorders at age 24 years, the presence of an early-onset Axis I disorder substantially increased the risk of personality disorders in young adulthood. Another community-based longitudinal study examined the bidirectional influence of risk between Axis I and Axis II disorders. Kasen and colleagues (1999) reported that prior major depression, as well as disruptive disorders and anxiety disorders, significantly increased the odds of personality disorder in young adulthood when controlling for the presence of adolescent personality disorder. Conversely, in the same study, adolescents with personality disorders were more than twice as likely as those without personality disorders to have mood disorders as well as anxiety, disruptive, and substance abuse disorders during early adulthood, even after controlling for comorbid Axis I disorders during adolescence (Johnson et al. 1999). This finding was validated in a different longitudinal adolescent community-sample study, in which subclinical Axis II symptoms were found to be risk factors for depressive symptomatology 3 years later (Daley et al. 1999). These studies seem to indicate a bidirectional influence of risk, in which having a personality disorder increases risk for subsequent development of a depressive disorder and vice versa. However, these studies suggest that the risk is not specific to depression or to particular personality disorders. Although these findings are consistent with the vulnerability model, it is also possible that some common pathological processes underlie the psychopathology across Axis I and II, as in a common-cause or spectrum model. This possibility highlights once again the point that despite the consistent findings of associations, even in longitudinal studies, it is difficult to determine the specific nature of the relationships (see Chapter 9 of this book for further discussion of adolescents).

Integration of Personality Traits and Disorders

An important direction of research on personality and psychopathology in the past decade is the focus on the relationship of personality disorders to dimensional models of personality traits, specifically the five-factor model of personality. In addition to the broad factor of NA/N and PA/E, discussed previously, the dimensions of (low) agreeableness (e.g., callousness, manipulativeness, suspiciousness) and (low) constraint or conscientiousness (e.g., impulsivity, disinhibition) have been related to personality disorders. Clark and colleagues (1996) examined the factor structures emerging from analyses of scores from two measures developed specifically to assess features or traits of personality disorder and then compared these structures to the factors of the five-factor model. Four of five factors that they identified showed close correspondence to the five-factor model dimensions of neuroticism, introversion, (dis)agreeableness, and (low) conscientiousness. Watson and colleagues (1994) also articulate the links of these dimensions to psychopathology common to the Axis I disorders. As discussed previously, the neuroticism or negative affectivity domain include traits that are relevant to a wide range of symptoms (e.g., depressed mood, guilt, self-blame) and disorders (e.g., depressive, anxiety, somatoform, and personality disorders). Low PA/E is linked to mood disorders more specifically, and low conscientiousness and low agreeableness are related to conduct disorder as well as antisocial personality disorder. Watson and colleagues further comment that many types of psychopathology, including depression and anxiety, are fairly stable and traitlike, with transient increases in level caused by stressful events. This integrative model offers a different explanation for the association of personality features and depression than has been postulated by various vulnerability or diathesis stress models: that conceptually distinct constructs such as dysfunctional cognitive schema, stress appraisals (reflected in reports of stressful life events), and dysphoric affect may all be components or lower order facets/expressions of the more general construct of NA/N. This view is thus more consistent with the common-cause or spectrum models of personality and depression.

Conclusions

The extensive amount of literature devoted to the topic of personality and depression speaks to the salience of the relationship between them. The literature has moved over time from theories and typologies based on clinical observations, to more empirically based studies of the relationships between various personality constructs and depression, to a more integrative model of lower and higher order trait structures that may underlie personality and psychopathology more broadly. What can be concluded from this vast literature?

It is clear that associations between personality traits/dimensions/disorders and depression exist. The "independence" model, which attributes any associations to treatment-seeking bias or chance factors, is untenable as a general explanation, although certainly treatment-seeking bias may result in higher rates of co-occurrence compared with nontreatment-seeking samples.

There is evidence that personality pathology has a broadly negative impact on the course of depression, particularly for neuroticism. The specific aspects of personality disorders, and the processes that underlie such negative effects both for neuroticism and for personality disorders, however, are far from clear. Neuroticism also increases risk for onset and recurrence of depressive episodes, although neuroticism also increases risk for other Axis I disorders, including anxiety and substance abuse disorders. The other personality traits with the strongest theoretical ties to depression, interpersonal dependency (SOC-DEP), and excessive autonomy and self-criticalness (AUT-SC), have also not shown specific associations with depression and, further, do not appear to increase risk for depression. There is also evidence that the Axis II personality disorders are a vulnerability to not only depression but to other Axis I disorders as well. Thus personality psychopathology can be viewed as a general vulnerability to a broad range of psychopathology. Pathological personality traits do not appear to be a residual complication of episodes of depression.

An important direction for the field has been the identification of higher order dimensions that underlie the domain of personality psychopathology and also the domain of what is currently defined as separate, Axis I disorders (Siever and Davis 1991). The conceptualization of these broad dimensions as underlying a wide range of psychopathology, currently categorized as distinct disorders, supports the common-cause/spectrum models. However, a key question for future research concerns how such core dimensions may represent vulnerabilities and what mechanisms are involved in their leading to "disorder." It will be important in future research to move beyond an exclusive focus on single disorders to understand the relationship between "personality" and "depression."

References

Akiskal HS, Hirschfeld RMA, Yerevanian BI: The relationship of personality to affective disorders. Arch Gen Psychiatry 40:801–810, 1983

Akiskal HS, Chen SE, Davis GC, et al: Borderline: an adjective in search of a noun. J Clin Psychiatry 46:41–48, 1985

American Psychiatric Association: Diagnostic and Statistical Manual of Mental Disorders, 3rd Edition. Washington, DC, American Psychiatric Association, 1980

American Psychiatric Association: Diagnostic and Statistical Manual of Mental Disorders, 4th Edition, Text Revision. Washington, DC, American Psychiatric Association, 2000

Andrews G, Neilson M, Hunt C, et al: Diagnosis, personality and the long-term outcome of depression. Br J Psychiatry 157:13–18, 1990

Angst J, Clayton P: Premorbid personality of depressive, bipolar, and schizophrenic patients with special reference to suicidal issues. Compr Psychiatry 27:511–532, 1986

Arieti S, Bemporad J: The psychological organization of depression. Am J Psychiatry 136:1360–1365, 1980

Beck AT: Cognitive therapy of depression: new perspectives, in Treatment of Depression: Old Controversies and New Approaches. Edited by Clayton PJ, Barrett JE. New York, Raven, 1983, pp 265–290

Blatt SJ: Levels of object representation in analytic and introjective depression. Psychoanal Study Child 29:105–157, 1974

Blatt SJ, D'Afflitti JP, Quinlan DM: Experiences of depression in normal adults. J Abnorm Psychol 85:383–389, 1976

Boyce P, Parker G, Barnett B, et al: Personality as a vulnerability factor to depression. Br J Psychiatry 159:106–114, 1991

Clark LA, Watson D: Tripartite model of anxiety and depression: psychometric evidence and taxonomic implications. J Abnorm Psychol 100:316–336, 1991

Clark LA, Watson D, Mineka S: Temperament, personality, and the mood and anxiety disorders. J Abnorm Psychol 103:103–116, 1994

Clark LA, Livesley WJ, Schroeder ML, et al: Convergence of two systems for assessing specific traits of personality disorder. Psychol Assess 8:294–303, 1996

Cloninger CR: A unified biosocial theory of personality and its role in the development of anxiety states. Psychiatr Dev 3:167–226, 1986

Cloninger CR: A systematic method for clinical description and classification of personality variants: a proposal. Arch Gen Psychiatry 44:573–588, 1987

Coyne JC, Whiffen VE: Issues in personality as diathesis for depression: the case of soiotropy-dependency and autonomy-self-criticism. Psychol Bull 118:358–378, 1995

Daley SE, Hammen C, Burge D, et al: Depression and Axis II symptomatology in an adolescent community sample: concurrent and longitudinal associations. J Personal Disord 13:47–59, 1999

Depue RA, Iacono WG: Neurobehavioral aspects of affective disorders. Annu Rev Psychol 40:457–492, 1988

Digman JM: Personality structure: emergence of the five-factor model. Annu Rev Psychol 41:417–440, 1990

Duggan CF, Lee AS, Murray RM: Does personality predict long-term outcome in depression? Br J Psychiatry 157:19–24, 1990

Duggan CF, Sham P, Lee AS, et al: Does recurrent depression lead to a change in neuroticism? Psychol Med 21:985–990, 1991

Eysenck HJ: Biological dimensions of personality, in Handbook of Personality: Theory and Research. Edited by Pervin LA. New York, Guilford, 1990, pp 244–276

Fowles DC: A motivational theory of psychopathology, in Nebraska Symposium on Motivation: Integrated Views of Motivation—Cognition and Emotion, Vol 41. Edited by Spaulding W. Lincoln, NE, University of Nebraska Press, 1994, pp 181–238

Gray JA: The Neuropsychology of Anxiety: An Inquiry Into the Functions of the Septa-Hippocampal System. Oxford, UK, Clarendon Press, 1982

Gunderson JG, Elliott GR: The interface between borderline personality disorder and affective disorder. Am J Psychiatry 142:277–288, 1985

Gunderson JG, Phillips KA: A current view of the interface between borderline personality disorder and depression. Am J Psychiatry 148:967–975, 1991

Hirschfeld RMA, Klerman GL, Gough HG, et al: A measure of interpersonal dependency. J Pers Assess 41:610–618, 1977

Hirschfeld RMA, Klerman GL, Andreasen N, et al: Psycho-social predictors of chronicity in depressed patients. Br J Psychiatry 148:648–654, 1986

Hirschfeld RMA, Klerman GL, Lavori P, et al: Premorbid personality assessments of first onset of major depression. Arch Gen Psychiatry 46:345–350, 1989

Johnson JG, Cohen P, Skodol AE, et al: Personality disorders in adolescence and risk of major mental disorders and suicidality during adulthood. Arch Gen Psychiatry 56:805–811, 1999

Jorm AF, Christensen H, Henderson AS, et al: Predicting anxiety and depression from personality: Is there a synergistic effect of neuroticism and extraversion? J Abnorm Psychol 109:145–149, 2000

Kasen S, Cohen P, Skodol AE, et al: Influence of child and adolescent psychiatric disorders on young adult personality disorder. Am J Psychiatry 156:1529–1535, 1999

Kendler KS, Neale MC, Kessler RC, et al: A longitudinal twin study of personality and major depression in women. Arch Gen Psychiatry 50:853–862, 1993

Klein MH, Wonderlich S, Shea MT: Models of relationships between personality and depression: toward a framework for theory and research, in Personality and Depression: A Current View. Edited by Klein MH, Kupfer DJ, Shea MT. New York, Guilford, 1993, pp 1–54

Koenigsberg JW, Anwunah I, New AS, et al: Relationship between depression and borderline personality disorder. Depress Anxiety 10:158–167, 1999

Krueger RF: Personality traits in late adolescence predict mental disorders in early adulthood: a prospective-epidemiological study. J Pers 67:39–65, 1999

Kwon P, Whisman MA: Sociotropy and autonomy as vulnerabilities to specific life events: issues in life event categorization. Cognit Ther Res 22:353–362, 1998

Lewinsohn PM, Rohde P, Seeley JR, et al: Axis II psychopathology as a function of Axis I disorders in childhood and adolescence. J Am Acad Child Adolesc Psychiatry 36:1752–1759, 1997

Mulder RT: Personality pathology and treatment outcome in major depression: a review. Am J Psychiatry 159:359–371, 2002

Nietzel MT, Harris MJ: Relationship of dependency and achievement/autonomy to depression. Clin Psychol Rev 10:279–297, 1990

Nystrom S, Lindegard B: Predisposition for mental syndrome: a study comparing predispositions for depression, neurasthenia, and anxiety state. Acta Psychiatr Scand 51:69–76, 1975

Perry JC, Lavori PW, Pagano CJ, et al: Life events and recurrent depression in borderline and antisocial personality disorders. J Personal Disord 6:394–407, 1992

Phillips KA, Hirschfeld RMA, Shea MT, et al: Depressive personality disorder, in The DSM-IV Personality Disorders. Edited by Livesley WJ. New York, Guilford, 1995, pp 287–302

Rohde P, Lewinsohn PM, Seeley JR: Are people changed by the experience of having an episode of depression? A further test of the scar hypothesis. J Abnorm Psychol 99:264–271, 1990

Shea MT, Widiger TA, Klein MH: Comorbidity of personality disorders and depression: implications for treatment. J Consult Clin Psychol 60:857–868, 1992

Shea MT, Leon AC, Mueller TI, et al: Does major depression result in lasting personality change? Am J Psychiatry 153:1404–1410, 1996

Siever LJ, Davis KL: A psychobiological perspective on the personality disorders. Am J Psychiatry 148:1647–1658, 1991

Spitz RA: Anaclitic depression. Psychoanal Study Child 2:313–342, 1946

Tellegen A: Structures of mood and personality and their relevance to assessing anxiety, with an emphasis on self-report, in Anxiety and the Anxiety Disorders. Edited by Tuma AH, Maser JD. Hillsdale, NJ, Erlbaum, 1985, pp 681–706

Watson D, Clark LA: On traits and temperament: general and specific factors of emotional experiences and their relations to the five-factor model. J Pers 60:443–476, 1992

Watson D, Clark LA, Harkness AR: Structures of personality and their relevance to psychopathology. J Abnorm Psychol 103:18–31, 1994

Widiger TA, Verheul R, Van Den Brink W: Personality and psychopathology, in Handbook of Personality: Theory and Research. Edited by Pervin LA, John OP. New York, Guilford, 1999, pp 347–366

Winokur G: Depression spectrum disease: description and family study. Compr Psychiatry 13:3–8, 1972

Winokur G, Behar D, VanValkenberg C, et al: Is a familial definition of depression both feasible and valid? J Nerv Ment Dis 166:764–768, 1978

THE DEPRESSIVE PERSONALITY

Psychopathology, Assessment, and Treatment

Andrew G. Ryder, Ph.D.

R. Michael Bagby, Ph.D.

Margarita B. Marshall, B.Sc.

Paul T. Costa Jr., Ph.D.

The concept of depressive personality (DP), despite a long history in the clinical literature, continues to have an uncertain nosological status. Over the past 10 years there has been a move toward including a depressive personality disorder (DPD) category in the *Diagnostic and Statistical Manual of Mental Disorders*, and research criteria for further study are included in DSM-IV-TR (American Psychiatric Association 2000, pp. 732–733). These provisional criteria led to renewed interest in researching DP, much of which was devoted to evaluating the new category. The research accumulated to this end has been deemed sufficient by several commentators to allow the inclusion of a new personality disorder in future editions of DSM (e.g., Huprich 1998; McDermut et al. 2003; Phillips and Gunderson 1999).

At the same time, other researchers have suggested that there is insufficient evidence of construct validity to allow DPD to be considered an official diagnostic category (e.g., Clark and Watson 1999; McLean and Woody 1995; Ryder and Bagby 1999). Ryder and colleagues (2002) evaluated DPD according to the criteria suggested by Robins and Guze (1970) for establishing the validity of a psychiatric disorder and concluded that although depressive personality traits are both valid and measurable, there is little evidence to suggest that they are best captured by a categorical diagnosis. Importantly, although dysthymic disorder does describe many patients who clearly do not fit into the DPD category, the reverse does not appear to be the case. Ryder and colleagues also noted that similar difficulties are found with many of the other personality disorders, taking a position with other writers who have proposed that personality disorders are perhaps better conceptualized as extremes along dimensions of normal personality functioning (e.g., Krueger and Tackett 2003; Lynam and Widiger 2001; Widiger and Trull 1992).

Although we continue to side with this second perspective, this chapter has more modest ambitions. We aim here to introduce the DP construct by reviewing research on its psychopathology and then to offer suggestions regarding its assessment and treatment. Given the continued uncertainty, we will describe both DPD and DP traits when discussing these topics. Thus, we begin by summarizing the history and research on DPD, which will inevitably include some discussion of the problematic overlap with dysthymic disorder. We then move to a brief description of proposed dimensional alternatives to the personality disorders and the ways in which DP traits might be situated within such a system. As previously noted by Ryder and colleagues (2002), consideration of these issues is important to the accurate assessment of DP, a topic on which we pick up explicitly in the third part of this chapter. We conclude with a discussion of treatment options.

Psychopathology: Categorical Approach

Historical Development of Depressive Personality Disorder

One of the earliest descriptions of DPD was provided by Kraepelin (1921), who used the term *depressive temperament* to refer to a predisposition to manic-depressive illness. Kraepelin characterized people with this temperament as being predominantly depressed, gloomy, and despairing, as well as overly serious, guilt-ridden, self-reproaching, self-denying, and lacking in confidence. A few decades later, Schneider (1959) added a number of additional characteristics to this list, including hypohedonia, quietness, worry, skepticism, and dutifulness. The

TABLE 4–1. Historical development of depressive personality disorder

Source	Contribution
Kraepelin (1921)	Describes *depressive temperament* as a predisposition to manic-depressive illness, present in individuals who are predominantly depressed, gloomy, despairing, overly serious, guilt-ridden, self-reproaching, self-denying, and lacking in confidence
Schneider (1959)	Adds additional traits to Kraepelin's description, namely hypohedonia, quietness, worry, skepticism, and dutifulness
American Psychiatric Association (1952)	Includes a category for *depressive reaction* as well as a depressive subtype under the more general category of *cyclothymic personality disorder*
American Psychiatric Association (1968)	Renames *depressive reaction* as *depressive neurosis* while adding an additional category called *neurasthenic neurosis; cyclothymic personality disorder* is maintained, and *asthenic personality disorder* is added
American Psychiatric Association (1980)	Retains only depressive neurosis, renaming this construct *dysthymic disorder*
Akiskal (1983)	Develops research criteria for *depressive personality disorder,* using Schneider's descriptions
American Psychiatric Association (1994)	Introduces *depressive personality disorder* as a diagnosis in need of further study, with criteria similar to those proposed by Akiskal

modern DPD criteria were based on those developed by Akiskal (1983), which are ultimately derived from Schneider's work (see Table 4–1).

The notion that DPD and dysthymic disorder should be allowed to exist side by side has a precedent in the early editions of DSM. In DSM-I (American Psychiatric Association 1952), depressive reaction was classified as a psychoneurosis, whereas the depressive subtype of cyclothymic personality was considered a personality disorder. DSM-II (American Psychiatric Association 1968) altered the names of these categories and added two more, neurasthenic neurosis and asthenic personality disorder. Only one of these four categories, however, survived into the next edition. Depressive reaction, relabeled as depressive neurosis in DSM-II, settled into its most recent permutation as dysthymic disorder in DSM-III (American Psychiatric Association 1980) and survived through DSM-III-R (American Psychiatric Association 1987) to DSM-IV (American Psychiatric Association 1994) and DSM-IV-TR. The decision to retain a chronic and low-grade depressive diagnosis on Axis I while eliminating the personality disorder on Axis II aroused some controversy (Frances 1980; Gunderson 1983; Kernberg 1984). Moreover, the DSM-III manual confusingly asserted that the affective symptoms of dysthymic disorder might be secondary to personality pathology (Widiger 1999). Current efforts to advance DPD as a "new" personality disorder are based in part on a desire to fill what is seen as a hole in the current system, namely, the lack of an explicitly characterological diagnosis primarily involving depressive traits.

At the present time, dysthymic disorder continues to be the only official diagnostic category for a chronic depressive presentation, requiring the presence of clinically significant depressed mood for at least 2 years accompanied by at least two of six symptoms. This list includes two "psychological" symptoms—low self-esteem and feelings of hopelessness—reminiscent of DPD traits (Ryder and Bagby 1999). Indeed, one of the reasons for the overlap between DPD and dysthymic disorder may be that relatively few patients with clinically significant impairment can meet criteria for DPD without also having these two symptoms plus chronic depressed mood (Ryder et al. 2001). In contrast, the other symptoms are primarily somatic and vegetative; they include insomnia/hypersomnia, aphagia/hyperphagia, fatigue, and concentration/decision-making difficulties.

Although at present the Appendix B–based DPD category has been primarily of interest to researchers, this relative inattention will surely change if DPD is included in the main text of DSM, which it would likely do with traits similar to those under investigation. The current research criteria are as follows: 1) usual mood is dominated by dejection, gloominess, cheerlessness, joylessness, and unhappiness; 2) self-concept centers around beliefs of inadequacy, worthlessness, and low self-esteem; 3) is critical, blaming, and derogatory toward self; 4) is brooding and given to worry; 5) is negativistic, critical, and judgmental toward others; 6) is pessimistic; and 7) is prone to feeling guilty or remorseful (American Psychiatric Association 2000, p. 789) (see Table 4–2). Individuals who meet the general criteria for personality disorders who have five or more of these seven traits and who do not meet criteria for dysthymic disorder are considered to have DPD. The dysthymic disorder exclusion criterion is not always applied in research, especially when the objective is to study diagnostic overlap or to compare "pure" samples with the two disorders. Note that older studies using the criteria developed by Akiskal (1983) and Hirschfeld and Holzer (1994) demonstrated that this definition describes a similar but somewhat narrower group of people as compared with DSM-IV.

TABLE 4–2. DSM-IV diagnostic criteria for depressive personality disorder

A. A pervasive pattern of depressive cognitions and behaviors beginning by early adulthood and present in a variety of contexts, as indicated by five (or more) of the following:
   (1) usual mood is dominated by dejection, gloominess, cheerlessness, joylessness, unhappiness
   (2) self-concept centers around beliefs of inadequacy, worthlessness, and low self-esteem
   (3) is critical, blaming, and derogatory toward self
   (4) is brooding and given to worry
   (5) is negativistic, critical, and judgmental toward others
   (6) is pessimistic
   (7) is prone to feeling guilty or remorseful
B. Does not occur exclusively during major depressive episodes and is not better accounted for by dysthymic disorder

Source. Reprinted from American Psychiatric Association: *Diagnostic and Statistical Manual of Mental Disorders*, 4th Edition, Text Revision. Washington, DC, American Psychiatric Association, 2000. Used with permission.

Reliability and Stability

DPD researchers have largely been successful in establishing reliability for this diagnosis to at least the level obtained for other personality disorders. Four studies have established adequate agreement between separate clinicians rating the presence versus absence of DPD (Gunderson et al. 1994; Klein 1990; Klein and Miller 1993; Klein et al. 1998), and three studies have demonstrated modest agreement over time using 6-month (Klein 1990), 12-month (Gunderson et al. 1994), and 30-month (Klein et al. 1998) intervals.

Meanwhile, Klein (1990) found that there were no significant differences in the number of DPD traits in a group of outpatients assessed during a major depressive episode and assessed again after 2 months of full recovery. These findings suggest that DPD can be measured at least as reliably as can the other personality disorders and that this reliability is not unduly compromised by changes in acute mood state. This last point is important because it shows that endorsement of DPD traits is not simply a product of being depressed at a particular time.

Diagnostic Validity

Studies have demonstrated that the features of DPD include several core traits, including self-criticism, gloominess and joylessness, pessimism, low self-esteem and feelings of inadequacy, and frequent brooding (Gunderson et al. 1994; Klein 1990; Klein and Miller 1993). Secondary features include introversion and passivity, and there is some suggestion that chronic loss of interest might also be a feature (Klein and Vocisano 1999). Features of conscientiousness that were once thought to be a part of DP have not been empirically supported and have thus been dropped. Klein and Vocisano (1999) note that the current definition of DPD focuses on those traits associated with negative affectivity, with only one trait having even a partial relation to low positive affectivity. The effect here may be to increase internal consistency at the cost of discriminant validity, especially as negative affectivity cuts across a large number of clinical conditions, with low positive affectivity being more specific to depression (Clark et al. 1994).

Comorbidity

The issue of comorbidity has thus far been the most contentious part of the debate surrounding DPD, and even proponents of the category generally agree that this issue is an important one to resolve. DPD has a certain degree of conceptual overlap with several of the other personality disorders, especially with the borderline, dependent, avoidant, and obsessive-compulsive categories (Bagby et al. 2003; McDermut et al. 2003; Ryder and Bagby 1999), although ways of distinguishing specific aspects of these shared traits have been articulated (Phillips et al. 1992). Nevertheless, concerns regarding these descriptive similarities are warranted given the available empirical evidence. Although Phillips and colleagues (1992) found minimal overlap with Cluster A and Cluster B personality disorders, a 48% overlap between DPD and Cluster C was identified. Two other studies found that 58% of individuals with DPD met criteria for another personality disorder (Klein and Shih 1998; Lyoo et al. 1998). Although overlap rates are increased when disorders are combined, these findings still demonstrate that the personality disorders as a group suffer from excessive overlap (Bagby et al. 2003). Moreover, even though this overlap is in the same range as that found for other personality disorders, it does not therefore follow that Axis II should be further complicated by the addition of another problematic category (Ryder and Bagby 1999). The clinician wishing to make a diagnosis of DPD will have many difficult distinctions to make if overdiagnosis involving many personality disorder categories is to be avoided.

More than the personality disorders, the overlap with dysthymic disorder has been central to the debate over the current status of DPD. Ryder and colleagues (2002) reviewed a number of studies designed to answer this question and found a wide range of overlap rates, ranging from a low of 19% to a high of 95%, with an average of around 50% (Bagby and Ryder 1999; R.M. Bagby, A.G. Ryder, D.R. Schuller, "Depressive Personality Disorder and Dysthymic Disorder: Evaluating Trait/Symptom and Syndrome Overlap," unpublished manuscript, 2005; Hirschfeld and Holzer 1994; Huprich 2001; Klein and Miller 1993; Klein and Shih 1998; Phillips et al. 1998; Ryder et al. 2001; Skodol et al. 1999). Although the highest rate should be interpreted with caution, given the presence of major depression in all of the participants, we believe these findings speak to the difficulty of separating these two diagnoses. Admittedly, the largest and most recent study of this question (McDermut et al. 2003), published since the earlier review, has shown a particularly low overlap.

Two of these studies also used statistical modeling techniques to investigate several theoretically plausible configurations of DPD traits and dysthymic disorder symptoms (R.M. Bagby et al., unpublished manuscript, 2005; Ryder et al. 2001). Results in both studies indicated that these two criterion sets could indeed be separated but also that the best results were obtained when the psychological symptoms of dysthymic disorder—low self-esteem and feelings of hopelessness—were allowed into *both* categories, in keeping with previous predictions (Ryder and Bagby 1999). The overwhelming majority of people with DPD in these studies reported both of these symptoms, which, along with reporting sufficient depressed mood, explained much of the reported overlap. These results have been interpreted as demonstrating that DP traits are indeed distinct and separable from the core of dysthymic disorder but are not ideally captured by the DPD category (Ryder et al. 2002).

Epidemiology

At present there are no data on the prevalence of DPD in the general population, and Klein (1990) noted that prevalence estimates in an outpatient sample were highly dependent on the cut-score used. Moreover, there has been a failure to find consistent differences between DPD and non-DPD samples on a range of demographic variables, including sex, age, race, marital status, education, and socioeconomic status (Hirschfeld and Holzer 1994; Klein 1990; Klein and Miller 1993; Perugi et al. 1990; Phillips et al. 1992). Klein and Vocisano (1999) linked the lack of a sex difference between DPD and non-DPD groups, which differs from numerous studies of major depressive disorder and dysthymic disorder, to Kretschmer's (1925) observation that individuals with DPD may be unhappy without actually experiencing sad mood.

Family History

Four studies have used the family history method to study lifetime rates of Axis I disorders in relatives of probands with and without DPD (Cassano et al. 1990; Klein 1990; Klein and Miller 1993; Kwon et al. 2000), and two other studies have examined the relatives of probands with and without mood disorders for the presence of DPD (Klein 1999b; Klein et al. 1988). Klein (1990) found that first-degree relatives of outpatients with DPD had significantly higher rates of bipolar disorder and severe major depression (see Table 4–3). Klein and Miller (1993) found that first-degree relatives of undergraduates with DPD had higher rates of major depression. Cassano and colleagues (1992) reported that relatives of probands with both DPD and major depression had higher rates of mood disorders than did relatives of those with major depression alone. Kwon and colleagues (2000) demonstrated that undergraduates with DPD alone were significantly more likely to have a family history of mood disorders than were healthy control subjects. Klein and colleagues (1988) found a greater prevalence of DPD in the offspring of inpatients with major depression than did either the offspring of inpatients with chronic medical conditions or the offspring of healthy control subjects. Finally, Klein (1999b) found a higher rate of DPD in first-degree relatives of outpatients with early-onset dysthymic disorder versus relatives of outpatients with episodic major depression or relatives of healthy control subjects. These studies all suggest that DPD shares more than just descriptive similarity with Axis I mood disorders.

Impairment and Treatment

Given that personality disorders should by definition result in impaired functioning, there is an unfortunate dearth of research looking at the effects of meeting criteria for DPD. Indeed, only two studies to date have studied individuals with DPD alone and not with the frequently co-occurring dysthymic disorder. Klein and Miller (1993) found that undergraduates with DPD alone, compared with a healthy control group, reported greater subjective distress even after controlling for a past history of mood disorder. At the same time, they found that such individuals are unlikely to seek treatment unless a mood disorder is part of their presentation. Kwon and colleagues (2000) found that undergraduates with DPD alone reported state depression in the mild range, showing also that the course of DPD includes a higher rate of unipolar mood disorders compared with healthy control subjects. Finally, Phillips and colleagues (1998) found that patients with DPD do not respond

TABLE 4–3. Family history of lifetime rates of Axis I disorders in relatives of probands with and without depressive personality disorder (DPD)

Authors	Sample	Findings
Cassano et al. (1992)	Relatives of probands with both DPD and major depressive disorder (MDD)	Higher rates of mood disorders than relatives with MDD alone
Klein (1990)	First-degree relatives of outpatients with DPD	Significantly higher rates of bipolar disorder and severe major depression
Klein (1999b)	First-degree relatives of outpatients with early-onset dysthymic disorder; relatives of outpatients with episodic MDD or relatives of healthy control subjects	Higher rate of DPD in first-degree relatives of outpatients with early-onset dysthymic disorder vs. relatives of outpatients with episodic MDD or relatives of healthy control subjects
Klein and Miller (1993)	First-degree relatives of undergraduates with DPD	Higher rates of MDD
Klein et al. (1988)	Offspring of inpatients with MDD Offspring of inpatients with chronic medical conditions or offspring of healthy control subjects	Greater prevalence of DPD in offspring of inpatients with MDD than either offspring of inpatients with chronic medical conditions or offspring of healthy control subjects
Kwon et al. (2000)	Undergraduates with DPD alone	Significantly more likely to have family history of mood disorders than healthy control subjects

well to treatment. These findings await confirmation in community or patient samples, preferably with a wider range of impairment and outcome variables.

Psychopathology: Dimensional Approach

Historical Development of Depressive Personality Traits

Traits describing DP were first articulated by psychoanalytic and psychodynamic writers who were less interested in developing categorical diagnoses and more focused on identifying the premorbid traits that increased the risk of depression. Most theories focused on orality/dependence and anality/obsessiveness, with some attention also paid to low self-esteem, helplessness, guilt, dependence, inability to love, hypercriticism, self-deprecation, hopelessness, emptiness, and hypochondriasis (Arieti and Bemporad 1980; Berliner 1966; Kahn 1975). Blatt (1974) described these two cardinal aspects as separate etiological pathways leading to depression, with dependency involving deep longing to be cared for coupled with a fear of abandonment and obsessiveness (in Blatt's language, self-criticism) involving harsh self-scrutiny coupled with a fear of disapproval. Kernberg (1987) folded both elements into his description of the depressive-masochistic personality disorder, linking them to the Freudian concept of moral masochism. Ryder and Bagby (1999) noted that an emphasis on these two core features has been made by writers from diverse traditions, providing converging evidence for their importance and potentially providing common ground for the identification of specific traits.

Although much of the work on DP over the past two decades has been on the DPD category, Ryder and colleagues (2002) recently suggested that one way of dealing with the problems with that category might be to consider dimensional alternatives. In so doing, they have joined with several other researchers who argue that the personality disorders are deeply flawed, with the same problems repeating themselves across the individual diagnoses. Concerns include difficulties with differentiating the traits of the various disorders, low levels of interrater agreement, unacceptable overlap rates, a lack of utility and comprehensiveness in the system as a whole, and even the fundamental assumption that personality disorders are discrete categories (Clark et al. 1993, 1997; Livesley 1985; Tyrer 1988; Widiger 1993; Widiger and Frances 1985). Ryder and colleagues argue that many of these problems are the result of opposing a categorical diagnostic system on phenomena that have predominantly dimensional characteristics. Research demonstrating that the key assumptions of a categorical model are not met by the DSM-IV personality disorder system, and that personality disorders are best captured dimensionally, is also reviewed elsewhere (Ryder et al. 2002).

Although a single-dimensional system for personality psychopathology has yet to be formally identified or even widely and universally accepted, the five-factor model of personality (FFM) has emerged as the dominant trait model of personality. The five core personality characteristics were first described by Allport (1937), who proposed that the most socially relevant and salient personality characteristics should be encoded in everyday language (John 1990). In the initial work, research assistants were asked to comb through English-language dictionaries in order to identify adjectives describing personality traits. Numerous research teams have since studied the resulting list using factor analysis, a statistical technique allowing identification of higher order dimensions underlying the individual traits. Although early efforts in this direction yielded various numbers of factors, the last few decades have seen a convergence on five broad domains as multivariate statistical techniques have improved.

Some researchers have argued that the approach just described would not be expected to capture many crucial features of personality (e.g., Block 1995). Numerous studies have therefore been conducted to examine the factor structure shared by a wide range of personality measures developed by psychologists operating independently of the lexical-semantic approach. The same five factors are consistently identified (McCrae and John 1992). These broad dimensions have been described most completely in the work of Costa and McCrae (1985) and are briefly defined in Table 4–4. The full version of this model subdivides each broad domain into six narrower facets (Costa and McCrae 1992).

Appropriateness of the Five-Factor Model for Personality Psychopathology

Despite the success of the FFM in capturing normal personality traits, it does not necessarily follow that this system is appropriate for personality psychopathology. Research has been conducted over the past decade to determine whether the FFM should indeed be used in this way, and the results have for the most part been positive. Bagby and colleagues (1999a) have demonstrated that the FFM structure can be derived from a sample of patients with Axis I psychopathology, suggesting that the same traits found in nonpsychopathological samples are also evident in clinical samples. Lynam and Widiger (2001), meanwhile, demonstrated that experts can describe all of the official DSM-IV personality disorders with the exception of the schizotypal disorder using the 30 facets of the FFM. O'Connor and Dyce (1998) used a meta-analytic procedure to test the extent to which a variety of personality models capture the 11 DSM-III-R personality disorder diagnoses and found that the best-fitting model involved four dimensions corresponding to *neuroticism, extraversion, agreeableness,* and *conscientiousness.* A review of 17 studies (Clark and Harrison 2001) concluded that there are systematic relationships between the personality disorders and the dimensions and facets of the FFM. Finally, two independent attempts to derive dimensional systems by factor analyzing pathological personality traits from DSM and from

TABLE 4–4. Domains of the five-factor model of personality

Dimension	Characteristics	High scorers	Low scorers
Neuroticism	Emotional instability, proneness to distress, excessive cravings or urges, unrealistic ideas Tendency to experience negative affect and psychological distress Fearfulness, sadness, embarrassment, anger, guilt, disgust	Prone to irrational ideas Less control of impulses Cope less effectively with stress Worrying, insecure, high anxiety, easily tempted	Calm, secure, relaxed, stable
Extraversion	Capacity for joy, need for stimulation, interest in other people and external events Sociality Liking people	Talkative, optimistic, sociable, affectionate Assertive, active, talkative, cheerful, upbeat, energetic, optimistic Enjoy excitement and stimulation	Reserved, comfortable being alone, stay in the background Introverts, not necessarily the opposite of extraverts
Openness	Toleration for and exploration of the unfamiliar	Creative, artistic, curious, imaginative, nonconformist Curious about inner experience and external world Willing to consider novel ideas and unconventional values Experience emotions more intensely than more closed individuals	Conventional and conservative Preserving the status quo Prefer familiarity to novelty Experience emotion less intensely

TABLE 4–4. Domains of the five-factor model of personality *(continued)*

Dimension	Characteristics	High scorers	Low scorers
Agreeableness	Measure of an individual's interpersonal tendencies. Orientation along a continuum from compassion to antagonism in thoughts, feelings, and actions	Altruistic, cooperative, sympathetic. Expect agreeable behavior from others	Disagreeable, antagonistic, egocentric, aggressive, irritable, competitive. Expect the worst from others
Conscientiousness	Measure of the ability to plan, organize, and carry out tasks	Degree of organization, persistence, and motivation in goal-directed behavior. Purposeful, strong-willed, and determined. Associated with success. Annoying rigidity, compulsive neatness. Scrupulous, punctual, and reliable	Unreliable, lazy, careless, negligent, spontaneous. Not amoral. Less goal driven, more hedonistic

the clinical literature showed marked convergence, both with one another and again with neuroticism, extraversion, agreeableness, and conscientiousness (Clark et al. 1996).

Although the exact form taken by an official dimensional system
may not exactly resemble the FFM, whatever model is chosen will likely
involve at least four of the five broad dimensions (Widiger 2001). Deviations from the FFM are most likely to occur with the *openness* dimension and with the various narrower constructs. Openness was not only
the smallest factor to emerge from the original lexical studies but is also
the factor that appears least related to psychopathology, although its
potential relation to somatoform disorders is just beginning to be examined, and it may have some implications for treatment. Similarly, it will
be necessary to establish the suitability of each facet, and not just each
domain, as well as to consider the addition of more narrow-band facets
targeting clinical constructs left out of the FFM. There is some evidence,
for example, that the current formulation of the FFM does not adequately measure psychoticism (Harkness and McNulty 1994), and the
same may be true of other traits. Regardless of these outstanding issues,
it seems increasingly likely that the FFM will form the backbone for
whatever dimensional model ultimately emerges (Ryder et al. 2002).

Positioning Depressive Personality Traits Within a Dimensional Model

Ryder and colleagues (2002) described three sources of data that can
help us to determine the best placement of DP traits within a dimensional model such as the FFM: 1) explicit descriptions of depressive tendency as a lower order dimension in several models, including the
FFM; 2) comparisons of DPD and healthy samples on personality measures; and 3) studies of personality traits in individuals thought to be at
risk for depression. Among the lower order dimensions, traits theoretically consistent with DP are captured in the depression dimension of
neuroticism in the FFM. A similar construct, anhedonia, is found in
Clark's (1993) dimensional model and itself has a strong correlation
with neuroticism.

Studies examining the relation between DPD and other personality
measures have shown links with hostility, self-consciousness, stress reactivity, self-criticism, harm avoidance, neuroticism, negative attributional style, low gregariousness, low novelty seeking, low extraversion,
and low openness (Ryder et al. 2002). Expected correlations with negative affectivity and low positive affectivity have been confirmed in at
least two studies (Klein and Shih 1998; Reynolds and Clark 2001). The

latter study also showed correlations between DPD and the neuroticism facets of depression, anxiety, and vulnerability, along with the agreeableness facet of (low) tender-mindedness. Psychiatric outpatients with DPD have been distinguished from psychiatric control subjects by virtue of having higher levels of interpersonal loss, negative perceptions of parents, and perfectionism (Huprich 2003a), and have been found to have higher levels of harm avoidance than patients with major depressive disorder or dysthymic disorder (Abrams et al. 2004). Finally, high self-consciousness and low tender-mindedness have been shown to predict increased scores on three different measures of DPD; these trait constructs also predicted variance above and beyond other personality disorder traits in a psychiatric outpatient sample (Huprich 2003b).

In a study of FFM personality traits in depressed individuals, Bagby and colleagues (1995) assessed depressed patients at treatment entry and again 3 months later. The neuroticism score for patients who ultimately recovered was almost two standard deviations higher at treatment entry as compared with the mean score of healthy control subjects and remained more than one standard deviation higher at the time of the second assessment. A corresponding, albeit weaker, relation was found for low extraversion scores, and subsequent regression analyses showed that low extraversion interferes with treatment. Interestingly, these individuals also had low scores on conscientiousness, contrary to the suggestion of some of the earlier theorists. A subsequent study with a larger sample of recovered depressed patients reported nearly identical results, with neuroticism scores one standard deviation higher, extraversion scores half a standard deviation lower, and conscientiousness scores one standard deviation lower than the healthy control sample. The same pattern of elevations was obtained in a later study using informant ratings (Bagby et al. 1997). Finally, Harkness and colleagues (2002) compared individuals with remitted unipolar and nonpsychotic depression alone compared with those meeting both the diagnosis and research diagnostic criteria for remitted chronic minor depression. This latter construct encompasses aspects of both dysthymic disorder and DPD. Individuals in this second group had significantly lower agreeableness scores and a trend toward higher neuroticism scores.

Assessment

Presentation and Differential Diagnosis

Regardless of whether DP is conceptualized as a category or as a dimension, assessment of these traits in the clinical setting is challenging.

Recognition of DP during a clinical interview first requires that the clinician be aware that it may be present in the absence of depressed mood and/or the somatic symptoms common in mood disorders. That said, the absence of an official diagnosis has naturally led to relative inattention to the ways in which these patients present. Bagby and colleagues (2003) have provided a brief clinical description of DPD:

> Individuals with DPD exhibit affective, cognitive, and interpersonal attributes that deviate substantially from the surrounding cultural norms. Emotionally, such patients are predominantly dejected, gloomy, worrying, and all but devoid of happiness. They often find it difficult to relax and to find enjoyment, to be in anything but "work mode." A marked sense of personal inadequacy, with harsh self-judgments, is a common feature of the construct. Depressive thoughts are also central to this diagnosis; individuals with DPD often brood over the past, feel remorse or regret about things they have or have not done, and often hold strongly to the belief that they have no right to be happy. They are as negative about and judgmental of other people as they are of themselves. Persons with DPD view their future as negatively as they do their present and their past—although, ironically, they often take some pride in their ability to make "realistic" judgments. The text of DSM-IV suggests that, interpersonally, they may exhibit a tendency to be introverted and underassertive, but some patients with DPD will also present in an overassertive, aggressive, manner. Their humorlessness and negativity will often make them less appealing to others, in turn reinforcing their negative beliefs about themselves and their interpersonal world. (p. 17)

Although this description is keyed to the categorical definition of the disorder, many of the traits described by Bagby and colleagues would also be applicable to the dimensional system. A long-standing pattern of such traits across a wide range of situations suggests that DP traits might form an important part of the clinical picture.

The next challenge for the clinician is to distinguish the particular pattern described by these traits from other clinical constructs. Differential diagnosis of the DPD category from other personality disorder categories is often difficult because of the problems discussed previously regarding the high degree of conceptual and empirical overlap between these categories. Such problems are far less apparent when using a dimensional approach because it is not necessary to place each patient within a predefined category. Assessment of DP traits in the context of dysthymic disorder, meanwhile, is complicated regardless of whether a categorical or a dimensional model is used. The remainder of this section briefly summarizes Klein and Vocisano's (1999) guidelines for making some of the more difficult distinctions. Although they are helpful, keep in mind that most of these descriptions are based on theoretical speculation and interpretation of clinical descriptions rather than on empirical research. Also, these descriptions are based on a categorical understanding of personality disorders and are discussed here primarily to aid clinicians attempting to make DSM-type distinctions.

Avoidant Personality Disorder

DPD often presents with social inhibition, interpersonal avoidance, feelings of inadequacy, and hypersensitivity. Compared with the avoidant personality disorder patient, however, the DPD patient is less reluctant to enter into relationships with others and is more likely to have a relatively larger social network (Klein and Vocisano 1999). Moreover, affects such as gloominess and joylessness rather than nervousness and fear predominate, and their feeling of inadequacy extends to a wider range of situations.

Dependent Personality Disorder

DPD often presents with dependence on others for approval and self-worth, a presentation that would also be expected from the dimension of orality/dependence (Kernberg 1987). Compared with dependent personality disorder, however, the DPD patients usually are not overtly clingy and are less likely to remain in relationships where their dependency needs are not being met (Klein and Vocisano 1999). Also, loss of relationships is less likely to lead to fearful and desperate attempts to retain connection and more likely to involve apathy and withdrawal.

Obsessive-Compulsive Personality Disorder

Although some earlier descriptions of DP included obsessive-compulsive personality traits such as conscientiousness, dutifulness, and excessive self-discipline, research has not supported the relation between these features and core DP traits. Whereas individuals with obsessive-compulsive personality disorder are affectively constricted and interpersonally controlling, the DPD patient is generally dejected and unassertive (Kernberg 1987; Klein and Vocisano 1999).

Borderline Personality Disorder

Although individuals with borderline personality disorder may at times enter into mood states that resemble those found with DPD, the former category describes people who experience marked reactive mood shifts. Individuals with DPD have a stable self-concept and most often turn inward when they experience aggression and hostility, in contrast with frequent and impulsive "acting out" of such emotions (Klein and Vocisano 1999).

Dysthymic Disorder

The assessment of DP, whether conceived categorically or dimensionally, is rendered most difficult by the conceptual and empirical overlap with dysthymic disorder. According to DSM-IV, DPD should not be diagnosed when dysthymic disorder is present (American Psychiatric Association 2000). Certain clinical presentations can be easily identified as dysthymic disorder if they contain features that are not permitted within the narrower confines of DPD. For example, patients whose clinical history involves a later onset and/or a pattern of remission and relapse are probably more characteristic of dysthymic disorder. Similarly, the presence of clinically significant and chronic somatic symptoms, such as insomnia or lack of appetite, strongly suggests dysthymic disorder even when DP traits are also present. Klein (1999a) has argued that the critical distinction between the two diagnoses is the presence of depressed mood in dysthymic disorder and raises the possibility that chronic anhedonia may be a feature of DPD. This distinction may, however, be difficult to make in practice; one DPD trait specifies that usual mood is dominated by dejection and gloominess, and several of the other traits (e.g., feelings of inadequacy or self-deprecation) suggest that such patients would likely present themselves in ways similar to individuals with clinically depressed mood.

Given the substantial interplay of personality traits and mood disorders, it is still useful to assess carefully for the presence of DP traits even when dysthymic disorder is the eventual diagnosis (Bagby and Ryder 2000). One advantage of the dimensional approach here is that it allows the clinician to explore thoroughly the personality of the individual patient without an undue—and perhaps an unnecessary—concern with differential diagnosis. Future research will be necessary to determine the various trait personality profiles that might be associated with different presentations of dysthymic disorder (e.g., dysthymic disorder with versus without the traitlike symptoms also associated with DPD).

Normality

On the other end of the continuum from the diagnostic challenges described previously is the issue of ensuring that normal variation in particular personality traits is not confused with a psychiatric diagnosis (Ryder and Bagby 1999). Although many individuals will exhibit the requisite number of traits, they may not necessarily be impaired to a degree that would warrant a diagnosis of DPD. To this end, it is important that the clinician keep in mind the general criteria for personality disorders in addition to the specific DPD criteria; specifically, a diagnosis should not be made unless the patient exhibits a marked deviation leading to clinically significant distress. A similar standard should be used before determining that a statistical deviation along a dimension of DP traits is indicative of psychopathology.

Instruments

Although it is important for clinicians to keep in mind these subjective clinical descriptions and guidelines for differential diagnosis when assessing for DP traits, instruments expressly designed for this purpose can help in increasing precision. There are a number of instruments that can aid in the assessment of DP. These tools can be broadly classified into three categories: 1) instruments that assess for the presence versus absence of DPD, 2) instruments that assess DP as a single dimension based on the DPD category, and 3) instruments that include assessment of DP traits among other interrelated constructs.

Assessment of the Depressive Personality Disorder Category

Two interview measures that assess for presence versus absence of DPD in the context of DSM-IV personality disorders are the *Structured Clinical Interview for DSM-IV Axis II Personality Disorders* (SCID-II) (First et al. 1997a) and the *Diagnostic Interview for DSM-IV Personality Disorders* (DIPD) (Zanarini et al. 1996). The SCID-II is a semistructured interview assessing the diagnostic criteria for the 10 personality disorders listed in the main text of DSM-IV as well as the unofficial depressive and passive-aggressive personality disorders. In addition, there is a self-report personality questionnaire that accompanies the SCID-II (First et al. 1997b) that is used as a screening instrument to identify the potential presence of personality psychopathology. This questionnaire assesses the 10 personality disorders that correspond to Axis II of DSM-IV and DSM-IV-TR. The DIPD is a 108-item, semistructured clinical interview also designed to categorically assess the personality disorders as outlined in DSM-IV and DSM-IV-TR, and it includes both the depressive and the passive-aggressive categories.

Two additional interviews, which include both DSM and ICD personality disorders, are the *Structured Interview for DSM-IV Personality* (SIDP-IV) (Pfohl et al. 1997), and the *International Personality Disorder Examination* (IPDE) (see Loranger 1997). Like the SCID-II, the SIDP-IV is a semistructured interview assessing the presence of the 10 main text personality disorders of DSM-IV as well as those from the *International Statistical Classification of Diseases and Related Health Problems*, 10th Revision (ICD-10) (World Health Organization 1992). In addition, the SIDP-IV includes items to assess the unofficial depressive, passive-aggressive, and self-defeating categories; it was developed so that the categories can be assessed either categorically or dimensionally. The IPDE is a semistructured interview assessing the diagnostic criteria for personality disorders described in both systems. The IPDE provides both categorical and dimensional scoring for DSM categories, and, as with the SCID-II, it is accompanied by a parallel true-or-false format self-report questionnaire that can be used as a screening instrument before conducting the interview.

One self-report inventory that can also be used categorically to assess DPD, in addition to those described previously with their accompanying interviews, is the *Personality Diagnostic Questionnaire–4+* (PDQ-4+) (Hyler 1994). This 99-item questionnaire is designed to assess categorically and dimensionally the symptom criteria of the DSM-IV personality disorders as well as the depressive and passive-aggressive categories. Items are designed in a true-or-false format and appear to have low to moderate internal consistency (see Wilberg et al. 2000). Items can also be summed to create a total dimensional score representing overall personality psychopathology.

Assessment of Depressive Personality Traits

Several instruments have also been developed specifically to assess a dimension of DP based on the DPD category. The *Millon Clinical Multiaxial Inventory–III* (MCMI-III) (Millon et al. 1994) is a 175-item self-report questionnaire designed as a dimensional measure of general psychopathology. Although some scales are keyed to DSM-IV Axis I disorders, the major thrust of this instrument is designed to assess personality disorder dimensions. The *Coolidge Axis II Inventory* (CATI) (Coolidge and Merwin 1992), meanwhile, is a 200-item self-report questionnaire designed to assess personality psychopathology along dimensions consistent with the 13 personality disorders described in DSM-III-R. Each item is scored on a 4-point Likert scale, and there is some item overlap across the scales (Kalchev et al. 1997).

Two instruments have been developed to specifically measure DP traits. The *Diagnostic Interview for Depressive Personality* (DIDP) (Gunderson et al. 1994) assesses 30 traits associated with DP from the psychoanalytic and descriptive literatures. The traits are divided into four general areas: depressive/negativistic, introverted/tense, unassertive/passive, and masochistic. Cut scores have also been developed to facilitate categorical diagnosis. The *Depressive Personality Disorder Inventory* (DPDI) (Huprich et al. 1996), meanwhile, is a 41-item self-report instrument that assesses DP traits.

Broad Assessment of Personality Including Depressive Personality Traits

The *Revised NEO Personality Inventory* (NEO-PI-R) (Costa and McCrae 1992) measures the five basic personality domains of the FFM. In addition, this questionnaire includes 30 specific construct scales subsumed by each domain that are also assessed, thus providing a means to assess for DP traits in the context of a comprehensive assessment. The NEO-PI-R consists of 240 items presented in a five-point Likert format and has first-person self-report (Form S) and third-person informant (Form R) versions. Both forms have demonstrated good reliability and validity and stability in a number of studies. The FFM can also be assessed through interview by using the *Structured Interview for the Five Factor Model* (SIFFM) (Trull and Widiger 1997), a 240-item interview designed to assess the same 5 domain and 30 facet scales as the NEO-PI-R.

Treatment

Choosing the best approach to the treatment of DP depends in large part on the information available, which in turn depends on the way in which DP traits are assessed. There is a lack of established treatment methods in this area regardless how the disorder is conceptualized—as category or dimension, as mood disorder or personality disorder. Given that these fundamental questions have not yet been worked out, it is not surprising that there is as yet no research evaluating treatment effectiveness. This final section is therefore speculative.

Pharmacotherapy

Klein's (1990) spectrum hypothesis does provide the clinician with a potential avenue to empirically informed treatment planning by implying that DPD exists on a continuum with other Axis I mood disorders. The closest link, of course, is with dysthymic disorder, but unfortunately there is a lack of treatment research here as well. In lieu of further evidence, therefore, the spectrum hypothesis would suggest that pharmacotherapy would involve cautious administration of antidepressant medication when necessary. Although traditionally personality disorders are considered to be relatively impervious to medication, there are two reasons to be more optimistic. First, as described earlier, the status of DPD as a pure personality disorder—if such a concept even exists—is very much in doubt. Second, research on the more recent antidepressants, particularly selective serotonin reuptake inhibitors, indicates that they have effects on personality traits as well as with mood symptoms (Bagby et al. 1999b; Ekselius and Von Knorring 1999; Gelfin et al. 1998; Knutson et al. 1998). That said, caution remains the best policy because these medications have not explicitly been tested in this context. Also, the research literature on the extent to which individuals meeting DPD criteria experience distress and impairment to warrant such an approach remains unclear. The same problem pertains to DP traits in that the ideal cutoff point for deciding that a patient is sufficiently impaired to justify treatment has not yet been defined. Clinicians should be sure to assess the extent of social, occupational, or other impairment before proceeding.

Psychotherapy

Clinicians choosing to use psychotherapy with DP traits can draw on both the mood disorders and personality disorders literature in the absence of definitive evidence in favor of one or the other. In the former case it may make sense to consider treatments tailored to long-term and chronic depressive states. An example of such an approach is Mc-Cullough's (2000) Cognitive Behavioral Analysis System of Psychotherapy (CBASP). CBASP was developed in response to the poor outcomes for chronic depression that are often observed in traditional cognitive-behavioral therapy (CBT). The system was developed by integrating effective techniques for chronic depression from the behavioral, cognitive, interpersonal, and psychodynamic literatures. Early research indicates that the treatment is promising, especially in combination with medication (McCullough 2000). The treatment has not yet been specifically examined in the context of DP, however.

If treating DP as a personality disorder, the clinician should consider using an approach that can be flexibly applied to a range of personality disorder diagnoses, especially to mixed presentations or to personality disorder not otherwise specified (NOS). One possibility is Beck and Freeman's (1990) schema-focused approach. (Use of this modality in depressed patients complicated by personality disorder NOS can be found in Chapter 9 of this book.) Young and colleagues (2003) have also developed a schema-focused therapy; as with CBASP, it developed from the realization that chronic conditions are often not well served by traditional CBT. Rather than focusing on diagnostic categories, Young has instead outlined 18 specific cognitive schemas representing deep-seated ways of seeing and interacting with the world. Several of these schemas describe characteristics similar to DP traits, with examples including emotional deprivation, defectiveness/shame, and negativity. The therapist works with the patient to identify specific schemas and to elaborate on the ways they operate in a wide range of situations. A variety of techniques from CBT, interpersonal, and experiential traditions are then brought to bear on the identified schemas and on the patient's habitual ways of coping with them.

A creative yet empirically grounded approach to DPD can also be applied to DP traits more generally, with the additional benefit created by a more detailed knowledge of the specific traits involved. For example, the presence of traits such as low self-esteem, introversion, and quietness are predictive of nonresponse to treatment (Hirschfeld et al. 1998). A recent study by Shahar and colleagues (2003) found that among patients with major depression, the presence of DP traits was the most important predictor of treatment outcome, again in a negative direction. Such findings are promising but await replication and elaboration. An important question will be how best to work with these traits when conducting therapy targeting Axis I conditions.

Working With Depressive Personality Traits in the Overall Context of Personality

A further advantage of working with DP traits can be realized if these traits are assessed as part of the overall context of personality. Although there is at present little research on this topic, several articles have explored theoretically the ways in which knowledge of a patient's personality can inform treatment planning. Harkness and Lillienfeld (1997) began this process by arguing that responsible care of a patient requires a knowledge of the relevant scientific literature—and that the literature on personality and individual differences is particularly relevant (see also Harkness and McNulty 2002). A careful and comprehensive assessment of a wide range of traits, both functional and dysfunctional, can aid in clinician-patient collaboration and can even be therapeutic (MacKenzie 2002). Rather than a formulation unduly focused on a few narrow distressing traits, an overall picture of strengths and weaknesses can be developed, and therapy can be more carefully designed and implemented to suit individual patients (Sanderson and Clarkin

2002; Stone 2002). Unfortunately, whereas much of this emerging work is both promising and amenable to empirical testing, the research required to use these approaches with confidence has not yet been conducted. Although the FFM in particular is now supported by a large and diverse empirical database, the links between personality traits and treatment will require a similar effort before the potential of this approach can be fully realized.

Conclusions

Regardless of whether DP is approached as a personality disorder category or as a dimension within a comprehensive trait set, the practitioner is greatly in need of more research to ensure that these traits are dealt with competently. Our group has outlined previously the categorical-dimensional debate as it applies to DP traits, and we have argued that a resolution of this issue will aid in the development of better clinical research (Ryder et al. 2002). Although we both agree with this position and have clearly articulated our perspective on how this debate should be resolved, our objective in this chapter has been to step back and survey our current knowledge of DP traits. The database on DP psychopathology is steadily growing, and improved methods of assessment continue to be developed; at the same time, the treatment literature lags far behind. It is our hope that this research will be done so that clinicians can work with these traits in scientifically and clinically informed ways.

References

Abrams KY, Yune SK, Kim SJ, et al: Trait and state aspects of harm avoidance and its implication for treatment in major depressive disorder, dysthymic disorder, and depressive personality disorder. Psychiatry Clin Neurosci 58:240–248, 2004

Akiskal HS: Dysthymic disorder: psychopathology of proposed chronic depressive subtypes. Am J Psychiatry 140:11–20, 1983

Allport GW: Personality: A Psychological Interpretation. New York, Holt, Rinehart, & Winston, 1937

American Psychiatric Association: Diagnostic and Statistical Manual: Mental Disorders. Washington, DC, American Psychiatric Association, 1952

American Psychiatric Association: Diagnostic and Statistical Manual of Mental Disorders, 2nd Edition. Washington, DC, American Psychiatric Association, 1968

American Psychiatric Association: Diagnostic and Statistical Manual of Mental Disorders, 3rd Edition. Washington, DC, American Psychiatric Association, 1980

American Psychiatric Association: Diagnostic and Statistical Manual of Mental Disorders, 3rd Edition, Revised. Washington, DC, American Psychiatric Association, 1987

American Psychiatric Association: Diagnostic and Statistical Manual of Mental Disorders, 4th Edition. Washington, DC, American Psychiatric Association, 1994

American Psychiatric Association: Diagnostic and Statistical Manual of Mental Disorders, 4th Edition, Text Revision. Washington, DC, American Psychiatric Association, 2000

Arieti S, Bemporad JR: The psychological organization of depression. Am J Psychiatry 137:1360–1365, 1980

Bagby RM, Ryder AG: Diagnostic discriminability of dysthymia and depressive personality disorder. Depress Anxiety 10:41–49, 1999

Bagby RM, Ryder AG: Personality and the affective disorders: past efforts, current models, and future directions. Curr Psychiatry Rep 2:465–472, 2000

Bagby RM, Joffe RT, Parker JDA, et al: Major depression and the five-factor model of personality. J Personal Disord 9:224–234, 1995

Bagby RM, Costa PT Jr, McCrae RR, et al: Replicating the five-factor model of personality in a psychiatric sample. Pers Individ Dif 27:1135–1139, 1999a

Bagby RM, Levitan RD, Kennedy SH, et al: Selective alteration of personality in response to noradrenergic and serotonergic antidepressant medication in depressed sample: evidence of nonspecificity. Psychiatry Res 86:211–216, 1999b

Bagby RM, Ryder AG, Schuller DR: Depressive personality disorder: a critical overview. Curr Psychiatry Rep 5:16–22, 2003

Beck AT, Freeman A: Cognitive Therapy of Personality Disorders. New York, Guilford, 1990

Berliner B: Psychodynamics of the depressive character. Psychoanalytic Forum 1:244–251, 1966

Blatt SJ: Levels of object representation in anaclitic and introjective depression. Psychoanal Stud Child 29:109–157, 1974

Block J: A contrarian view of the five-factor approach to personality description. Psychol Bull 117:187–215, 1995

Cassano GB, Dell'Osso L, Frank E, et al: The bipolar spectrum: a clinical reality in search of diagnostic criteria and an assessment methodology. J Affect Disord 54:319–328, 1992

Clark LA: Schedule for Nonadaptive and Adaptive Personality (SNAP). Minneapolis, MN, University of Minnesota Press, 1993

Clark LA, Harrison JA: Assessment instruments, in Handbook of Personality Disorders: Theory, Research, and Treatment. Edited by Livesley WJ. New York, Guilford, 2001, pp 277–306

Clark LA, Watson D: Personality, disorder, and personality disorder: towards a more rational conceptualization. J Personal Disord 13:142–151, 1999

Clark LA, McEwan JL, Collard LM, et al: Symptoms and traits of personality disorder: two new methods for their assessment. Psychol Assess 5:81–91, 1993

Clark LA, Watson D, Mineka S: Temperament, personality, and the mood and anxiety disorders. J Abnorm Psychol 103:103–116, 1994

Clark LA, Livesley WJ, Schroeder ML, et al: Convergence of two systems for assessing specific traits of personality disorder. Psychol Assess 8:294–303, 1996

Clark LA, Livesley WJ, Morey L: Personality disorder assessment: the challenge of construct validity. J Personal Disord 11:205–231, 1997

Coolidge FL, Merwin MM: Reliability and validity of the Coolidge Axis II Inventory: a new inventory for the assessment of personality disorders. J Pers Assess 59:223–238, 1992

Costa PT Jr, McCrae RR: The NEO Personality Inventory Manual. Odessa, FL, Psychological Assessment Resources, 1985

Costa PT Jr, McCrae RR: Revised NEO Personality Inventory (NEO-PI-R) and NEO Five-Factor Inventory (NEO-FFI): Professional Manual. Odessa, FL, Psychological Assessment Resources, 1992

Ekselius L, Von Knorring L: Changes in personality traits during treatment with sertraline or citalopram. Br J Psychiatry 174:444–448, 1999

First MB, Gibbon M, Spitzer RL, et al: Structured Clinical Interview for DSM-IV Axis II Personality Disorders (SCID-II). Washington, DC, American Psychiatric Press, 1997a

First MB, Gibbon M, Spitzer RL, et al: Structured Clinical Interview for DSM-IV Axis II Personality Disorders (SCID-II), Interview and Questionnaire. Washington, DC, American Psychiatric Press, 1997b

Frances A: The DSM-III personality disorders section: a commentary. Am J Psychiatry 137:1050–1054, 1980

Gelfin Y, Gorfine M, Lerer B: Effect of clinical doses of fluoxetine on psychological variables in health volunteers. Am J Psychiatry 155:290–292, 1998

Gunderson JG: DSM-III diagnoses of personality disorders, in Current Perspectives on Personality Disorders. Edited by Frosh JP. Washington, DC, American Psychiatric Press, 1983, pp 20–39

Gunderson JG, Phillips KA, Triebwasser J, et al: The Diagnostic Interview for Depressive Personality. Am J Psychiatry 151:1300–1304, 1994

Harkness AR, Lilienfeld SO: Individual differences science for treatment planning: personality traits. Psychol Assess 9:349–360, 1997

Harkness AR, McNulty JL: The personality Psychopathology Five (PSY-5): issues from the pages of a diagnostic manual instead of a dictionary, in Differentiating Normal and Abnormal Personality. Edited by Strack S, Lorr M. New York, Springer, 1994, pp 291–315

Harkness AR, McNulty: Implications of personality individual differences science for clinical work on personality disorders, in Personality Disorders and the Five-Factor Model of Personality. Edited by Costa PT Jr, Widiger TA. Washington, DC, American Psychological Association, 2002, pp 391–404

Harkness KL, Bagby RM, Joffe RT, et al: Major depression, chronic minor depression, and the neuroticism personality dimension. European Journal of Personality 16:271–281, 2002

Hirschfeld RM, Holzer CE III: Depressive personality disorder: clinical implications. J Clin Psychiatry 55 (suppl):10–17, 1994

Hirschfeld RM, Russell JM, Delgado PL, et al: Predictors of response to acute treatment of chronic and double depression with sertraline or imipramine. J Clin Psychiatry 59:669–675, 1998

Huprich SK: Depressive personality disorder: theoretical issues, clinical findings, and future research questions. Clin Psychol Rev 18:477–500, 1998

Huprich SK: Object loss and object relations in depressive personality analogues. Bull Menninger Clin 65:549–559, 2001

Huprich SK: Depressive personality and its relationship to depressed mood, interpersonal loss, negative parental perceptions, and perfectionism. J Nerv Ment Dis 191:73–79, 2003a

Huprich SK: Evaluating facet-level predictions and construct validity of depressive personality disorder. J Personal Disord 17:219–232, 2003b

Huprich SK, Margrett JE, Barthelemy KJ, et al: The Depressive Personality Disorder Inventory: an initial investigation of its psychometric properties. J Clin Psychol 52:153–159, 1996

Hyler SE: Personality Diagnostic Questionnaire–4+ (PDQ-4+). New York, New York State Psychiatric Institute, 1994

John OP: The "Big Five" factor taxonomy: dimensions of personality in the natural language and in questionnaires, in Handbook of Personality: Theory and Research. Edited by Pervin LA. New York, Guilford, 1990, pp 66–100

Kahn E: The depressive character. Folia Psychiatr Neurol Jpn 29:291–303, 1975

Kalchev P, Balev J, Coolidge F: The Coolidge Axis II Inventory (CATI): evidences for psychometric and factorial validity for Bulgarian nonclinical sample. Pers Individ Dif 22:363–369, 1997

Kernberg O: Severe Personality Disorders: Psychotherapeutic Strategies. New Haven, CT, Yale University Press, 1984

Kernberg O: Clinical Dimensions of Masochism. Hillside, NJ, Analytic Press, 1987

Klein DN: Depressive personality: reliability, validity, and relation to dysthymia. J Abnorm Psychol 99:412–421, 1990

Klein DN: Commentary on Ryder and Bagby's "Diagnostic Viability of Depressive Personality Disorder: Theoretical and Conceptual Issues." J Personal Disord 13:118–127, 1999a

Klein DN: Depressive personality in the relatives of outpatients with dysthymic disorder and episodic major depressive disorder and normal controls. J Affect Disord 55:19–27, 1999b

Klein DN, Miller GA: Depressive personality in nonclinical subjects. Am J Psychiatry 150:1718–1724, 1993

Klein DN, Shih JH: Depressive personality: associations with DSM-III-R mood and personality disorders and negative and positive affectivity, 30-month stability, and prediction of course of Axis I depressive disorders. J Abnorm Psychol 107:319–327, 1998

Klein DN, Vocisano C: Depressive and self-defeating (masochistic) personality disorders, in Oxford Textbook of Psychopathology. Edited by Millon P, Blaney P. New York, Oxford University Press, 1999, pp 653–673

Klein DN, Clark DC, Dansky L, et al: Dysthymia in the offspring of parents with primary unipolar affective disorder. J Abnorm Psychol 97:265–274, 1988

Klein DN, Norden KA, Ferro T, et al: Thirty-month naturalistic follow-up study of early onset dysthymic disorder: course, diagnostic stability, and prediction of outcome. J Abnorm Psychol 107:338–348, 1998

Knutson B, Wolkowitz OM, Cole SW, et al: Selective alteration of personality and social behavior by serotonergic intervention. Am J Psychiatry 155:373–379, 1998

Kraepelin E: Manic Depressive Insanity and Paranoia. Edinburgh, UK, Livingstone, 1921

Kretschmer E: Physique and Character. New York, Harcourt Brace, 1925

Krueger RF, Tackett JL: Personality and psychopathology working toward the bigger picture. J Personal Disord 17:109–128, 2003

Kwon JS, Kim YM, Chang CG, et al: Three-year follow-up of women with the sole diagnosis of depressive personality disorder: subsequent development of dysthymia and major depression. Am J Psychiatry 157:1966–1972, 2000

Livesley WJ: The classification of personality disorder; I: the choice of category concept. Can J Psychiatry 30:353–358, 1985

Loranger AW: International Personality Disorder Examination (IPDE), in Assessment and Diagnosis of Personality Disorders: The ICD-10 International Personality Disorder Examination (IPDE). Edited by Loranger AW, Janca A, Sartorius N. Cambridge, UK, Cambridge University Press, 1997, pp 43–51

Lynam DR, Widiger TA: Using the five-factor model to represent the DSM-IV personality disorders: an expert consensus approach. J Abnorm Psychol 110:401–412, 2001

Lyoo K, Gunderson JG, Phillips KA: Personality dimensions associated with depressive personality disorder. J Personal Disord 12:46–55, 1998

MacKenzie KR: Using personality measurements in clinical practice, Personality Disorders and the Five-Factor Model of Personality. Edited by Costa PT Jr, Widiger TA. Washington, DC, American Psychological Association, 2002, pp 377–390

McCrea RR, John OP: An introduction to the five-factor model and its applications. J Pers 60:175–215, 1992

McCullough JP: Treatment for Chronic Depression: Cognitive Behavioral Analysis System of Psychotherapy (CBASP). New York, Guilford, 2000

McDermut W, Zimmerman M, Chelminski I: The construct validity of depressive personality disorder. J Abnorm Psychol 112: 49–60, 2003

McLean P, Woody S: Commentary on depressive personality: a false start, in The DSM-IV Personality Disorders. Edited by Livesley WJ. New York, Guilford, 1995, pp 303–311

Millon T, Davis R, Millon C: Manual for the Millon Clinical Multiaxial Inventory–III (MCMI-III). Minneapolis, MN, National Computer Systems, 1994

O'Connor BP, Dyce JA: A test of models of personality disorder configuration. J Abnorm Psychol 107:3–16, 1998

Perugi G, Musetti L, Simonini E, et al: Gender-mediated clinical features of depressive illness: the importance of temperamental differences. Br J Psychiatry 157:835–841, 1990

Pfohl B, Blum N, Zimmerman M: Structured Interview for DSM-IV Personality (SIDP). Washington, DC, American Psychiatric Press, 1997

Phillips KA, Gunderson JG: Depressive personality disorder: fact or fiction? J Personal Disord 13:128–134, 1999

Phillips KA, Gunderson JG, Kimball CR, et al: An empirical study of depressive personality, in 1992 CME Syllabus and Proceedings Summary, 145th Annual Meeting. Washington, DC, American Psychiatric Association, 1992

Phillips KA, Gunderson JG, Triebwasser J, et al: Reliability and validity of depressive personality disorder. Am J Psychiatry 155:1044–1048, 1998

Reynolds SK, Clark LA: Predicting dimensions of personality disorder from domains and facets of the Five-Factor Model. J Pers 69:199–222, 2001

Robins E, Guze SB: Establishment of diagnostic validity in psychiatric illness: its application to schizophrenia. Am J Psychiatry 126:983–987, 1970

Ryder AG, Bagby RM: Diagnostic viability of depressive personality disorder: theoretical and conceptual issues. J Personal Disord 13:99–117, 1999

Ryder AG, Bagby RM, Dion KL: Chronic, low-grade depression in a nonclinical sample: depressive personality or dysthymia? J Personal Disord 15:84–93, 2001

Ryder AG, Bagby RM, Schuller DR: Differentiating depressive personality disorder and dysthymia: a categorical problem with a dimensional solution. Harv Rev Psychiatry 10:337–352, 2002

Sanderson C, Clarkin JF: Further use of the NEO-PI-R personality dimensions in differential treatment planning, in Personality Disorders and the Five-Factor Model of Personality. Edited by Costa PT Jr, Widiger TA. Washington, DC, American Psychological Association, 2002, pp 351–376

Schneider K: Clinical Psychopathology. London, Grune & Stratton, 1959

Shahar G, Blatt SJ, Zuroff DC, et al: Role of perfectionism and personality disorder features in response to brief treatment for depression. J Consult Clin Psychol 71:629–633, 2003

Skodol AE, Stout RL, McGlashan TH, et al: Co-occurrence of mood and personality disorders: a report from the Collaborative Longitudinal Personality Disorders Study (CLPS). Depress Anxiety 10:175–182, 1999

Stone MH: Treatment of personality disorders from the perspective of the Five-Factor model, in Personality Disorders and the Five-Factor Model of Personality. Edited by Costa PT Jr, Widiger TA. Washington, DC, American Psychological Association, 2002, pp 405–430

Trull TJ, Widiger TA: Structured Interview for the Five-Factor Model of Personality (SIFFM): Professional Manual. Odessa, FL, Psychological Assessment Resources, 1997

Tyrer P: What's wrong with the DSM-III personality disorders? J Personal Disord 2:281–291, 1988

Widiger TA: Personality and Depression: Assessment Issues. New York, Guilford, 1993

Widiger TA: Depressive personality traits and dysthymia: a commentary on Ryder and Bagby. J Personal Disord 13:135–141, 1999

Widiger TA: Official classification system, in Handbook of Personality Disorders: Theory, Research, and Treatment. Edited by Livesley WJ. New York, Guilford, 2001, pp 60–83

Widiger TA, Frances A: The DSM-III personality disorders: perspectives from psychology. Arch Gen Psychiatry 42:615–623, 1985

Widiger TA, Trull TJ: Personality and psychopathology: an application of the five-factor model. J Pers 60:363–393, 1992

Wilberg T, Dammen T, Friis S: Comparing Personality Diagnostic Question-naire–4+ with Longitudinal, Expert, All Data (LEAD) standard diagnoses in a sample with a high prevalence of Axis I and Axis II disorders. Compr Psychiatry 41:295–302, 2000

World Health Organization: International Statistical Classification of Diseases and Related Health Problems, 10th Revision. Geneva, World Health Organization, 1992

Young JE, Klosko JS, Weishaar ME: Schema therapy: a practitioner's guide. New York, Guilford, 2003

Zanarini MC, Frankenburg FR, Sikel AE, et al: The Diagnostic Interview for DSM-IV Personality Disorders. Belmont, MA, McLean Hospital, Laboratory for the Study of Adult Development, 1996

PART II

TREATMENT IMPLICATIONS

THE IMPACT OF PERSONALITY ON THE PHARMACOLOGICAL TREATMENT OF DEPRESSION

Sidney H. Kennedy, M.D.

Peter Farvolden, Ph.D.

Nicole L. Cohen, M.A.

R. Michael Bagby, Ph.D.

Paul T. Costa Jr., Ph.D.

Major depressive disorder (MDD) is the most common mood disorder, with a prevalence rate of 5% worldwide (Weissman et al. 1996). MDD and dysthymia are distinguished from bipolar spectrum disorders by the absence of manic, mixed, or hypomanic episodes (Murray and Lopez 1997). MDD occurs approximately twice as frequently in women as in men (Weissman et al. 1996). The average age at onset of MDD is in the third and fourth decade of life, and the length of an untreated major depressive episode can range from 6 to 24 months (Weissman et al. 1996). There are also considerable variations in the symptom constellation, rate of recurrence, and response to psychological and pharmacological treatments.

In addition to a genetic vulnerability, adverse early life experiences appear to predispose susceptible individuals to MDD. Vulnerabilities may be activated later in life as a result of negative life events, including chronic social stress, social isolation, and social defeat. In the absence of negative life events, people with the diathesis may avoid developing MDD. In short, current evidence suggests that the pathophysiology of nonbipolar MDD is related to how individuals respond to stress and perhaps more specifically how they respond to loss, social challenge, and social defeat (Akiskal and McKinney 1975; Kendler et al. 2003). Variations in risk for the development of MDD, its clinical presentation, response to treatment, and risk of recurrence are likely influenced by a number of other inherent individual differences, including personality traits and dimensions that influence how individuals respond to stress and social challenge. Cultural factors can be important in patients' experience and perception of depression, and racial and ethnic issues can be factors in the metabolism of medications (Lin et al. 1995; Strakowski et al. 1996).

The goal of this chapter is to review the relationship between personality and various aspects of the treatment process for depressed patients, including help seeking, treatment selection, treatment compliance, and response to treatment with a focus on pharmacotherapy.

Personality Disorders and Depression

Maladaptive personality functioning has long been considered a risk factor for psychiatric disorders, including MDD (Maher and Maher 1994). However, the precise nature of the relations between personality functioning and MDD remains unknown (e.g., Clark et al. 1994; Frank et al. 1987; Klein et al. 1993; see also Chapter 3 of this book). Current barriers to a better understanding include the heterogeneous presentation and course of mood disorders, the limitations of the current multiaxial DSM-IV-TR classification system (American Psychiatric Association 2000), and the variety of proposals for modeling these relationships.

Certainly the heterogeneity of mood disorders (including the bipolar spectrum disorders and dysthymia as well as the comorbidities including depressive personality disorder) complicates the task of understanding the etiology and personality correlates of these conditions (McCullough 2000; Sloman et al. 2003; Thase and Howland 1995; Van Praag 1998). Although the DSM-IV-TR Axis I system represents a great advance, it is also associated with significant diagnostic shortcomings (Widiger 2003). For example, the imperfection of the Axis I system makes it difficult to discriminate specific risk factors for mood versus anxiety disorders (Kendler et al. 2003). In addition, there are considerable methodological challenges in separating depressed "state" from personality "trait" (Bagby and Ryder 2000; Santor et al. 1997).

As previously discussed, there are a number of different ways to conceptualize the relations between personality and MDD (Klein et al. 1993; see also Chapters 3 and 4 of this book). Initially, investigators focused on the relations between personality traits and depression, but after the introduction of the categorical Axis II classification of personality disorders, the focus switched to examining relations between categorical personality disorders and the Axis I disorders. Limitations of the Axis II system have been well documented, including the multiple comorbidities across these Axis II disorders and the failure to take into account the extent to which Axis I diagnoses can inflate Axis II diagnoses (Widiger 2003). Indeed, as a result of the problems with the current Axis II system and some fundamental problems with categorical conceptualizations of personality disorders, a number of authors have argued that future versions of the Axis II system should be dimensional rather than categorical (e.g., Clark et al. 1997; Livesley 1998; Livesley and Jang 2000; McCrae et al. 2001; Westen and Arkowitz-Westen 1998; Widiger and Frances 2002).

Despite these problems, certain personality characteristics are associated with vulnerability to depression as well as response to pharmacological treatment. Individual differences in personality likely influence the course of depression and response to treatment in various ways, including help-seeking behavior, illness detection, treatment selection, side-effect reporting, and treatment adherence or compliance. Finally, the pharmacological treatment of depression has been associated with changes in specific personality characteristics, suggesting a potential for better understanding the mechanism of action of pharmacological treatments.

Dimensional Models of Personality and Their Relationships to Depression

Personality disorders are conceptualized as maladaptive sets of traits that are qualitatively distinct from "normal" personality. In contrast, according to dimensional conceptualizations of personality pathology, there is a continuous relationship between adaptive (healthy) and maladaptive (unhealthy) personality traits. In addition to the well-described limitations of current categorical approaches to understanding personality, dimensional approaches to personality pathology make sense from an evolutionary perspective. If one assumes that temperament is largely inherited and that personality evolves as a result of the interaction between temperament and environment, then evolutionary theory would predict variation along a continuum for both temperament and personality traits. Indeed, from a Darwinian perspective, the more successful and widespread a species, the more one observes continuous gradations in features and behavior. In contrast, if one considers personality disorders to be typologically distinct from normal personality, then from an evolutionary perspective they should be relatively rare "monstrosities" (Darwin 1859/1979) rather than fairly commonly observed deviations from the norm.

There have been a number of dimensional models of temperament and personality applied to understanding the relations between temperament, personality, and MDD, leading to mixed results (Bagby et al. 1995). However, despite the variability in measures, models, and sample characteristics, there is considerable support for relations between MDD and two broad dimensions of temperament often referred to as "The Two": *neuroticism* (negative temperament, negative affectivity) and *extraversion* (positive temperament, positive affectivity). These two broad traits appear to be correlated with a diagnosis of MDD and symptom severity (Watson et al. 1988). Although the data are more compelling for negative than positive temperament, both broad traits appear to constitute vulnerability factors for MDD, predict prognosis, and may be affected by the course of the disorder (Bagby and Ryder 2000; Clark et al. 1994). Dimensional models of personality that have been applied to understanding the relations between temperament, personality, and MDD include the psychobiological models proposed by Eysenck (Eysenck and Eysenck 1964) and Cloninger (1986) as well as the five-factor model (FFM) for traits (Digman 1990).

Personality and Psychobiology

Prominent among models of personality and personality disorders is the psychobiological model of personality and personality disorders proposed by Eysenck (Eysenck and Eysenck 1964). This model posits three super factors of *psychoticism, extraversion,* and *neuroticism.* The extraversion dimension reflects cortical arousal. Introverts are characterized by chronic overarousal (anxious), whereas extraverts are chronically underaroused (bored). Neuroticism is a reflection of individual differences in the activation thresholds of the sympathetic nervous system (fight/flight response). Neurotic people are characterized by a low activation threshold and experience negative affect (fight/flight) in the context of minor stressors, whereas emotionally stable people have a high activation threshold and generally remain calm in the face of stress. Finally, psychoticism is a complex construct associated with risk for having psychotic experiences and aggression. Each of these three superfactors is comprised of several lower order factors. The superfactors and factors are derived from the Eysenck Personality Inventory (Eysenck and Eysenck 1964). Neuroticism has been identified as a risk factor for MDD as well as recurrence (Berlanga et al. 1999; Roberts and Kendler 1999).

The Seven-Factor Model of Temperament and Character

Cloninger (1986) has proposed a psychobiological theory of temperament and character composed of four components: *harm avoidance, novelty seeking, reward dependence,* and *persistence.* Novelty seeking describes approach motivation or behavioral activation and encompasses extraversion. Harm avoidance reflects a tendency to be fearful, shy, and nervous; it is associated with behavioral inhibition and is similar to neuroticism. Reward dependence is described as sensitivity to cues for reward, especially social reward and social attachment, whereas persistence has to do with ambitiousness, eagerness, and sensitivity to cues for partial reinforcement.

Each temperament is theorized to be associated with specific monoaminergic activity (Cloninger et al. 1993, 1998). In addition, three character dimensions, including *self-directedness, cooperativeness,* and *self-transcendence,* have been added to help capture personality psychopathology not adequately accounted for by the four temperaments. An earlier version of the model, the unified biosocial model (Cloninger 1986), included only three temperaments (persistence originally being a part of reward dependence) that were measured using the Tridimensional Personality Questionnaire (TPQ), whereas the Temperament and Character Inventory (TCI) assesses four temperaments and three characters (Cloninger et al. 1998).

In general, the results of studies using the TPQ suggest that MDD is associated with elevated scores on harm avoidance as well as average scores on novelty seeking and reward dependence. Harm avoidance scores have been found to be correlated with symptom severity and somewhat reduced with treatment, although remitted MDD patients have higher scores after treatment compared with nonpatient control subjects (Bagby and Ryder 2000; Brown et al. 1992; Chien and Dunner 1996; Hansenne et al. 1998, 1999; Joffe et al. 1993; Mulder et al. 1994; Nelson and Cloninger 1995; Sauer et al. 1997; Strakowski et al. 1992, 1995; Young et al. 1995). Using the TCI, Hansenne and colleagues (1999) reported that patients with MDD have higher scores on self-transcendence and lower scores on self-directedness and cooperativeness, with self-directedness, cooperativeness, and harm avoidance correlating positively with severity of depression.

The Five-Factor Model

It has been argued that the predictive power of the FFM in psychiatric contexts is limited because its content does not extend sufficiently into the pathological realm (e.g., Clark 1993; Haigler and Widiger 2001). However, other dimensional models of personality psychopathology (e.g., Livesley 1987) that selected personality disorder traits and symptoms as the sources for their models have been highly correlated with and similar in predictive power to the FFM (Miller et al. 2001; Reynolds and Clark 2001; Trull et al. 1995).

In a study using the Revised NEO Personality Inventory (NEO-PI-R) to assess the five factors (Costa and McCrae 1992), acutely ill patients with MDD scored significantly higher on neuroticism and significantly lower on extraversion (Bagby and Ryder 2000). Whereas neuroticism scores decrease and extraversion scores increase with treatment, they remain significantly different from community norms (Bagby and Ryder 2000; Bagby et al. 1995, 1997; Petersen et al. 2001) (P. T. Costa Jr., R. M. Bagby, J. H. Herbst, et al.: "Evidence for the Validity of Personality Traits Measured During Major Depressive Disorder: Reinterpretation of the State Artifact Issue." Unpublished manuscript, 2005).

Personality and Treatment

Help-Seeking Behavior and Illness Detection

Only a minority of people who have a diagnosable mental disorder receive professional help. This has been repeatedly shown across major epidemiological surveys (Kessler et al. 1994, 1997; Lin et al. 1996; Regier et al. 1993). In both the European Depression Epidemiological Survey (DEPRES) (Lepine et al. 1997) and in the Ontario Health Survey (Parikh et al. 1997), fewer than 50% of detected cases of MDD in the community had been identified by a health care professional, and fewer than half of those identified had received psychiatric treatment. Similarly, only 28% of those in the Epidemiologic Catchment Area study who met DSM-III-R (American Psychiatric Association 1987) criteria for a psychiatric disorder during the previous year had sought help from a mental health professional, and only 21% of those diagnosed with a mental disorder in the last year in the National Comorbidity Survey had sought help (Kessler et al. 1994). Overall, a systematic literature review on treatment-seeking rates for individuals with various types of depressive illness ranged from 21% to 61% (Bristow and Patten 2002), yet very few investigators have measured the effect of personality variables on treatment seeking. More often demographic and clinical variables have been examined in epidemiological surveys (Bland et al. 1997; Lefebvre et al. 1998; Rabinowitz et al. 1999). For example, being male, living alone, and living in a large urban community adversely affected help-seeking behavior. Among men, low neuroticism scores and an external attributional style have also been linked to a reduced rate of help-seeking behavior (Moller-Leimkuhler 2002).

Personality and Symptom Presentation

The relationship between personality dimensions and symptom presentation has also been evaluated. Using the TCI (Cloninger et al. 1998) to assess personality dimensions and the Center for Epidemiologic Studies Depression Scale (CES-D) (Radloff 1977) to evaluate depressive symptoms, Grucza and colleagues (2003) examined relationships between various depression parameters and the four personality dimensions, including symptom severity, comorbidity, and suicidality (see Table 5–1). In brief, Grucza et al. (2003) reported that 1) high harm avoidance was associated with panic attacks and total severity of depressive symptoms; 2) high novelty seeking alone was associated with suicide attempts, inability to concentrate, and alcohol use; 3) high harm avoidance with high novelty seeking was associated with the number of psychiatric admissions; 4) high reward dependence with high persistence was associated with restless sleep; 5) high reward dependence with low persistence was associated with appetite loss and low energy; and 6) high harm avoidance with low novelty seeking was associated with a lack of positive affect.

Treatment Preference and Selection

Bedi and colleagues (2000) addressed two issues relevant to treatment effectiveness for MDD in primary care. Although the study was primarily designed to compare the effectiveness of counseling and pharmacotherapy under randomized controlled conditions, a secondary aim was to compare outcomes in the group who agreed to be randomly assigned and the group who opted for personal selection of treatment. No differences were observed across patient variables in the self-selection and randomized groups, including scores on the Eysenck Personality Inventory. Similarly, Ward and Colleagues (2000) found no differences in outcome between self-selection and randomized subjects in a compari-

TABLE 5–1. Personality predictors of depressive symptoms

	Level associated with symptom			
	Harm avoidance	Novelty seeking	Reward dependence	Persistence
Severity of depressive symptoms	↑	-	-	-
Presence of panic attacks	↑	-	-	-
Psychiatric admission	↑	↑	-	-
Suicide attempts	-	↑	-	-
Gastrointestinal complaints	↑	-	↑	-
Alcohol symptoms	-	↑	↓	-
Restless sleep	-	-	↑	↑
Subjective symptoms	-	-	↑	↑
Appetite loss	-	-	↑	↓
Low energy	↑	-	↑	↓
Lack of positive affect	↑	↓	-	-
Inability to concentrate	-	↑	-	-
Total score	↑	-	-	-

Note. ↑=high; ↓=low; –=no association.
Source. Adapted from Grucza RA, Przybeck TR, Spitznagel EL, et al.: "Personality and Depressive Symptoms: A Multi-Dimensional Analysis." *Journal of Affective Disorders* 74:123–130, 2003.

son of nondirective counseling, cognitive-behavioral therapy, and usual general practitioner care for the treatment of MDD. In summary, although more research is needed, personality dimensions do not appear to influence treatment preference or selection.

Compliance With Treatment Recommendations

In a review of patient adherence or compliance during randomized controlled trials in the treatment of MDD, Pampallona and associates (2002) concluded that one in every three patients did not complete the investigational treatment. Even higher dropout rates have been reported in other settings. Fifty-three percent of patients who were treated in primary care practices with antidepressant medication had discontinued treatment before the end of 12 weeks (Maddox et al. 1994). Rates of discontinuation and the reasons provided in this study were remarkably similar to those reported by Demyttenaere and colleagues (2001) across family practice units in Europe (see Table 5–2).

TABLE 5–2.   Reasons cited for antidepressant medication discontinuation

Maddox (1994)		Demyttenaere et al. (2001)	
Feeling better	35%	Feeling better	55%
Adverse events	30%	Adverse events	23%
Other reasons	17%	Fear of dependence	10%
Physician instruction	15%	Stigma	10%
Lack of effect	15%	Lack of effect	10%

Side effects are one reason for discontinuation. Using the Eysenck Personality Inventory, Davis and colleagues (1995) investigated the influence of personality variables on side-effect reporting in a group of healthy volunteer subjects during a randomized placebo-controlled trial involving the reversible inhibitor of monoamine oxidase-A, moclobemide. The authors confirmed a positive relationship between neuroticism score at baseline and subsequent side-effect reporting. By the end of the study the relations between neuroticism and side-effect reporting had increased in the placebo group and declined in the moclobemide group. In summary, these results underscore the interindividual variability in side-effect reporting, which is usually neglected in clinical trials. The following case illustrates the importance of individual differences in side effect reporting:

Case Example

Ms. A, a 25-year-old patient with MDD, panic disorder, and comorbid borderline personality disorder, was repeatedly unable to complete even a minimum trial of numerous antidepressants. After agreeing to participate in a randomized placebo-controlled trial of a novel antidepressant with potentially fewer side effects, the patient arrived at the emergency room 2 days later. She reported severe nausea and panic symptoms, which she attributed to the new medication. She discontinued the trial, and the double-blind medication turned out to be placebo.

This experience was discussed with Ms. A in terms of her expectancy effects and fear of losing control when she took any medication. It became a defining experience and allowed her to be rechallenged with gradually increasing doses of a previously intolerable antidepressant. She responded to this medication.

Medication Compliance

Despite an increased awareness that noncompliance with antidepressant treatment is a major contributing factor to suboptimal therapeutic outcomes (Demyttenaere 1997), there has been very little empirical research conducted in the area of personality and relationship variables and compliance with antidepressant medication (Book 1987). Sirey and colleagues (2001), using the Inventory of Interpersonal Problems (Horowitz et al. 1988) to screen for personality pathology, reported that antidepressant compliance was associated with the absence of personality pathology. However, the Inventory of Interpersonal Problems has not been validated against more frequently used measures. Ekselius and colleagues (2000) used the Karolinska Scales of Personality (Schalling et al. 1987) to investigate the relationship between personality traits and compliance with antidepressant medication. Ekselius et al. reported that medication noncompliance, defined as out-of-range plasma levels of medication, was associated with elevated scores on the sensation-seeking subscale of this instrument. Similarly, Wingerson and colleagues (1993) found early discontinuation from clinical trials was positively associated with the novelty-seeking dimension on the Tridimensional Personality Questionnaire in patients with panic disorder and generalized anxiety disorder.

Although other researchers have proposed that personality factors may be associated with medication noncompliance in psychiatric populations (Fawcett 1995; Kusumakar and Kennedy 1996; Stein and Hackerman 1991), there are virtually no evaluations. On the basis of the combined use of the Minnesota Multiphasic Personality Inventory (MMPI-2) clinical and content scales and the NEO PI, Stein and Hackerman (1991) proposed that low conscientiousness scores and high neuroticism scores, combined with the MMPI-2 content scale "work interference" and "negative indicators," are indicative of the potential for poor treatment compliance. However, as these conclusions were drawn from a single case study, a prospective controlled approach is required to test the hypothesis.

Demyttenaere (1997) also recognized anecdotal and theoretical literature addressing personality factors and compliance, including psychodynamic literature by Book (1987), who discussed the implications of projection, denial, identification, and transference in understanding medication compliance in psychiatric patients. Demyttenaere noted that noncompliance may reflect an individual's attempt to deny having depression or to avoid identifying with another family member who may also have the disorder.

Cohen and colleagues (2004) evaluated the relationship between personality (FFM) and compliance in depressed outpatients. Compliance was measured using an electronic bottle-cap device designed to record openings and closings of medication bottles, the Medication

Event Monitoring System (MEMS). High extraversion was found to be a significant negative predictor of compliance to antidepressant medication. At the level of NEO facets, *activity* (extraversion) and *feelings* (openness) were negatively correlated with compliance, whereas modesty (agreeableness) was positively associated with compliance.

Although excitement seeking as measured by the NEO-PI-R was not significantly related to medication compliance, the elevation in extraversion is consistent with the findings of Ekselius and colleagues (2000), who found that noncompliance with antidepressant medication was associated with impulsive sensation seeking. The extraversion equivalent, *novelty seeking,* in patients with panic disorder and generalized anxiety disorder was also associated with early discontinuation in clinical trials (Wingerson et al. 1993).

The feelings facet of openness, characterized by excitable, spontaneous, insightful, imaginative, affectionate, talkative, and outgoing attributes, was also inversely related to compliance. Taken together, the characteristics associated with feelings coupled with the characteristics associated with activity, particularly being energetic, hurried, quick, excitable, and spontaneous, are somewhat related to characteristics of excitement seeking. From a clinical perspective, this suggests that people who have elevated levels of extraversion and openness are more likely to experience early (although potentially transient) symptomatic improvement followed by a reduction in medication compliance. This is illustrated in the case of Mr. T.

Case Example

Mr. T worked in the sales department of an office supply company. He was a particularly gregarious individual. Over a 6-year period, he had been seen for approximately 2 months at three different psychiatric clinics. On each occasion he presented with typical symptoms of major depression. For him, the most prominent symptom was losing interest in his normally active social life.

There was also a pattern to his antidepressant usage. On each occasion, he responded very quickly, often during the first week. He would regain interest in social activities and increase his success in sales. Unfortunately, this is also the time when he would skip his antidepressant medication for days at a time and eventually stop altogether.

Only after a detailed discussion about the potential negative relationship between his personality style and medication compliance did Mr. T agree to comply with antidepressant therapy and he has remained well for the past 2 years.

Personality and Response to Antidepressant Medication

Personality Disorders

Although the general consensus among clinicians is that patients who present with comorbid depression and personality disorders have a worse outcome, this is not always supported by research findings. Several large clinical investigations did find evidence to support an adverse outcome in depressed patients with comorbid personality disorders.

In a study designed to examine the effects of personality traits (as determined by the Structured Clinical Interview for DSM-III Personality Disorders [SCID]) in depressed patients receiving desipramine over 4–5 weeks, responders had a significantly lower total personality trait score and a significantly lower Cluster C personality trait score than nonresponders (Peselow et al. 1992). Those with a sustained response after 6 months were found to have significantly lower Cluster B, Cluster C, and total personality scores. In a study assessing predictors of response and remission, Ezquiaga and colleagues (1998) found that the presence of a personality disorder, as assessed by DSM-III-R criteria, was a strong predictor of outcome and was associated with significantly less likelihood of response or remission. Bschor and colleagues (2001) examined retrospectively predictors of a good response to lithium augmentation in a group of depressed patients who failed to respond to tricyclic antidepressants (TCAs). Absence of comorbid personality disorders was a significant predictor of response to lithium augmentation.

In a large tertiary-based study involving over 600 patients and designed to investigate predictors of response to sertraline or imipramine in patients with chronic or double depression, Hirschfeld and colleagues (1998) reported that the presence of a comorbid personality disorder (measured by the SCID-II, based on DSM-III-R criteria) did not predict treatment response. When individual personality disorders were examined, however, a diagnosis of passive-aggressive personality disorder was predictive of a positive response to treatment. Similarly, Fava and colleagues (1994) evaluated the predictive value of personality disorder comorbidity in a group of patients who received fluoxetine treatment. Based on the Personality Diagnostic Questionnaire-Revised (PDQ-R), the presence of a Cluster B diagnosis before treatment predicted positive antidepressant response. However, no differences in response were found in patients with or without a Cluster A or C diagnosis.

In contrast, Joyce and colleagues (1994) found that neither individual personality disorders nor clusters (DSM-III-R) were predictive of treatment outcome, although there was a trend toward those with a borderline personality disorder having a poorer outcome.

Almost a decade later, Mulder (2002) published the most comprehensive review to date on the influence of both personality disorders and dimensions on pharmacotherapy and psychotherapy outcomes. This review of 27 studies using DSM Axis II criteria to examine the relation between personality comorbidity in MDD and treatment outcome found conflicting results. Fifteen studies reported a worse outcome, five reported a partially worse outcome, and seven reported no difference in treatment outcome. Overall, the author concluded that the best-designed studies reported the least effect of personality pathology on depression treatment outcome. With the same group of studies, Mulder and colleagues (2003) also examined the interaction between antidepressant class (selective serotonin reuptake inhibitor [SSRI; fluoxetine] and TCA [nortriptyline]), personality disorder, and outcome. They reported that the presence or absence of a comorbid personality disorder (assessed by the SCID-II, based on DSM-III-R criteria) did not significantly affect outcome. However they confirmed an interaction between presence of a comorbid personality disorder, drug type, and outcome. Although there was a trend for all patients treated with nortriptyline to have a less favorable outcome, those patients with a Cluster B personality disorder who received nortriptyline demonstrated significantly less improvement. These findings support the idea that individuals with Cluster B personality disorders, in particular those with borderline personality disorder, respond better to SSRIs than to TCAs. The findings are also consistent with previous reports that patients with a Cluster B diagnosis at baseline assessment demonstrated a significantly greater decrease in Hamilton Rating Scale for Depression (Ham-D) scores with fluoxetine treatment compared with those without a Cluster B diagnosis (Fava et al. 1994).

Personality Dimensions

The Seven-Factor Model of Temperament and Character

Several investigators have examined the influence of TPQ- and TCI-derived dimensions and temperament types on treatment response. Using the TPQ, Joyce and colleagues (1994) predicted differential treatment responses to clomipramine and desipramine in depressed outpatients. Although none of the dimensions of the Eysenck Personality Inventory predicted outcome, temperament as measured by the TPQ accounted for 35% of the variance in treatment outcome, which increased to 49% when the sample was limited to the severely depressed group. By contrast, less than 5% of the variance was predicted by clinical variables. Depressed patients with high reward dependence and harm avoidance scores, or both, had a good outcome regardless of sex or drug. However, in women high reward dependence was associated with a better response to clomipramine, whereas high harm avoidance was associated with a better response to desipramine. The authors speculated that reward dependence is related to features of atypical depression, including interpersonal sensitivity, and that patients with these temperamental traits may preferentially respond to serotonergic-acting medications, including clomipramine.

Unfortunately, these findings have proven difficult to replicate. Nelson and Cloninger (1997) evaluated more than 1,000 depressed subjects receiving open-label treatment with nefazodone. Although they also found that the levels of reward dependence and harm avoidance and their interaction had significant predictive value, this accounted for only 1.1% of the variance.

Similarly, Newman and colleagues (2000) failed to replicate these results in a study involving fluoxetine treatment for depressed outpatients. There was no correlation between harm avoidance, reward dependence, or novelty seeking and percent improvement in depression score. These authors state that their failure to replicate previous findings may in large part be because of the use of different classes of antidepressants (SSRIs as opposed to TCAs) as well as not maximizing fluoxetine dosages. Using the TCI to determine possible predictors of response to the heterocyclic antidepressant maprotiline, Sato and colleagues (1999) were also unable to confirm that any of the seven personality dimensions had predictive value.

In summary, although the original results of the Joyce and colleagues (1994) study are thought provoking, these findings have been difficult to replicate.

Neuroticism and Extraversion

The relationship between neuroticism and treatment response in MDD has received considerable attention. In a comprehensive review of 13 studies that have examined the relation between neuroticism and treatment outcome, Mulder (2002) found that high neuroticism scores generally predicted worse treatment outcome in depressed patients, although he also concluded that in the best-designed studies, personality pathology has the least effect on depression treatment outcome. In a large randomized, controlled trial involving over 300 patients in primary care who met criteria for dysthymia, those with high neuroticism scores, as assessed by the NEO PI (Costa and McCrae 1989), were less likely to achieve remission (Katon et al. 2002). This finding applied to both problem-solving and paroxetine treatment groups. The authors cite literature suggesting that individuals with high neuroticism report lower tolerance for stress, lower self-esteem, and a greater likelihood of feeling victimized and resentful. They also report that high neuroticism has been shown to be predictive of adverse life events and is associated with an increased perception of severity of life stressors (Katon et al. 2002).

Some have shown neuroticism to be a predictor of poor long-term outcome, whereas others have failed to confirm such a relationship. Petersen and colleagues (2002) found that neuroticism was not a significant predictor of clinical response in a 6-week open trial of fluoxetine in depressed outpatients. Similarly, Bagby and colleagues (1995) did not find that neuroticism predicted treatment outcome. Consistent with previous research, the mean neuroticism score for depressed patients pretreatment was almost two standard deviations higher than scores in a normative sample. The authors also reported that neuroticism score was significantly correlated with severity of depression scores, and there was a significant drop in neuroticism scores with treatment, although neuroticism scores for recovered patients remained more than one standard deviation higher than the normative sample (Bagby et al. 1995). These results suggest that elevated neuroticism scores in a sample of depressed patients may not be explained entirely by depressive symptomatology at the time of the initial assessment.

A similar pattern of results was described for extraversion, although the magnitude of change and correlation with measures of depression was less than that observed for neuroticism scores. Patients who ultimately recovered were less than one standard deviation lower on extraversion compared with the normative sample and less than half a standard deviation lower compared with the normative sample following treatment. Such results suggest that low extraversion may not be a specific vulnerability factor for MDD. However, extraversion may have an important role to play in course and/or treatment outcome (Bagby and Ryder 2000; Bagby et al. 1995; Barnett and Gotlib 1988; Widiger and Trull 1992). Indeed, in a regression analysis using neuroticism and extraversion scores as predictors of treatment outcome, only extraversion scores predicted a significant reduction of depressive symptoms, with higher extraversion scores, in particular the "gregariousness" facet, predicting a greater reduction of symptoms. Moreover, extraversion scores at treatment entry for patients who did not recover were more than two standard deviations below the normative sample. These results were later replicated (Bagby et al. 1997; Du et al. 2002).

Other cognitive variables, including rumination and distraction, also have been linked to vulnerability and recovery from depression. Bagby and Parker (2001) investigated the relationship between neuroticism and extraversion as measured by the NEO-PI-R and the cognitive constructs, rumination and distraction, as measured by the Response Style Questionnaire (RSQ) (Nolen-Hoeksema and Morrow 1991), before the initiation of a 14-week trial of pharmacotherapy in 168 patients with major depression. They found that remission defined as both a decrease of at least 50% in Ham-D scores and a final score of less than 9 (after 14 weeks of treatment) was significantly associated with extraversion and distraction but not related to neuroticism or a ruminative response style. Partial correlations were calculated to determine whether the contributions of extraversion and distraction were independent of their shared variance with one another. After controlling for distraction, the relationship between extraversion and treatment outcome was preserved, although the correlation between distraction and outcome was no longer significant after controlling for extraversion.

Overall the above results suggest that neuroticism may be a vulnerability factor for MDD, whereas extraversion may moderate treatment outcome (Bagby and Ryder 2000). Differences across studies in the degree to which neuroticism predicts outcome may be partly explained by examining whether the investigators covaried out baseline depression. When baseline severity of depression is covaried from the predictor model, neuroticism does not predict outcome (Bagby et al. 1995). In summary, results of the relationship between personality comorbidity and MDD are quite mixed. In general, the better controlled the study, the less evidence there is for personality pathology affecting outcome (Bagby et al. 2002; Mulder 2002).

Conclusions

Maladaptive personality functioning has long been considered a risk factor for MDD. Despite a wide variety of different models investigated in the context of a variety of experimental designs, treatments, and samples, current evidence suggests that personality traits have important implications for help seeking as well as for treatment compliance and response.

Clinicians in the meantime should consider the following when assessing and treating patients with depression. In addition to demographic variables, the personality dimensions of neuroticism and harm avoidance predict treatment seeking. More specifically, in men lower neuroticism scores and an external attributional style have also been linked to a reduced rate of help-seeking behavior. Individual differences in personality dimensions may also influence symptom presentation. For example, high neuroticism (harm avoidance) appears to be associated with the presence of comorbid anxiety symptoms, whereas high neuroticism (harm avoidance) and low extraversion (novelty seeking) may be associated with a low positive affect. Such findings support the notion that whereas anxiety is characterized by high harm avoidance (neuroticism), depression is characterized by high harm avoidance (neuroticism) and low positive affect (low novelty seeking, low extraversion). These distinctions may have psychobiological and treatment implications. For example, the interventions employed to reduce harm avoidance (e.g., reducing fear-based avoidance, treatment with serotonergic- and norepinephrine-acting agents) may be somewhat different from the interventions used to increase novelty seeking (e.g., scheduling pleasant activities, treatment with dopaminergic-acting agents).

Recognizing the level of neuroticism in depressed patients has important implications in planning optimal pharmacotherapy. Given that neuroticism is positively and significantly associated with side-effect reporting, the clinician should pay particular attention to slow medication titration (start low, go slow) for patients with comorbid anxiety (essentially high neuroticism). For depressed patients with high extraversion, additional attention needs to be paid to compliance, particularly when they begin to experience subjective symptomatic improvement.

Comorbid personality pathology should not necessarily be assumed to be an impediment to good treatment response (Mulder 2002). This appears to be especially true for diagnoses of DSM-IV-TR personality disorders. With respect to personality dimensions, it may be that high harm avoidance in combination with high reward dependence is a positive predictor of treatment outcome. It may be that differences across studies in the degree to which neuroticism (harm avoidance) predicts outcome may be partly explained by examining whether the investigators covaried out baseline depression. In general, although the best-designed studies reported the least effect of personality pathology on depression treatment outcome (Mulder 2002), it appears likely that relatively high extraversion (positive emotion) may prove to be a reasonably good positive predictor of treatment response. Once again, these data suggest that interventions targeting high neuroticism may be more effective when combined with interventions that target low extraversion.

Brief rating scales, such as the NEO short version (NEO-FFI) (Costa and McCrae 1992), offer promise as a practical application for clinicians to use in routine practice. In the meantime, clinicians need to keep in mind that personality pathology, whether assessed in terms of dimensions or disorders, can affect the patient's capacity to seek, be engaged in, and be compliant with treatment. Thinking about personality issues can help clinicians formulate interventions to engage their patients in treatment, whether by addressing and countering maladaptive attributional styles, helping patients overcome denial of their depression, or keeping them from overfocusing on side effects.

Although research on personality and treatment outcome in depression is not without controversy, the presence of personality psychopathology, in terms of maladaptive dimensions or disorders, should not preclude patients from experiencing robust trials of pharmacotherapy, psychotherapy, or both.

References

Akiskal HS, McKinney WT Jr: Overview of recent research in depression: integration of ten conceptual models into a comprehensive clinical frame. Arch Gen Psychiatry 32:285–305, 1975

American Psychiatric Association: Diagnostic and Statistical Manual of Mental Disorders, 3rd Edition, Revised. Washington, DC, American Psychiatric Association, 1987

American Psychiatric Association: Diagnostic and Statistical Manual of Mental Disorders, 4th Edition, Text Revision. Washington, DC, American Psychiatric Association, 2000

Bagby RM, Parker JDA: Relation of rumination and distraction with neuroticism and extraversion in a sample of patients with depression. Cognit Ther Res 25:91–102, 2001

Bagby RM, Ryder AG: Personality and the affective disorders: past efforts, current models, and future directions. Curr Psychiatry Rep 2:465–472, 2000

Bagby RM, Joffe RT, Parker JDA, et al: Major depression and the five-factor model of personality. J Personal Disord 9:224–234, 1995

Bagby RM, Bindseil KD, Schuller DR, et al: Relationship between the five-factor model of personality and unipolar, bipolar, and schizophrenic patients. Psychiatry Res 70:83–94, 1997

Bagby RM, Ryder AG, Cristi C: Psychosocial and clinical predictors of response to pharmacotherapy for depression. J Psychiatry Neurosci 27:250–257, 2002

Barnett PA, Gotlib IH: Psychosocial functioning and depression: distinguishing among antecedents, concomitants, and consequences. Psychol Bull 104:97–126, 1988

Bedi N, Chilvers C, Churchill R, et al: Assessing effectiveness of treatment of depression in primary care: partially randomised preference trial. Br J Psychiatry 177:312–318, 2000

Berlanga C, Heinze G, Torres M, et al: Personality and clinical predictors of recurrence of depression. Psychiatr Serv 5:376–380, 1999

Bland RC, Newman SC, Orn H: Help-seeking for psychiatric disorders. Can J Psychiatry 42:935–942, 1997

Book HE: Some psychodynamics of non-compliance. Can J Psychiatry 32:115–117, 1987

Bristow K, Patten S: Treatment-seeking rates and associated mediating factors among individuals with depression. Can J Psychiatry 47:660–665, 2002

Brown SL, Svrakic DM, Przybeck TR, et al: The relationship of personality to mood and anxiety states: a dimensional approach. J Psychiatr Res 26:197–211, 1992

Bschor T, Canata B, Muller-Oerlinghausen B, et al: Predictors of response to lithium augmentation in tricyclic antidepressant-resistant depression. J Affect Disord 64:261–265, 2001

Chien AJ, Dunner DL: The tridimensional personality questionnaire in depression: state versus trait issues. J Psychiatr Res 30:21–27, 1996

Clark LA: Personality disorder diagnosis: limitations of the five-factor model. Psychological Inquiry 4:100–104, 1993

Clark LA, Watson D, Mineka S: Temperament, personality, and the mood and anxiety disorders. J Abnorm Psychology 103:103–116, 1994

Clark LA, Livesley WJ, Morey L: Personality disorder assessment: the challenge of construct validity. J Personal Disord 11:205–231, 1997

Cloninger CR: A unified biosocial theory of personality and its role in the development of anxiety states. Psychiatr Dev 4:167–226, 1986

Cloninger CR, Svrakic DM, Przybeck TR: A psychobiological model of temperament and character. Arch Gen Psychiatry 50:975–990, 1993

Cloninger CR, Bayon C, Svrakic DM: Measurement of temperament and character in mood disorders: a model of fundamental states as personality types. J Affect Disord 51:21–32, 1998

Cohen NL, Ross EC, Bagby RM, et al: The five-factor model of personality and antidepressant medication compliance. Can J Psychiatry 49:106–113, 2004

Costa PT Jr, McCrae RR: The NEO-PI/NEO-FFI manual supplement. Odessa, FL, Psychological Assessment Resources, 1989

Costa PT Jr, McCrae RR: Revised NEO Personality Inventory (NEO-PI-R) and NEO Five-Factor Inventory (NEO-FFI): Professional Manual. Odessa, FL, Psychological Assessment Resources, 1992

Darwin CR: The Origin of Species (1859). New York, Random House, 1979

Davis C, Ralevski E, Kennedy SH, et al: The role of personality factors in the reporting of side effect complaints to moclobemide and placebo: a study of healthy male and female volunteers. J Clin Psychopharmacol 15:347–352, 1995

Demyttenaere K: Compliance during treatment with antidepressants. J Affect Disord 43:27–39, 1997

Demyttenaere K, Enzlin P, Dewe W, et al: Compliance with antidepressants in a primary care setting, 1: beyond lack of efficacy and adverse events. J Clin Psychiatry 62 (suppl 22):30–33, 2001

Digman JM: Personality structure: emergence of the five-factor model. Annu Rev Psychol 41:417–440, 1990

Du L, Bakish D, Ravindran AV, et al: Does fluoxetine influence major depression by modifying five-factor personality traits? J Affect Disord 71:235–241, 2002

Ekselius L, Bengtsson F, von Knorring L: Non-compliance with pharmacotherapy of depression is associated with a sensation seeking personality. Int Clin Psychopharmacol 15:273–278, 2000

Eysenck SB, Eysenck HJ: An improved short questionnaire for the measurement of extraversion and neuroticism. Life Sci 305:1103–1109, 1964

Ezquiaga E, Garcia A, Bravo F, et al: Factors associated with outcome in major depression: a 6-month prospective study. Soc Psychiatry Psychiatr Epidemiol 33:552–557, 1998

Fava M, Bouffides E, Pava JA, et al: Personality disorder comorbidity with major depression and response to fluoxetine treatment. Psychother Psychosom 62:160–167, 1994

Fawcett J: Compliance: definitions and key issues. J Clin Psychiatry 56 (suppl 1): 4–8, 1995

Frank E, Kupfer DJ, Jacob M, et al: Personality features and response to acute treatment in recurrent depression. J Personal Disord 1:14–26, 1987

Grucza RA, Przybeck TR, Spitznagel EL, et al: Personality and depressive symptoms: a multi-dimensional analysis. J Affect Disord 74:123–130, 2003

Haigler ED, Widiger TA: Experimental manipulation of NEO-PI-R items. J Pers Assess 77:339–358, 2001

Hansenne M, Pitchot W, Gonzalez Moreno A, et al: The tridimensional personality questionnaire and depression. Eur Psychiatry 13:101–103, 1998

Hansenne M, Reggers J, Pinto E, et al: Temperament and character inventory (TCI) and depression. J Psychiatr Res 33:31–36, 1999

Hirschfeld RM, Russell JM, Delgado PL, et al: Predictors of response to acute treatment of chronic and double depression with sertraline or imipramine. J Clin Psychiatry 59:669–675, 1998

Horowitz LM, Rosenberg SE, Baer BA, et al: Inventory of interpersonal problems: psychometric properties and clinical applications. J Consult Clin Psychol 56:885–892, 1988

Joffe RT, Bagby M, Levitt AJ, et al: The tridimensional personality questionnaire and major depression. Am J Psychiatry 150:959–960, 1993

Joyce PR, Mulder RT, Cloninger CR: Temperament predicts clomipramine and desipramine response in major depression. J Affect Disord 30:35–46, 1994

Katon W, Russo J, Frank E, et al: Predictors of nonresponse to treatment in primary care patients with dysthymia. Gen Hosp Psychiatry 24:20–27, 2002

Kendler KS, Hettema JM, Butera F, et al: Life event dimensions of loss, humiliation, entrapment, and danger in the prediction of onsets of major depression and generalized anxiety. Arch Gen Psychiatry 60:789–796, 2003

Kessler RC, McGonagle KA, Zhao S, et al: Lifetime and 12-month prevalence of DSM-III-R psychiatric disorders in the United States: results from the National Comorbidity Survey. Arch Gen Psychiatry 51:8–19, 1994

Kessler RC, Zhao S, Blazer DG, et al: Prevalence, correlates, and course of minor depression and major depression in the National Comorbidity Survey. J Affect Disord 45:19–30, 1997

Kendler KS, Hettema JM, Butera F, et al: Life event dimensions of loss, humiliation, entrapment, and danger in the prediction of onsets of major depression and generalized anxiety. Arch Gen Psychiatry 60:789–796, 2003

Klein MH, Wonderlich SA, Shea MT: Models of the relationship between personality and depression: toward a framework for theory and research, in Personality and Depression: A Current View. Edited by Klein MH, Kupfer DJ, Shea MT. New York, Guilford, 1993, pp 1–54

Kusumakar V, Kennedy SH: Promoting therapeutic alliance and adherence to medication treatment in depression. Canadian Journal of Diagnosis (suppl):2–9 1996

Lefebvre J, Lesage A, Cyr M, et al: Factors related to utilization of services for mental health reasons in Montreal, Canada. Soc Psychiatry Psychiatr Epidemiol 33:291–298, 1998

Lepine JP, Gastpar M, Mendlewicz J, et al: Depression in the community: the first pan-European study DEPRES (Depression Research in European Society). Int Clin Psychopharmacol 12:19–29, 1997

Lin E, Goering P, Offord DR, et al: The use of mental health services in Ontario: epidemiologic findings. Can J Psychiatry 41:572–577, 1996

Lin KM, Anderson D, Poland RE: Ethnicity and psychopharmacology: bridging the gap. Psychiatr Clin North Am 18:635–647, 1995

Livesley WJ: A systematic approach to the delineation of personality disorders. Am J Psychiatry 144:772–777, 1987

Livesley WJ: Suggestions for a framework for an empirically based classification of personality disorder. Can J Psychiatry 43:137–147, 1998

Livesley WJ, Jang KL: Toward an empirically based classification of personality disorder. J Personal Disord 14:137–151, 2000

Maddox JC, Levi M, Thompson C: The compliance with antidepressants in general practice. J Psychopharmacol 8:48–53, 1994

Maher BA, Maher WB: Personality and psychopathology: a historical perspective. J Abnorm Psychol 103:72–77, 1994

McCrae RR, Yang J, Costa PT Jr, et al: Personality profiles and the prediction of categorical personality disorders. J Pers 69:155–174, 2001

McCullough JP Jr: Treatment for Chronic Depression: Cognitive Behavioral Analysis System of Psychotherapy (CBASP). New York, Guilford, 2000

Miller JD, Lynam DR, Widiger TA, et al: Personality disorders as extreme variants of common personality dimensions: can the Five Factor Model adequately represent psychopathology? J Pers 69:253–276, 2001

Moller-Leimkuhler AM: Barriers to help-seeking by men: a review of sociocultural and clinical literature with particular reference to depression. J Affect Disord 71:1–9, 2002

Mulder RT: Personality pathology and treatment outcome in major depression: a review. Am J Psychiatry 159:359–371, 2002

Mulder RT, Joyce PR, Cloninger CR: Temperament and early environment influence comorbidity and personality disorders in major depression. Compr Psychiatry 35:225–233, 1994

Mulder RT, Joyce PR, Luty SE: The relationship of personality disorders to treatment outcome in depressed outpatients. J Clin Psychiatry 64:259–264, 2003

Murray CJ, Lopez AD: Alternative projections of mortality and disability by cause 1990–2020: Global Burden of Disease Study. Lancet 349:1498–1504, 1997

Nelson EC, Cloninger CR: The tridimensional personality questionnaire as a predictor of response to nefazodone treatment of depression. J Affect Disord 35:51–57, 1995

Nelson E[C], Cloninger CR: Exploring the TPQ as a possible predictor of antidepressant response to nefazodone in a large multi-site study. J Affect Disord 44:197–200, 1997

Newman JR, Ewing SE, McColl RD, et al: Tridimensional personality questionnaire and treatment response in major depressive disorder: a negative study. J Affect Disord 57:241–247, 2000

Nolen-Hoeksema S, Morrow J: A prospective study of depression and posttraumatic stress symptoms after a natural disaster: the 1989 Loma Prieta Earthquake. J Pers Soc Psychol 61:115–121, 1991

Pampallona S, Bollini P, Tibaldi G, et al: Patient adherence in the treatment of depression. Br J Psychiatry 180:104–109, 2002

Parikh SV, Lin E, Lesage AD: Mental health treatment in Ontario: selected comparisons between the primary care and specialty sectors. Can J Psychiatry 42:929–934, 1997

Peselow ED, Fieve RR, Difiglia C: Personality traits and response to desipramine. J Affect Disord 24:209–216, 1992

Petersen T, Bottonari K, Alpert JE, et al: Use of the five-factory inventory in characterizing patients with major depressive disorder. Compr Psychiatry 42:488–493, 2001

Petersen T, Papakostas GI, Bottonari K, et al: NEO-FFI factor scores as predictors of clinical response to fluoxetine in depressed outpatients. Psychiatry Res 109:9–16, 2002

Rabinowitz J, Gross R, Feldman D: Correlates of a perceived need for mental health assistance and differences between those who do and do not seek help. Soc Psychiatry Psychiatr Epidemiol 34:141–146, 1999

Radloff LS: The CES-D scale: a self-report depression scale for research in the general population. Applied Psychological Measurement 1:385–401, 1977

Reynolds SK, Clark LA: Predicting dimensions of personality disorder from domains and facets of the Five-Factor Model. J Pers 69:199–222, 2001

Regier DA, Farmer ME, Rae DS, et al: One-month prevalence of mental disorders in the United States and sociodemographic characteristics: the Epidemiologic Catchment Area study. Acta Psychiatr Scand 88:35–47, 1993

Roberts SB, Kendler KS: Neuroticism and self-esteem as indices of the vulnerability to major depression in women. Psychol Med 29:1101–1109, 1999

Santor DA, Bagby RM, Joffe RT: Evaluating stability and change in personality and depression. J Pers Soc Psychol 73:1354–1362, 1997

Sato T, Hirano S, Narita T, et al: Temperament and character inventory dimensions as a predictor of response to antidepressant treatment in major depression. J Affect Disord 56:153–161, 1999

Sauer H, Richter P, Czernik A, et al: Personality differences between patients with major depression and bipolar disorder: the impact of minor symptoms on self-ratings of personality. J Affect Disord 42:169–177, 1997

Schalling D, Asberg M, Edman G, et al: Markers for vulnerability to psychopathology: temperament traits associated with platelet MAO activity. Acta Psychiatr Scand 76:172–182, 1987

Sirey JA, Bruce ML, Alexopoulos GS, et al: Perceived stigma as a predictor of treatment discontinuation in young and older outpatients with depression. Am J Psychiatry 158:479–481, 2001

Sloman L, Gilbert P, Hasey G: Evolved mechanisms in depression: the role and interaction of attachment and social rank in depression. J Affect Disord 74:107–121, 2003

Stein MB, Hackerman FR: The use of the MMPI-2 in conjunction with the NEO-Personality Inventory. Psychol Rep 69:955–958, 1991

Strakowski SM, Faedda GL, Tohen M, et al: Possible affective-state dependence of the tridimensional personality questionnaire in first-episode psychosis. Psychiatry Res 42:93–99, 1992

Strakowski SM, Dunayevich E, Keck PE, et al: Affective state dependence of the tridimensional personality questionnaire. Psychiatry Res 57:209–214, 1995

Strakowski SM, McElroy SL, Keck PE, et al: Racial influence on diagnosis in psychotic mania. J Affect Disord 39:157–162, 1996

Thase ME, Howland RH: Biological processes in depression: an updated review and integration, in Handbook of Depression, 2nd Edition. Edited by Beckham EE, Leber WR. New York, Guilford, 1995, pp 213–279

Trull TJ, Useda D, Costa PT, et al: Comparison of the MMPI-2 Personality Psychopathology Five (PSY-5) and the NEO-PI(-R). Psychol Assess 7:508–516, 1995

Van Praag HM: The diagnosis of depression in disorder. Aust N Z J Psychiatry 32:767–772, 1998

Ward E, King M, Lloyd M, et al: Randomised controlled trial of non-directive counselling, cognitive-behaviour therapy, and usual general practitioner care for patients with depression, I: clinical effectiveness. Br Med J 321:1383–1388, 2000

Watson D, Clark LA, Carey G: Positive and negative affectivity and their relation to anxiety and depressive disorders. J Abnorm Psychol 97:346–353, 1988

Westen D, Arkowitz-Westen L: Limitations of axis II in diagnosing personality pathology in clinical practice. Am J Psychiatry 155:1767–1771, 1998

Weissman MM, Bland RC, Canino GJ, et al: Cross-national epidemiology of major depression and bipolar disorder. JAMA 276:293–299, 1996

Widiger TA: Personality disorder and Axis I psychopathology: the problematic boundary of Axis I and Axis II. J Personal Disord 17:90–108, 2003

Widiger TA, Frances AJ: Toward a dimensional model for the personality disorders, in Personality Disorders and the Five-Factor Model of Personality, 2nd Edition. Edited by Costa PR Jr, Widiger TA. Washington DC, American Psychological Association, 2002, pp 23–44

Widiger TA, Trull TJ: Personality and psychopathology: an application of the five-factor model. J Pers 60:363–393, 1992

Wingerson D, Sullivan M, Dager S, et al: Personality traits and early discontinuation from clinical trials in anxious patients. J Clin Psychopharmacol 13:194–197, 1993

Young LT, Bagby RM, Cooke RG, et al: A comparison of Tridimensional Personality Questionnaire dimensions in bipolar disorder and unipolar depression. Psychiatry Res 58:139–143, 1995

CHAPTER 6

CLINICAL STRATEGIES FOR EFFICIENT TREATMENT OF MAJOR DEPRESSIVE DISORDER COMPLICATED BY PERSONALITY DISORDER

Ari Zaretsky, M.D.

Michael Rosenbluth, M.D.

Daniel Silver, M.D.

Although mood disorders with comorbid personality disorder have been traditionally associated with a poorer prognosis, recent research suggests that such therapeutic nihilism is not warranted. In this chapter, we describe a detailed case of mixed personality disorder (DSM-IV-TR personality disorder not otherwise specified [NOS] [American Psychiatric Association 2000]) in order to highlight a multimodal, phased treatment approach that involves targeted pharmacotherapy and integrative individual psychotherapy. The focus of this chapter is mixed personality disorder, which tends to be much more common in both clinical practice and research than one specific personality disorder in isolation. Working with an actual case of a subject with major depression with comorbid mixed personality disorder will facilitate a review of the issues related to diagnostic assessment, formulation, and treatment.

Case of Mixed Personality Disorder and Major Depression

History of Present Illness

Ms. C is a 30-year-old single woman who was referred for outpatient treatment for depression 5 days after coming to the emergency room and reporting an intense urge to cut her wrists with razor blades, an urge that both disturbed and frightened her. She had cut herself on three previous occasions in her life, but the last time had been 5 years ago. It became clear after taking a detailed history that Ms. C had had major depression for the last month, with symptoms of sadness, tearfulness, low energy, hypersomnia, muscle fatigue, binge eating, poor concentration, poor motivation, social withdrawal, self-criticism, hopelessness, and passive suicidal ideation.

Past Psychiatric History

Ms. C described chronic low-grade depression since her early teens, with frequent exacerbations approximately once a year that met full criteria for a major depressive episode that typically lasted 3–6 months. She had been treated with an array of antidepressant medications over the last decade, which included paroxetine, bupropion, desipramine, and tranylcypromine. Ms. C usually responded to these medications but relapsed during maintenance treatment. It was not clear whether some of these relapses were precipitated by medication nonadherence. Since her teens, she had been in and out of therapy with both male and female therapists. These treatments often began with the patient developing an intense emotional attachment and erotic feelings toward the therapist. Unfortunately, Ms. C typically terminated treatment prematurely (after 3–6 months) when she either feared that she was frustrating her therapist by not making progress or feared she was developing an intense attachment to the therapist and "becoming too dependent."

Psychiatric Functional Inquiry

Ms. C denied any manic or psychotic symptoms but did describe an intense suspiciousness of people, who she feared were judging her negatively. She had also felt unreal and disconnected from her body during two previous depressive episodes. Ms. C admitted that during her depressive exacerbations she tended to binge drink, which was often associated with promiscuous sexual behavior. She also drank excessively to cope with social anxiety when she was at parties or social gatherings. Ms. C binged on food episodically and had been bulimic for 2 years in her early 20s. Although her purging behavior has abated, she has continued to binge eat, particularly before her menstrual period.

It was initially unclear whether Ms. C's behavior was truly caused by a personality disturbance. However, more detailed information gathering, which included interviewing her mother in a second session, revealed problems since young adulthood that were largely independent of her major depressive episodes. Ms. C manifested an enduring and pervasive pattern of low self-esteem and affective instability with marked mood reactivity and chronic feelings of emptiness and boredom, as well as problems tolerating frustration associated with impulsive binging on food, sexual promiscuity, and drug and alcohol abuse. In addition, her history revealed long-standing rejection sensitivity and a fear that she would be abandoned if she revealed her true self to others. She typically avoided intimate relationships with other people and was inhibited in social situations because of her profound fear of shame and ridicule. On a few isolated occasions Ms. C had engaged in superficial cutting after she experienced rejection. In the past, she had developed very intense, dependent relationships with men who were often exploitive and controlling in the hope that they would "rescue" her or take care of her. Sometimes Ms. C experienced intense anxiety if she had to be alone, and often she would look to her family and few friends to make her decisions for fear that she would make the wrong choice.

Diagnostic Assessment

Unlike more homogeneous Axis I patients who are the subjects of clinical drug trials (Davidson et al. 2001; Mundo et al. 2000; Zimmerman et al. 2002), this particular patient is quite typical of the more complex patients that psychiatrists see in general practice. Ms. C has a chronic mood disorder but also appears to exhibit a chronic, enduring pattern of feeling, thinking, and behaving that is dysfunctional and associated with distress.

When working with a patient who has both a personality disorder and major depressive disorder, it is important to be clear conceptually and clinically about the relationship between these two entities. From a conceptual perspective there has been considerable research trying to elucidate this relationship. The theories can be summarized by considering three major hypotheses: that 1) certain personality features predispose a person to major depression; 2) personality modifies major depression; and 3) personality disturbances are a complication of or are simply an attenuated expression of major depression (Akiskal et al. 1983).

It has been suggested that certain traits such as obsessionality, dependency, neuroticism, and interpersonal sensitivity are more associated with depression. Boyce and Mason (1996) and Skodol and colleagues (1999) have suggested that certain personality disorders such as borderline and avoidant dependent personality disorders are more associated with depression. Zimmerman (Zimmerman and Mattia 1999) has indicated that patients with borderline personality disorders are more likely than those without such personality disorders to have multiple Axis I diagnoses. Fava and colleagues (1996) suggested that early-onset depression has more associated personality disorders than late-onset depression. Ilardi and Craighead (1995) reported that 35%–65% of patients with major depression have comorbid personality disorders. Pepper and colleagues (1995) have suggested that patients with early-onset dysthymia have more personality disorders and episodic depression.

Another approach to examining the relationship between personality disorders and depression has been to explore whether personality disorders are state dependent. Mullen and colleagues (1999) have noted that the treatment of major depression results in an improvement in maladaptive defenses. Hirschfeld and colleagues (1998) have suggested the treatment of major depression results in improvement in personality disorder, and Fava and colleagues (2002) have described a significant reduction in the proportion of comorbid personality disorders in unipolar depressed patients after only 8 weeks of fluoxetine treatment.

Fifty percent of patients with dysthymic disorder have comorbid personality disorders (Keller et al. 2000). Hirschfeld (1998) has suggested that comorbid borderline personality disorder predicts a decrease in likelihood of response to treatment in patients who have chronic depression. Thus, there are interesting conceptual issues with regard to borderline personality disorder and affective disorder.

Implications for Ms. C

The clinical implication for our work with this patient is to clarify in the assessment phase whether 1) the patient is experiencing major depression only or 2) experiencing major depression that is amplifying personality traits in an individual who when not depressed does not have a personality disorder, or 3) whether there is coexistent personality disorder and depression. Ways of clarifying this question are to get a collateral history so that a history of long-standing interepisode personality function can be clarified. When the longitudinal history is suggestive but not conclusive for personality disorder, it is important to reserve final judgment regarding the presence of a personality disorder until after the major depressive disorder has been robustly treated. Once treated, if the personality features remain, then it suggests that there is a personality disorder that exists in addition to the Axis I disorder.

Finally, it is important to recognize that from a pragmatic therapeutic perspective, diagnostic precision and delineation of which behaviors constitute Axis I versus Axis II disorders is very often not critical. Clinically, patients with chronic depression whose dysfunctional pattern of thinking, feeling, and behaving was acquired secondary to refractory affective illness will require the same types of treatment interventions as those patients whose recurrent and chronic affective illness developed in tandem or as a consequence of dysfunctional personality traits.

Borderline Personality Disorder and the Bipolar Spectrum

When dealing with borderline personality symptomatology in particular, it is important to carefully consider the possibility of a bipolar diathesis or a bipolar spectrum disorder (Benazzi 2002; Benazzi and Akiskal 2003; Ghaemi et al. 2002) because this recently proposed diagnostic entity may not only provide a more parsimonious explanation of the patient's symptoms but also has implications for pharmacotherapy. It should also be noted that it is not uncommon for patients with bipolar disorder to have comorbid personality disorders (MacQueen and Young 2001; Vieta et al. 2000). In Ms. C's case, there were a number of features consistent with a bipolar spectrum disorder. Ms. C experienced her first depressive episode prior to age 25 years, had recurrent depression, displayed atypical depressive features, and had a history of suboptimal response to antidepressant medication. Her interpersonal sensitivity and demanding behavior are features that Akiskal and colleagues (1995) described as characteristic of depressed individuals who later convert into bipolar II presentations. Ms. C's sister actually had been diagnosed with bipolar II disorder. Ms. C had no history of antidepressant-induced rapid cycling or hypomania, spontaneous mania or hypomania, seasonal affective disorder, or postpartum depression. Although Ms. C's affective illness is clearly encompassed by DSM-IV-TR unipolar depression, Ghaemi and colleagues (2002) have suggested that such patients have more diagnostic features in common with bipolar disorder than unipolar depression and have suggested the term *bipolar spectrum disorder* for this group. Ms. C's bipolar spectrum diagnosis will be revisited in the context of discussing her pharmacotherapy.

From a DSM-IV-TR diagnostic perspective, it is valid to conclude that Ms. C has a mixed personality disorder that is comorbid with her chronic unipolar affective illness (recurrent major depression superimposed on dysthymic disorder). Additional Axis I conditions that should be identified are binge-eating disorder and alcohol abuse. From a DSM-IV-TR perspective, she would meet criteria for borderline personality disorder, but in addition to the patient's classic borderline symptoms (e.g., affective instability, chronic emptiness, impulsive self-destructive behavior, self-harm through mutilation, micropsychotic episodes), it is also clinically relevant to recognize that she has some dependent and avoidant personality features.

Beginning Treatment: Empirical Evidence for Cautious Therapeutic Optimism

Although depressed patients with comorbid personality disorders often have been viewed as having a much worse prognosis, recent outcome research suggests that far more optimism is warranted. In a recent review of the literature on unipolar depression complicated by Axis II pathology, Mulder (2002) concluded that Axis II pathology did not worsen the treatment outcome of major depressive disorder if optimal medication and psychotherapy were used. This contradicts conventional wisdom that Axis II comorbidity negatively affects depression treatment. Other studies suggest that personality disorders respond to psychotherapy and improve over time. In a recent meta-analysis of seven published psychotherapy studies, Perry and colleagues (1999) found that 50% of patients with Axis II disorders lost their diagnosis within 93 sessions, and psychotherapy accelerated remission in personality disorders sevenfold. In a recent 6-year naturalistic follow-up of 290 relatively young inpatients with borderline personality disorder treated with intensive psychotherapy and medication, it was found that although 70% continued to experience depression, anger, boredom, and loneliness, only 30% experienced persistent quasipsychotic thoughts, substance use, self-mutilation, and manipulative suicidal behavior (Zanarini et al. 2003).

Our psychotherapy treatment approach is also informed by recent outcome research. Although only 25 studies were included in a recent meta-analysis of contemporary higher quality research studies conducted on psychotherapy for patients with personality disorders, the general conclusion was that psychodynamic and cognitive-behavioral therapy (CBT) were quite comparable in their effectiveness, with moderate overall effect sizes ranging between 1.00 and 1.50 for both modalities (Leichsenring and Leibing 2003). Two randomized controlled trials of psychodynamic therapy (Bateman and Fonagy 1999; Winston et al. 1994) and three randomized controlled trials of CBT demonstrated superiority over the control treatment (Alden 1989; Linehan et al. 1994, 1999).

General Principles of Treatment for Depression Complicated by Axis II Pathology

In treating patients with depression complicated by Axis II pathology, we suggest a strategic, staged, multimodal approach. By *strategic* we mean "working smart" rather than just "working hard." The clinician should view him- or herself as a "tactician of change," deliberately applying treatment interventions that will yield the greatest therapeutic outcome for the effort involved. *Staged* refers to the concept of therapy unfolding in distinct phases and the clinician attempting to move the patient sequentially to higher developmental levels. Although a discussion of developmental considerations in psychotherapy is beyond the purview of this chapter, this concept has been previously addressed by other authors (Greenspan and Benderly 1998; McCullough 2000). McCullough, for example, describes his Cognitive Behavioral Analysis System of Psychotherapy (CBASP) treatment for chronic depression as a psychological intervention that specifically remediates the chronically depressed person's developmental arrest at the Piagetian preoperational stage and gradually moves the person to acquire the skills to address interpersonal problems at the Piagetian stage of formal operations (McCullough 2000). Therapy for patients with Axis II disorders should therefore be developmentally informed. Finally, optimal treatment of depressed patients with Axis II comorbidity requires many different modalities that extend beyond pharmacotherapy and individual psychotherapy. Many patients require group therapy, family psychoeducation/therapy, and occupational therapy. Ms. C's treatment unfolded in the following manner:

Stage I: Thorough Assessment Including Self-Report Instruments

Before initiating treatment, the clinician gathered sufficient information not only to arrive at a DSM-IV diagnosis but also to understand Ms. C's personality in order to generate a tentative formulation. We generally suggest up to two and not more than three sessions for assessment. At the beginning of the assessment, it is critical to provide the patient with realistic and accurate expectations about the assessment process and to take special care to ensure that the patient does not conclude that the clinician performing the assessment will be providing the treatment if this is not the case. Patients with personality disorders have particular difficulties with trust, boundaries, and frustration tolerance, and these vulnerabilities must be considered during the assessment procedure. We suggest that the clinician not explore painful details of sexual or physical trauma, especially if he or she will not be providing the subsequent treatment. Although initial assessments should evaluate trauma histories cautiously, we do suggest that the clinician routinely ask pointed questions about the impact of particular life events and relationships on the patient's view of him- or herself and the world. This information provides a context that helps the clinician understand the patient's latent pathogenic beliefs, which will ultimately become the major target of therapy. What follows is a sample of an early session:

Psychiatrist: How did your relationship with your father and mother affect the way you feel about yourself as a person and see the world?

Ms. C: I don't think it was very positive. My dad was very busy looking after my older sister. She is manic-depressive and had serious problems in her early teens. He never really spent any time with me, and whenever he did, he was very frustrated and critical. He would tell me I was stupid when I made mistakes. He yelled a lot at my mother and could be very controlling with money. He used to hit me whenever I got angry. I think I actually hated him when I was a kid.

Psychiatrist: What kind of beliefs about yourself or the world do you think developed from your relationship with your dad?

Ms. C: I don't know...I guess I'm not very worthwhile and that I can't really depend on myself to make the right decisions. I also think that I learned to distrust people and felt that people close to you can really hurt you.

Psychiatrist: What about your mother? How has she influenced you in terms of how you feel about yourself as a woman and how you see the world?

Ms. C: My mom spent a lot of time with my brother because he had a learning disability and she was a teacher. She never stood up to my father when he yelled at her. She just took it. I never wanted to be like her in relationships, but I think I pretty much follow in her footsteps. I never think it's safe to express what I really want from someone else, and I just get angry and resentful until I totally lose it. My mom also would get really frustrated with me for being so emotional. She would always tell me that I was way too sensitive and that I should just "get over it" whenever I was upset. I never learned how to deal with my feelings, and even today when I get upset about something, I feel out of control and ashamed at the same time that I'm getting so upset.

The patient should be asked not only about past relationships/ events, but in order to generate an accurate and comprehensive case formulation the clinician should also try to assess carefully how the patient interprets two or three discrete situations/events that are intimately associated with the current depressive episode. The patient's thoughts about these situations should be delineated after first assessing the patient's emotional reaction to the event:

Psychiatrist: You described how the depression started a month ago in the context of accidentally getting pregnant and then having an abortion. Can you describe how this all happened?

Ms. C: I met a guy at a bar and I ended up sleeping with him. It was just a one-night stand, but I ended up pregnant.

Psychiatrist: I see. This may be hard to talk about, but I want to understand how it was that you got pregnant. Did you forget to use birth control? I ask this question not to criticize you in any way but simply to try to understand your experience. My hunch is that it may have been hard for you to speak up for what you wanted.

Ms. C: No, I didn't actually forget to use birth control. You're right. I just didn't feel I could say no when this guy said he didn't want to use condoms.

Psychiatrist: Can you describe that situation more fully to me? Try to slow it down like a film happening in slow motion. I want to understand what you were feeling and thinking just at that second.

Ms. C: The guy that I met at the bar is over at my apartment, and we're starting to have sex. I ask him to use a condom, and he says that he doesn't want to and that I don't need to worry about diseases.

Psychiatrist: And what were you feeling at that moment?

Ms. C: I felt kind of anxious.

Psychiatrist: Anything else?

Ms. C: Well, come to think about it, I think I was probably angry too.

Psychiatrist: What do you think was going through your mind just at that second when you felt anxious and angry?

Ms. C: I was thinking: "If I say no, he'll leave and I'll be all alone tonight." I think I must have also been thinking: "You selfish bastard, you guys are all the same, you just want one thing!"

Psychiatrist: So it sounds like it was a really difficult situation for you. Here you were thinking that if you stood up for yourself, he would abandon you. It also sounds like you were angry at him because he confirmed some of your worse fears about men. Is that right?

Ms. C: Yes, exactly.

The Role of Rating Scales in Therapy

Part of the assessment process includes self-report instruments. In our clinic, we have found that a number of simple, brief, clinically oriented self-report instruments can provide additional information that helps to guide therapy and measure the impact of treatment. The Beck Depression Inventory II (BDI-II) (A. Beck et al. 1996) provides a simple measure of depressive symptomatology, including atypical symptoms, and is more sensitive than the clinician-administered Hamilton Depression Rating Scale (Hamilton 1960) in terms of detecting the psychological symptoms of depression. We find it very useful to ask our Axis II patients who have had a partial response to antidepressant treatment to identify the residual symptoms that still need to be addressed with psychotherapy by examining the items that they continue to endorse on the

BDI-II. The Beck Anxiety Inventory (BAI) (A. Beck et al. 1988) is a simple, self-report measure of anxiety symptoms, although it is most sensitive for panic/physiological arousal. The Beck Hopelessness Inventory (A. Beck et al. 1989), which is derived from a 20-item self-report, true or false questionnaire, may not change for some time, even if the patient's depressive symptoms improve. The Dysfunctional Attitudes Scale (DAS) (Weissman and Beck 1978) is a 40-item self-report inventory that measures depressogenic beliefs, which are thought to confer cognitive vulnerability to relapse.

Stage II: Generation of a Tentative Case Formulation Using the Cognitive Model

Before beginning treatment, Ms. C's psychiatrist generated a tentative case formulation. Although this formulation borrowed heavily from Linehan (1993) as well as Young (Young et al. 2003), McCullough (2000), and object relations and self-psychology psychodynamic theory (Hingley 2001; Kernberg et al. 1989; Shaver and Mikulincer 2002), it was based primarily on A. Beck's model of personality psychopathology (A. Beck et al. 1990, 2004), which is shown in Figure 6–1. Many psychological models exist and offer distinct though often converging perspectives on the etiology of personality disorder. For pragmatic reasons J. Beck's (1995) cognitive case conceptualization diagram is used because in our experience it demystifies complex behavior and can be readily shared and understood by patients. The treating psychiatrist, in collaboration with Ms. C, was able to generate the cognitive case conceptualization and show her the entire diagram after only 10 therapy sessions. Ms. C's case conceptualization is represented in Tables 6–1 through 6–4. J. Beck's formulation is concise, clear, simple, relatively comprehensive, and has the distinct advantage of being able to delineate clearly the fluid interrelationship between Axis I and Axis II disorders. At the bottom of the diagram in Figure 6–1, the basic cognitive model is illustrated by the triangles, which correspond to specific situations. In each triangle, thoughts, feelings, and behavior are depicted as interrelated and interacting. Situation-specific automatic thoughts are derivatives of deeper, more pervasive and enduring cognitive structures called *schemas*. Schemas are emotionally laden associative networks of meaning that actively guide an individual's information processing and construal of current events in the present. Schemas usually are formed early on in life but are modified and refined by later life events that either contradict or reinforce the original schema (Young et al. 2003).

TABLE 6–1. Ms. C's relevant life history

- Middle child
- Depressed mother
- Father rigid, controlling, sadistic
- Sister developed bipolar illness in her teens
- Adopted brother learning disabled
- Multiple moves as a child
- Very shy, anxious by temperament but prone to tantrums
- Beaten by father and berated for being emotional by mother
- Adolescent depression/cutting
- Sexual promiscuity/use of alcohol
- Academic underachievement
- Involvement with "losers"

TABLE 6–2. Ms. C's core beliefs

Negative core beliefs about self	Negative core beliefs about the world
• I am unlovable • I am worthless • I am invisible • I am a failure • I am helpless	• The world is cruel • People are abusive • People are uncaring • People cannot be trusted • People don't care about my feelings

---

TABLE 6–3. Ms. C's conditional assumptions

- If I don't get close to people, I won't be rejected
- If I do get close to someone, I will be rescued but ultimately abandoned
- If I don't try, I won't really fail
- If I depend on strong people, I will be rescued
- If I use alcohol, I can relax with people and not feel so awkward
- If I have sex with men, they will give me attention and stick around
- If I eat normally, I will get fat and will be rejected
- If I break my diet, I might as well "pig out"
- If I feel negative feelings, it will be intolerable
- If I use alcohol/food/sex, I can avoid negative feelings
- If I cut myself, I will be able to control my emotions
- If I go out with "losers," I won't be really hurt
- If I express my needs, I will be disappointed or rejected

TABLE 6–4. Ms. C's compensatory strategies

- Cognitive avoidance
- Mistrust
- Social avoidance
- Alcohol abuse
- Binge eating
- Self-mutilation
- Sexual promiscuity (when younger)
- Attraction to strong men
- Task procrastination/avoidance
- Self-handicapping
- Self-presentation as incompetent
- Submissiveness/unassertiveness

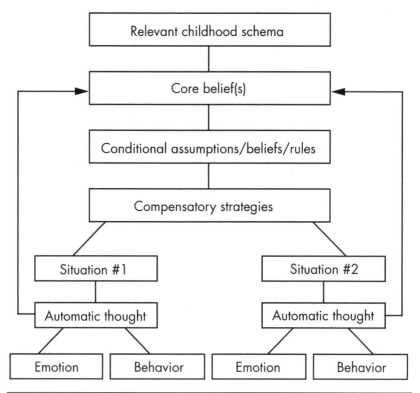

FIGURE 6–1. Cognitive conceptualization diagram.

Source. Adapted with permission from Judith S. Beck, Ph.D.: *Cognitive Therapy: Basics and Beyond.* New York, Guilford, © 1995.

A. Beck and Young's conceptualization of personality pathology (A. Beck et al. 1990; Young et al. 2003) helps to explain why personality disorders are refractory to change and why longer term treatment is indicated. Essentially, two phases of treatment have to proceed. The first phase corresponds to weakening the negative schemas of the patient. However, this process alone is insufficient. In the second phase, there must also be a nurturing and development of positive schemas about the self and the world, which may never have existed up until the present time.

Core beliefs are closely related to the concept of a schema. *Schema* refers to a broader concept and encompasses not only verbal statements, but also specific memories, emotions, and physical sensations. Ms. C's helplessness schema encompasses early memories of watching her sister going for chemotherapy, being disciplined physically by her father for not being able to control her temper, being shunned by her mother for days, feeling too depressed and apathetic to study in high school and then failing tests, and many painful memories of not being able to assert herself when she was dating emotionally and sexually exploitive men. Associated with these memories are feelings of anxiety and exhaustion as well as an intense sensation of heaviness in her limbs. The cognitive content of a schema is a core belief. Core beliefs should ideally be expressed in the patient's own words because these words will evoke more affect and resonate more emotionally. Ms. C's core belief that expresses her helplessness schema in words is, "I am powerless. I can't look after myself."

In the cognitive case conceptualization, intermediate beliefs about the self and world are expressed as conditional assumptions. Conditional assumptions are essentially two related "if..." rules for living that, although not overtly expressed, are easily accessible when the pattern of the patient's reactions to situations is monitored over time. Conditional assumptions compensate for the patient's negative core beliefs and allow the patient to cope with the world with less emotional distress despite having these negative beliefs. Ms. C's conditional assumption that derives directly from her core belief, "I can't look after myself," can be expressed as, "If I rely on myself to make decisions and assert my needs and try to look after myself, I won't survive." The related corollary can be expressed as, "If I depend on strong people, I will be rescued and looked after." The value of having the patient articulate his or her conditional assumptions is that they can be deliberately tested and evaluated throughout the course of therapy. This deliberate testing efficiently creates corrective emotional experiences that serve to modify the patient's dysfunctional belief system.

In addition to conditional assumptions, compensatory strategies are also delineated in the cognitive conceptualization diagram. These strategies represent the behavioral enactments of the patient's conditional assumptions and are pervasive across time and context. They are akin to the psychodynamic concept of defense mechanism and are often not completely conscious. Ms. C's compensatory strategies (see Table 6–4) that are derived from her core belief, "I can't look after myself," are avoidance of challenging tasks that require physical or mental exertion or effort, attraction to strong characters (particularly men), submissiveness in relationships with men, interpersonal self-presentation as incompetent, and self-handicapping manifested by retreating to her bed whenever she perceives any expectation to function well or cope independently.

A. Beck's case conceptualization provides a useful way of understanding the relationship between Axis I and Axis II disorders. According to the cognitive model of personality disorders (A. Beck et al. 1990, 2004), Axis I and Axis II disorders are not different categories as they appear to be in DSM-IV-TR but merely differ in their degree of schema activation. For example, a previously high-functioning adult who experiences a first episode of depression after a major career setback will likely experience an activation of a failure schema. However, this schema usually can be deactivated by basic cognitive-behavioral interventions or antidepressants. Treatment of such patients is usually straightforward and uncomplicated, and leads to deactivation of the patient's failure schema and reactivation of the patient's competence schema. Patients with Axis II conditions are different because *even when they are not severely depressed*, they still experience high activation of negative schema. These schemas serve to constantly filter and distort information processing such that all positive experiences are ignored or minimized and all neutral or negative experiences are magnified and attended to. Patients with Axis II disorders, therefore, have difficulty processing positive information or corrective emotional experiences because they lack any countervailing positive schema. This conceptualization of the Axis I/II relationship provides practical psychotherapy and medication intervention opportunities.

According to Young (Young et al. 2003), patients with Axis II disorders are impervious to change because of three processes: schema maintenance, schema avoidance, and schema compensation. *Schema maintenance* refers to the phenomenon whereby information is filtered in a manner such that only congruent negative experiences are attended to and remembered. Positive experiences that have the potential to contradict the original negative schema are ignored or minimized. Schema maintenance helps to explain the many cognitive distortions that are typically seen in patients with Axis II disorders. *Schema avoidance* refers to the phenomenon in which a patient will avoid thinking about something painful (cognitive avoidance), avoid feeling certain emotions (emotional avoidance), or avoid engaging in specific behaviors (behavioral avoidance).

Schema avoidance is a useful concept that helps to explain the deficits in affect recognition, affect intolerance, and skill deficits that are often seen in patients with Axis II disorders. Individuals who chronically avoid painful emotions by dysfunctional behavior (e.g., using drugs or engaging in high-risk behaviors) eventually lose the capacity to recognize and discriminate between emotional states. In addition, their chronic avoidance insulates them from corrective emotional experiences and leads to "disuse atrophy" of adaptive coping skills. Instead of coping with stress by drawing on a broad array of strategies, individuals with personality disorders have a rigid and restricted repertoire of compensatory strategies, which they overuse. One of the therapeutic goals with Axis II patients is to increase their repertoire of compensatory strategies and teach them to become more flexible rather than rigid in their response to stress.

Schema compensation refers to the phenomenon whereby individuals try to overcompensate for their negative views of themselves and the world. A patient with narcissistic personality traits may truly view him- or herself as inadequate but overcompensates for this painful core belief by trying to view and present him- or herself as better than others, which may also be associated with entitled behavior. In the end, however, the narcissistic individual's behavior inevitably leads to negative feedback from others, which paradoxically reinforces the original negative view of the self as inadequate.

Stage III: Socialize the Patient to the Structure of Treatment and Proactively Address Therapy-Interfering Behaviors

Ms. C's psychiatrist began by explaining how the treatment would unfold and the nature of the therapy sessions. In our experience, contracting to work together for approximately 16–20 sessions and then formally reevaluating the treatment is a worthwhile strategy. Many patients with depression associated with comorbid Axis II pathology will actually require a much longer active treatment, often lasting years. However, in today's cost-containment climate, treatment efficacy should be evaluated and carefully scrutinized. Even for patients with severe Axis II pathology, more treatment is not necessarily better. In our experience, it is advisable for the psychiatrist to discuss directly with the patient the progress of treatment after approximately three sessions. At this time, there is no real expectation that the patient's symptoms will have remitted; however, there should be some mutual sense that the treatment holds promise, based on a number of factors such as the patient's attendance, medication adherence, adherence with therapy tasks, and the quality of the therapeutic alliance.

In Ms. C's case, her psychiatrist devoted extra time anticipating how her beliefs and behaviors might inadvertently interfere with treatment. Proactively addressing therapy-interfering behavior and negative transference reactions is in keeping with Linehan's Dialectical Behavior Therapy (DBT) for borderline personality disorder (Linehan 1993) and McCullough's CBASP for chronic depression (McCullough 2000). Although Linehan's DBT was specifically developed to treat parasuicidal borderline personality disorder (Linehan et al. 1991, 1993) this highly influential, evidence-based treatment model has recently been expanded to treat other related conditions that share a propensity for affect dysregulation (Linehan et al. 1999; van den Bosch 1999). We find Linehan's biosocial model of a reciprocal interaction between a stressful invalidating environment and a diathesis toward affect dysregulation to be highly relevant in treating many depressed patients with Axis II comorbidity even if they are not strictly borderline. The term *affect dysregulation* reflects and distills a number of older psychodynamic concepts (e.g., Adler 1985; Kernberg et al. 1989; Masterson 1981), but this construct has the advantage of being more readily comprehended by the patient and is therefore more clinically useful. In the following dialog, Ms. C's psychiatrist devotes a lot of time to contract with her and anticipate treatment difficulties:

> Psychiatrist: Before we really begin treatment, I think it would be good for us to talk about what you should expect from me and what I should expect from you and how this will all unfold over time.
>
> Ms. C: Okay.
>
> Psychiatrist: I see your problems as related to difficulties in how you feel, difficulties in how you think, and difficulties in how you act, especially when under stress. Does this make sense to you?
>
> Ms. C: Yes. Sort of.
>
> Psychiatrist: Let's actually go over a recent situation that turned out badly for you, or a situation where you felt negative feelings, to illustrate this idea more clearly to you.

Ms. C's psychiatrist then illustrated the cognitive model by delving into a recent event associated with an interpersonal dispute. The psychiatrist helped her to see how in this specific problematic situation, her feelings were intimately connected with her thoughts and behaviors:

Psychiatrist: The goal of treatment will be to change your negative thoughts, feelings, and behaviors. I see you looking down as I speak, and I wonder if you are skeptical. What's going through your mind right now?

Ms. C: I've been this way my whole life. To be quite honest, I just don't think I can really change.

Psychiatrist: I understand that you are skeptical. You have a right to be, given your past experiences. What I want you to know right now are a few things. First, skepticism can be a good thing because it tells me that you don't take what anyone says at face value. It means you analyze things. I'm hoping that we can actually turn your innate skepticism on your negative thinking. Even though you are skeptical about this working, I would like you to try things that might make you feel better. For this treatment to work, you will need to suspend your disbelief long enough to actually try things that you haven't been doing up until now. After you try these different things for a set period of time, like 6 weeks, you can then evaluate whether they actually make some difference in terms of how you feel and decide if you want to continue. What reactions do you have to what I am saying?

Ms. C: I'm willing to try for 6 weeks and then see what happens.

Psychiatrist: Great. To change your negative thinking, feeling, and behavior, we're going to use a number of different things, and I think that over time these different things together will win the day. The goal of this treatment is not to cure you so that you never experience problems but to teach you how to become your own therapist. This treatment will require a commitment from you to work on your problems almost every day. Are you open to this?

Ms. C: I guess so. How much time will it take?

Psychiatrist: Not a long time. Do you think you could spend 15 to 20 minutes 4 or 5 days a week?

Ms. C's psychiatrist then addressed policies about confidentiality, missed appointments, and availability during crises. Special emphasis was placed on how to deal with suicidal behavior and any other therapy-interfering behavior:

Psychiatrist: One of the things that we might have to face during treatment is you feeling you want to kill yourself or harm yourself through mutilation. I would like to make one of our goals to be that we try to teach you alternative ways of handling your feelings so that you don't have to resort to this way of coping. How do you feel about what I'm suggesting?

Ms. C: I understand what you're saying, but I don't think that I can make a promise like that right now. Sometimes cutting myself comforts me. I don't think I want to give that up.

Psychiatrist: I understand your concern about what I'm asking. Sometimes when you're in a lot of emotional pain, fantasizing about suicide can actually comfort you because you know that you are not trapped forever. You know that if things get really bad and don't change, you ultimately have an "out." I don't ever want to take that away from you. What I do want you to think about very carefully is what exactly we're trying to do together in this treatment and how your cutting yourself or drinking will impact on those goals. I said earlier that what I want you to learn is to be your own therapist. What that means is that you will be able to talk to yourself and comfort yourself when you are feeling upset and overwhelmed. When you cut yourself or when you abuse alcohol or drugs, you are either trying to make yourself numb or to make yourself feel something because you are feeling numb. Does what I am saying resonate with you?

Ms. C: Yes, exactly.

Psychiatrist: Well, here's the problem. Even though the drinking and cutting works in the short term, it will prevent you from learning a different set of skills to regulate your emotions. So what we're trying to accomplish through this treatment, and the cutting and drinking, are actually working at cross purposes. They're canceling each other out. It's like driving with your foot on the gas pedal and the brake at the same time. What are your reactions to what I'm saying?

Through negotiation, Ms. C and her psychiatrist arrived at an agreement about how they will deal with her suicidal thoughts and urges, as well as her urges to harm herself and to drink and use drugs. They agreed that the first priority was safety and preventing Ms. C from doing something impulsive that she would later regret. They also agreed that in order for Ms. C to ultimately benefit from therapy and create what Linehan has referred to as "a life worth living," she needed to be alive (Linehan et al. 2001). As described by Linehan, certain behaviors would be labeled as "therapy-interfering behaviors," including missed appointments, self-mutilation, alcohol and drug use, and misusing prescribed medication or missing medication doses (Linehan et al. 2001). In Ms. C's case, her alcohol and drug use was not so severe that special treatment was required. In other cases, however, in which the substance abuse is severe and pervasive, it is advisable to place special emphasis on curtailing or eliminating the abuse through specialized treatment before actively addressing the patient's depressive disorder.

In addition to discussing overtly destructive behavior, Ms. C's psychiatrist also tried proactively to anticipate other more subtle interpersonal difficulties that could insidiously threaten the therapy and lead to premature termination. Reviewing the patient's past therapeutic experiences provides useful information about characteristic patterns and possible future challenges. In addition, the therapeutic alliance is enhanced by engaging the patient as a partner in reviewing what treatment worked or did not work in the past, what was learned from these experiences, and what the implications for the current treatment might be:

> Psychiatrist: Before we talk about medication options to help you with your depression, I'd like us to think about other problems that could develop during therapy. I'm aware of the fact that you have been in treatment before and that it often ended badly for you with you leaving the psychiatrist prematurely. What kind of problems do you think could interfere with this current treatment working?
>
> Ms. C: Well, I don't trust people very much.
>
> Psychiatrist: Anything else? Let's make a detailed list of all the negative scenarios that could arise between us so that we can then try to plan how we will deal with them right now.

In the ensuing frank discussion, Ms. C's psychiatrist gently explored how she tended to become emotionally attached to her previous therapists and would sometimes develop sexual feelings for them. Ms. C and her psychiatrist both hypothesized that these feelings may have not been completely related to the psychiatrist but instead to what he or she represented. Ms. C acknowledged that her core view of herself as helpless and in need of rescue might be a major impediment to treatment. The two hypothesized that Ms. C might fall back into a passive helpless stance in therapy and that her psychiatrist might even feel a pull to rescue her even though this would not be in Ms. C's best interest in the long-term.

In keeping with Leahy's comprehensive model of resistance to change in cognitive therapy (Leahy 2001), Ms. C and her psychiatrist proactively addressed her problems adhering to medication and her tendency to prematurely discontinue treatment. On deeper exploration, Ms. C acknowledged that there were many different reasons why she stopped taking medication. Sometimes it was because of hopelessness, whereas at other times the reasons for stopping were more complex. She sometimes stopped her medication when she felt she was becoming too dependent on her psychiatrist, feeling this was a way of reasserting independence. When she began to feel better and could actually imagine having the capacity to function as a "normal" person, Ms. C would become anxious about the demands that others might place on her, and she would fear failing and disappointing others and herself. At these times, she would stop medication as a self-handicapping protection from failing.

The open and empathic exploration of reasons for nonadherence with medication and premature termination of psychotherapy in the past allowed Ms. C's psychiatrist to reduce the likelihood that these types of problems would fully develop as treatment unfolded. In keeping with the cognitive therapy feedback form developed by J. Beck (1995) and the empathy scale questionnaire developed by Burns and Nolen-Hoeksema (1992), Ms. C agreed that she would try to write down her reactions to each therapy session so that this could be reviewed by her psychiatrist in the next session. By actively providing feedback throughout the session and between sessions, Ms. C learned how to practice more optimal ways of asserting her emotional needs within an interpersonal relationship. In addition, given the inherent unreliability of relying on countertransference alone to gauge the quality of the therapeutic relationship (Burns and Auerbach 1997; Strupp 1980), written feedback from the patient provided the psychiatrist with a much better understanding of problems that were developing during treatment, so that he was able to address these difficulties much earlier before they became a serious threat to the therapeutic alliance.

Stage IV: Treat the Acute Axis I Problems

Ms. C's psychiatrist proceeded to treat her depression, social anxiety, and binge eating with a combination of pharmacotherapy and psychodynamically informed CBT. Basic principles of pharmacotherapy will be reviewed before describing the psychotherapy treatment.

Principles of Pharmacotherapy for Depression With Comorbid Personality Disorder

Clinical lore suggests that medication treatment of major depression complicated by Axis II pathology is often associated with treatment nihilism. Bloch and colleagues (1988) reported that depressed patients with comorbid personality disorder are less likely to receive an adequate course of pharmacotherapy than depressed patients without comorbid Axis II pathology. In the case of Ms. C, in which Axis I and Axis II diagnoses are confirmed, the challenge is to reject treatment nihilism and develop a medication approach that is both acceptable and helpful to the patient. This goal depends critically on the treatment alliance. It is important to have mutual understanding regarding the role of medication when working with borderline or other patients with personality disorder who have Axis I issues. Exploring their experience and perception of medication is critical. Reviewing ambivalence and maladaptive attitudes about medication will improve adherence to a medication plan. Reviewing the past history of medication trials is important. It is important to clarify which medications have been used; which have been helpful; or whether they have been unhelpful, caused a partial response, or have been stopped because of side effects or "poop out."

In Chapter 7 of this book, Drs. Howland and Thase provide an in-depth discussion of pharmacotherapy for refractory and chronic depression complicated by personality disorder. A review of the mechanism of action of antidepressants that have been employed provides guidance in terms of selecting a current medication. Thus, if a patient has been tried on several serotonin agents, one might prefer to try a dual-action serotonin noradrenergic agent. With regards to dosing, it is important with patients with personality disorder to start low, go slow, and keep in mind that they may need more. Thus, the target usually is to go to the maximum dose required by the patient symptoms and tolerated by the patient before concluding that a drug trial has not been helpful. Frank and Kupfer (1990) have emphasized that the presence of personality disorder can influence the response time to antidepressant medications. When personality was evaluated after antidepressant response, the rapid responders had less personality pathology than slow responders. Poor responders had more personality issues. They suggested that the usual clinical standard of 8 weeks may be too short for patients with severe depression, particularly if they have personality pathology. In their sample, half the patients who ultimately responded would have been considered treatment resistant in 8 weeks. Thus, this emphasizes the importance of not only going to the maximum dose tolerated but also having a longer duration of trial before switching.

Sometimes a partial response is obtained with these patients. When considering augmenting or combination agents, it is important to keep safety in mind, recalling that the presence of personality disorder increases the likelihood of self-harm behavior. Special caution is advised for prescribing medications such as tricyclic antidepressants and agents such as lithium, which are toxic in overdose.

Treatment delivery is another issue that needs to be considered when combining antidepressant medication to psychotherapy for patients with Axis II comorbidity. Cost-containment pressures in contemporary mental health care delivery have made split treatment the rule rather than the exception today. Patients with depression and personality disorders typically see a psychopharmacologist for medication and a psychologist or a social worker for psychotherapy. This approach has advantages and disadvantages. It may be cost-effective if the psychiatrist is much more skilled in medication treatment than in the delivery of empirically supported psychotherapeutic approaches (which many but not all psychologists practice today). Split treatment may also be appropriate if the psychiatrist has concerns that a combination treatment may dilute the rigor of either the delivery of the psychotherapy or the pharmacotherapy. Nonetheless, a split-treatment approach is also associated with limitations. It requires close communication and mutual respect between the different clinicians in order to provide the patient with clear and consistent information. This need for close communication may be a problem for very busy psychopharmacologists, who treat a large number of patients. The allocation of regular time for communication is crucial for patients with personality disorders, who are prone to cognitive distortions such as dichotomous thinking. In situations where clinician communication and mutual respect are not present, it is not uncommon to observe splitting as well as devaluation of one of the therapies undermining the overall treatment. Our strong opinion, based on personal experience, is that psychiatrists who provide medication treatment combined with an active, skills-oriented, empirically supported psychotherapeutic approach offer the depressed Axis II patient the most satisfactory treatment. Future research should delineate whether this combined treatment is actually feasible and cost-effective.

Once a patient has responded to medication, it is very important to empower him or her by emphasizing that the patient gets the credit for the changes that have occurred, not the medications. It is critical for the clinician to emphasize that the medication allowed the patient to handle a specific stressful situation and to function in spite of the difficulties that were encountered. It is also important that patients see themselves as active participants who have the opportunity to become their own pharmacotherapists:

> Ms. C: Last night when I felt alone and discouraged, I felt like cutting again but didn't.
>
> Psychiatrist: Do you know why you didn't?
>
> Ms. C: I think the medications are making a big difference.
>
> Psychiatrist: Let's look at that. I'm glad that although you felt like cutting, you didn't. I agree that the medications may be helping. But I think that perhaps you're not taking enough credit for yourself. I think the work you've been doing, becoming more aware of the triggers that overwhelm you, is very important. The meds may be helping, but you're the one doing the work.

With regard to medication and major depression and personality disorder patients, it is important to target Axis I disorders primarily. However, if the patients do not meet the full criteria of Axis I, it is reasonable to target symptom clusters and treat appropriately. Augmentation strategies are worth considering as well. In some depressive patients who have personality disorder and micropsychotic episodes, atypical neuroleptics are worth considering. Atypical neuroleptics help as a third-line augmentation strategy for major depression (Kennedy et al. 2001), but they also may help with micropsychotic episodes, with mood stabilization, and as "ego glue" (a term loosely used clinically). Given the relationship between major depression and borderline personality disorder and the possibility that some such patients are bipolar spectrum disorder patients, atypical neuroleptics may have a mood-stabilizing function. Traditional mood stabilizers such as lithium and divalproex can be considered, although one is more hesitant using lithium because of its lower therapeutic index.

Thus, with regard to medication issues and depressed patients with personality disorder, it is important not to be blinded by conceptual frameworks that could cause clinicians to overlook Axis I or Axis II issues. Seeing only the Axis I issue deprives clinicians of considering the Axis II issues that need psychotherapeutic intervention. Seeing only Axis II issues deprives clinicians of using pharmacotherapy to help with negative affective states as well as with affective dysregulation.

In Ms. C's case, her psychiatrist was guided by the fact that Ms. C's sister had a history of bipolar II disorder, and Ms. C herself had many symptoms consistent with a bipolar spectrum disorder. Other important considerations were Ms. C's history of erratic medication adherence and her potential for impulsive self-destructive behavior. Ms. C's sister had a positive response to fluoxetine combined with lamotrigine, and this regimen was initiated with Ms. C. Unfortunately, despite very slow dosage titration, she developed a severe rash on lamotrigine and this was discontinued. A trial of fluoxetine combined with olanzapine was then initiated and after 12 weeks was successful in relieving much of the patient's depressive and anxiety symptoms.

Principles of Psychotherapy for Patients With Depression and Personality Disorder

As noted earlier, patients with depression and personality disorder generally require longer term treatment than patients with depression uncomplicated by severe personality dysfunction. One of the special

challenges of therapy for personality disorders in today's cost contain-
ment environment is ensuring that the longer term treatment retains the
focus and momentum that are associated with shorter term treatment
for depression such as interpersonal therapy (IPT) or CBT. We offer a
number of suggestions based on our experience and, as with Paris
(1992), view the treatment that we advocate as essentially psychodynamically informed CBT.

We acknowledge and use the rich contributions of dynamic theore-
ticians such as Kernberg (1989), Masterson (1981), and Kohut (see Gabbard 2001). However, readers wishing a more particular reading of
these authors are referred elsewhere. Michels (1992) provides a useful
description of the conceptual differences between Kernberg and Kohut
as to whether the patient's destructive rage is primary or secondary and
how to handle this in treatment. Levy (1992) describes how characterologically difficult patients may exert intense emotional demands on the
therapist, specifically when their powerful regressive transference
needs are reviewed in treatment. He advises therapists to seek consul-
tation in order to be away from the "heat" of the therapeutic interaction
and to contain and understand the transference-countertransference sequence that is coloring treatment.

In psychodynamically informed CBT, we begin by first emphasizing
that treatment should be accountable. The therapist and patient should
begin treatment by generating a written set of treatment goals based on
the patient's presenting problems. These goals should be explicit and
should be defined in operational or behavioral terms. For example,
rather than having a goal such as "I want to have better self-esteem,"
Ms. C delineated all of the signs that would demonstrate that she had
accomplished this particular goal. After defining treatment goals in behavioral terms, the patient and therapist should group the related goals
together and decide collaboratively on which to focus initially and on
which to focus later. In keeping with Linehan's DBT for borderline personality disorder (Linehan 1987, 1993), we suggest that after addressing
life-threatening behavior (such as self-mutilation, overdosing, and substance use), the therapist should then focus on therapy-threatening behavior and make these the goals that are addressed (e.g., missed
appointments, lateness, excessive contact between sessions, nonadherence with medication, and therapy homework tasks). Next on the hier-
archy are goals pertaining to the patient's quality of life. These would
broadly pertain to lessening anxiety and depression through increased
engagement with activities that promote a sense of pleasure and mastery, reducing negative and self-defeating patterns of thinking, improving assertiveness skills, and increasing interpersonal engagement and

capacity for intimacy. We suggest that treatment should be revisited every 3–6 months to evaluate the progress toward achieving the treatment goals. If possible, the patient and therapist should articulate objective anchor points that broadly define 25%, 50%, 75%, and 100% goal achievement so that treatment can be continually evaluated, refined, and recalibrated.

Second, we emphasize a treatment program that pragmatically teaches the patient specific skills while focusing on "here-and-now" issues. The goal of treatment should not be to solve all of the patient's problems but rather to teach the patient to become his or her own therapist by providing basic methods to solve emotional problems and deal effectively with distress in the face of adversity (Hollon et al. 1992). This emphasis on skill acquisition can be empowering for patients who have strong dependency needs, feelings of powerlessness and helplessness, and a perceived need for indefinite treatment. CBT-oriented interventions are ideally suited to a treatment orientation that emphasizes skill acquisition. In addition to skill acquisition, CBT has the advantage of being structured, which can be useful when working longer term with patients who because of affect dysregulation and multiple crises, tend to be unstructured. A CBT approach also tends to be more transparent and essentially demystifies the process of psychotherapy, which can be useful for patients who are prone to regression in unstructured therapeutic situations and have deficits in affect tolerance. In our clinic, we have found that patients presenting with depression and Axis II comorbidity have benefited from two particular self-help CBT manuals that can be used as references for each patient's individual therapy. *Mind Over Mood: Change How You Feel By Changing the Way You Think* (Greenberger and Padesky 1995) has the advantage of providing patients with basic CBT skills to master depression and anxiety, whereas *Reinventing Your Life: How to Break Free From Negative Life Patterns and Feel Good Again* (Young and Klosko 1994) focuses more attention on helping patients to understand the basis of their ingrained and often latent pathogenic beliefs and describes basic CBT strategies to alter these beliefs.

The following therapeutic exchange between Ms. C and her psychiatrist occurred after the 10th therapy session and illustrates the structure and skill-acquisition emphasis that we advocate:

Psychiatrist: Why don't we wrap up, since we only have 10 minutes left in the session. I want to review what we focused on today so that you'll be able to remember it and apply it by yourself in the future. What will you extract from today's session?

Ms. C: Well, I came in feeling really depressed and hopeless, and you helped me sort out why, so that I feel better now. You helped me to realize that after my boss called me to cancel one of my work shifts, I started to think that I was never going to make a decent living and that maybe this was jumping to conclusions.

Psychiatrist: Yes. Now how exactly did I do that? That's what I want you to take away from the session.

Ms. C: You had me focus on the specific moment during last week when my mood worsened.

Psychiatrist: Why do you think I keep stressing that?

Ms. C: Because this helps me to identify what I was feeling, and I often have difficulty knowing what the specific feelings are. I just feel bad without trying to sort out what "bad" means.

Psychiatrist: Exactly. Your feelings "mark the spot" that something important is happening for you. What do you need to do next after focusing on the situation and identifying your feelings?

Ms. C: I need to review all the thoughts that go with my feelings and try to identify the "hot thought"…the thought that causes me to feel the most distress.

In this vignette, Ms. C's psychiatrist was teaching her how to fill out the first three columns of the automatic thought record. Mastery of this basic skill is critical for patients with Axis II comorbidity because they often experience difficulty distinguishing between thoughts and feelings as well as with introspection, affect intolerance, and affect dysregulation. By learning how to decenter from their thoughts (Safran and Segal 1991) and view their thoughts as "ideas," patients with Axis II disorders can eventually learn to become observer-participants in their own experience. Mastery of this initial cognitive-behavioral skill helps to reduce impulsivity and affect dysregulation.

We emphasize a treatment approach that, in keeping with Linehan's DBT (Linehan 1987, 1993; Linehan et al. 2001), balances change interventions with unconditional acceptance. In working with patients with personality pathology, the therapist should constantly be sending the patient two seemingly incompatible messages: "I unconditionally accept you the way you are" and "You must change." At any one moment in time during therapy, the signal of one of these messages may be stronger than the other; however, both are critical for the patient to make progress. To accomplish this fine balance between acceptance and change, Ms. C's psychiatrist deliberately modified and reduced the structure of each therapy session. Although treatment goals were delineated and focused on, the sessions themselves were less structured than traditional, short-term CBT for depression or anxiety. In addition, in keeping with more psychodynamic therapeutic approaches, much more emphasis was placed on optimizing the health of the therapeutic alliance. Unlike traditional CBT for uncomplicated depression or anxiety, CBT for depression with significant comorbid Axis II pathology has a greater focus on the thoughts and feelings that emerge within the context of the therapeutic relationship (transference). The therapeutic alliance is not only a precondition for the teaching of cognitive and behavioral coping skills but also an active vehicle of change in and of itself.

Our treatment approach emphasizes understanding vulnerability and nurturing strengths. An important role of the therapist is to help the patient see the positive changes that are occurring as treatment unfolds. The therapist needs to be explicit about the nature of the change, for example, "A few months ago you would not have been able to do… "Let me know how that made you feel… "Deal with that disappointment in such a positive manner… "Resist taking out your feelings by cutting," and so on. This strategy not only highlights positive changes but also has a strong transferential and validating component that deepens the therapeutic alliance. Giving the patient, not the medication, credit for the positive changes has a similar function.

In treating Ms. C's multiple problems, her psychiatrist negotiated a strategy that he felt would efficiently yield the maximum benefit in the shortest period. This required that Ms. C and her psychiatrist agree on a general order in which basic problems, such as low energy, were addressed and thoroughly mastered before moving on to more complex problems, such as poor relationships with men. Table 6–5 illustrates the order in which Ms. C's complex and interacting problems were delineated and addressed using cognitive-behavioral principles.

The successful treatment of Ms. C's depression required a longer period than the 12–24 weeks typically seen in cases of depression uncomplicated by significant Axis II pathology. Over the course of the first year of treatment, Ms. C's psychiatrist successfully initiated antidepressant and atypical antipsychotic treatment, and after taking the time to build rapport and trust was also able to implement some of the CBT techniques that are traditionally used in treating depression. In addition, therapy techniques were also directed at the patient's social anxiety and her alcohol abuse and binge eating. In keeping with Linehan's (1993) emphasis on remediating affect dysregulation and Teasedale's (Teasedale et al. 2000) emphasis on mindfulness training to reduce relapse from depression, Ms. C was also referred for an intensive 8-week course of meditation after her level of acute depression diminished. At this point in time the focus of therapy turned more attention to addressing Ms. C's underlying core beliefs and her personality pathology in a more explicit manner.

TABLE 6–5. Treatment priorities and therapeutic interventions for Ms. C

Treatment priorities

- Suicidal ideation and urge to self-mutilate
- Lack of energy/amotivation/hopelessness
- Poor problem-solving skills secondary to emotional dysregulation
- Alcohol and drug use
- Unemployment
- Limited social network
- Binge eating
- Social skill deficits and poor assertiveness skills
- Chronic low self-esteem
- Dysfunctional relationships with men

Therapeutic interventions

- Prescribe atypical antipsychotic medication; examine advantages and disadvantages of suicide; implement distraction and self-soothing techniques; provide a written contract with list of coping strategies to try prior to telephone contact
- Prescribe antidepressant pharmacotherapy; schedule pleasurable activities; recommend self-monitor daily activities
- Prescribe antidepressant/atypical antipsychotic to reduce affect dysregulation; keep automatic thought records; teach general problem-solving techniques; attend mindfulness training/meditation course
- Examine advantages and disadvantages of drug/alcohol use; self-monitor consumption; prescribe distraction and self-soothing techniques; encourage involvement in Alcoholics/Narcotics Anonymous
- Examine advantages and disadvantages of working; examine thoughts associated with fears of working; attend vocational rehabilitation course; provide occupational therapy referral
- Graded social exposure to reduce social anxiety; involvement in volunteer work and hiking group; referral for interpersonal group therapy
- Examine advantages and disadvantages; keep daily self-monitoring log of food intake/thoughts/feelings; eat regular three meals and two snacks per day; teach stimulus control, and distraction and self-soothing techniques
- Use written cognitive therapy session feedback form; focus more on positive and negative feelings toward therapist; implement role-playing/ assertiveness training practice; provide interpersonal feedback and transparency from therapist; attend interpersonal group therapy
- Focus more on developmental underpinnings of negative beliefs; keep core belief worksheets to record daily positive experiences; provide interpersonal feedback and transparency from therapist
- Focus on relationship with male therapist as a paradigm for a healthier relationship with a man; encourage sexual abstinence in the very earliest stages of dating

Stage V: Treat the Personality Disorder and Facilitate Relapse Prevention

After approximately 6 months of treatment had elapsed, Ms. C's psychiatrist began to focus more and more attention on her personality disorder and restructuring the concomitant core beliefs associated with her personality problems. In addition to sharing his cognitive conceptualization diagram, Ms. C's psychiatrist provided her a considerable amount of psychoeducation about her personality problems in order to demystify why these patterns had become so ingrained. To help the patient understand her impulsivity and her problems tolerating frustration and negative feelings, the psychiatrist explained how invalidating a child's feelings when that child is very young creates a recipe for disaster when it comes to adult skills in both recognizing emotions and being able to soothe oneself. In addition, the psychiatrist also tried to explain how negative core beliefs act like a selective filter that only attend to negative events and ignore or devalue positive experiences:

> Psychiatrist: I'd like to share a hypothesis about why you find it so difficult to change your view of yourself and the world, and have difficulty looking at things more positively even though intellectually you have learned the skills to examine your initial reactions with more objectivity.
>
> Ms. C: Why do you think I have difficulty changing my basic outlook no matter whatever good happens to me?
>
> Psychiatrist: I think that in a lot of ways you are prejudiced against yourself.

The psychiatrist then used the analogy of prejudice to help Ms. C recognize how many of her beliefs about herself and the world functioned like prejudices. These negative beliefs, like prejudice, tended to be ingrained, emotionally laden, overgeneralized, and impervious to rational disputation. Asking her about what strategy she would employ to change the prejudice of a friend allowed Ms. C to recognize that logic alone would not be effective and that instead she would need to *deliberately create* repetitive "corrective emotional experiences" for her friend that disconfirmed her negative prejudice. This analogy was useful because Ms. C was readily able to understand the importance of her keeping a daily log of positive experiences and accomplishments that would over time help to build up a more positive view of herself.

In addition, during this later phase of treatment, Ms C's psychiatrist focused more attention on the therapeutic relationship and tried to use it in a more explicit manner as a source of therapeutic relearning. More emphasis was placed on activating negative affect in the sessions rather than simply containing negative affect, which had been the goal originally when Ms. C presented for treatment and was extremely depressed. In keeping with McCullough's (2000) concept of "disciplined personal involvement" and Young's (Young et al. 2003) concept of "limited reparenting," Ms. C's psychiatrist tried to incorporate more transparent comments about his reactions to the patient while carefully maintaining appropriate professional boundaries and ensuring that the comments that were shared did not overwhelm or overstimulate the patient:

> Ms. C: Sometimes I just feel like I should pack it in. Nobody cares about me anyways.
>
> Psychiatrist: You sound hopeless when you say that. What emotional impact do you think your comments have on me?
>
> Ms. C: What do you mean?
>
> Psychiatrist: What impact does your comment have on the way I feel about you right now?
>
> Ms. C: I don't know. I have no idea.
>
> Psychiatrist: I feel completely distanced from you. After 7 months of seeing you weekly and making an effort to see you when you were in crisis, you said that nobody cares about you. Your comment makes me feel like I'm invisible to you, like you are pushing me away. Your tone of voice when you just contemplated suicide was flippant, like nothing we worked on was of any importance in the end. Why would you want to send that kind of message to me?
>
> Ms. C: I had no idea I was coming across to you that way or that you cared about me as much as you do. I'm sorry. I think sometimes I try to hurt you on purpose whenever I fear I'm becoming too dependent on you.

In subsequent sessions, much time was devoted to exploring this interpersonal pattern and the developmental underpinnings in terms of Ms. C's history of abuse from both of her parents. After a year of weekly individual therapy, Ms. C was referred to concurrent interpersonal group therapy to help her develop more adaptive interpersonal styles of relating to others and also as a means of amplifying the interpersonal feedback that Ms. C's psychiatrist was trying to provide to her. Ms. C continued to be followed by her psychiatrist, but after 2 years of treatment she was able to see him no more than every 4–6 weeks. In her second year of individual therapy, she was referred for a course of interpersonal group psychotherapy, and over the course of the two years that she regularly attended group, Ms. C developed and refined more adaptive interpersonal skills. Her mood has remained stable and she has not relapsed. Her binge eating and alcohol abuse have attenuated, and she successfully went back to work and began to develop a healthier pattern of relating to other people, particularly men.

In our clinical experience, depressed patients with moderate personality disturbance typically improve over the course of 1–2 years of weekly treatment. This observation is consistent with Perry and colleagues (1999), who concluded that DSM-IV criteria for personality disorder were no longer met by the majority of Axis II patients after 1–2 years of weekly treatment. In keeping with the fact that patients with Axis II comorbidity often experience chronic or recurrent depression, we suggest that psychiatrists continue to follow these types of patients for long periods by providing regular booster sessions. Ideally, these less frequent booster sessions should avoid inadvertently creating excessive dependency in the patient and should emphasize reinforcing the gains that were achieved in the earlier period of more intensive therapy in order to prevent relapse.

Conclusions

We have presented a detailed case of depression complicated by a mixed personality disorder in order to realistically illustrate a pragmatic and integrative treatment approach that is based on diagnostic rigor; a concise, easily understood psychological formulation; pharmacotherapy; and a phasic approach to efficiently and strategically address the patient's complex symptoms and problems. By marrying powerful CBT change techniques with validation, unconditional acceptance, disciplined personal involvement, and targeted pharmacotherapy, the clinician can be successful in not only treating acute major depression but also modifying personality psychopathology.

References

Adler G: Borderline Psychopathology and Its Treatment. New York, Jason Aronson, 1985

Alden L: Short-term structured treatment for avoidant personality disorder. J Consult Clin Psychol 56:756–764, 1989

American Psychiatric Association: Diagnostic and Statistical Manual of Mental Disorders, 4th Edition, Text Revision. Washington, DC, American Psychiatric Association, 2000

Akiskal HS, Hirschfield RM, Yerevanian BI: The relationship of personality to affective disorders. Arch Gen Psychiatry 40:801–810, 1983

Akiskal HS, Maser JD, Zeller PJ, et al: Switching from "unipolar" to bipolar II: an 11-year prospective study of clinical and temperamental predictors in 559 patients. Arch Gen Psychiatry 52:115–123, 1995

Bateman A, Fonagy P: Effectiveness of partial hospitalization in the treatment of borderline personality disorder: a randomized controlled trial. Am J Psychiatry 156:1563–1569, 1999

Beck A, Epstein N, Brown G, et al: An inventory for measuring clinical anxiety: psychometric properties. J Consult Clin Psychol 56:893–897, 1988

Beck A, Brown G, Steer R: Prediction of eventual suicide in psychiatric inpatients by clinical ratings of hopelessness. J Consult Clin Psychol 57:309–310, 1989

Beck A, Freeman A, Associates: Cognitive Therapy of Personality Disorders. New York, Guilford, 1990

Beck A, Steer R, Ball R, et al: Comparison of Beck Depression Inventories -IA and -II in psychiatric outpatients. J Pers Assess 67:588–597, 1996

Beck A, Freeman A, Associates: Cognitive Therapy of Personality Disorders, 2nd Edition. New York, Guilford, 2004

Beck J: Cognitive Therapy: Basics and Beyond. New York, Guilford, 1995

Benazzi F: Highly recurrent unipolar may be related to bipolar II. Compr Psychiatry 43:263–268, 2002

Benazzi F, Akiskal H: Refining the evaluation of bipolar II: beyond the strict SCID-CV guidelines for hypomania. J Affect Disord 73:33–38, 2003

Bloch D, Bell S, Hulbert J, et al: The importance of axis II in patients with major depression: a controlled study. J Affect Disord 14:115–122, 1988

Boyce P, Mason C: An overview of depression-prone personality traits and the role of interpersonal sensitivity. Aust N Z J Psychiatry 30:90–103, 1996

Burns D, Auerbach A: Therapeutic empathy in cognitive therapy, in Frontiers of Cognitive Therapy. Edited by Salkovskis P. New York, Guilford, 1996, pp 135–164

Burns D, Nolen-Hoeksema S: Therapeutic empathy and recovery from depression in cognitive-behavioral therapy: a structural equation model. J Consult Clin Psychol 60:441–449, 1992

Davidson J, Rothbaum B, van der Kolk B, et al: Multicenter, double-blind comparison of sertraline and placebo in the treatment of posttraumatic stress disorder. Arch Gen Psychiatry 58:485–492, 2001

Fava M, Alpert JE, Borus JE, et al: Patterns of personality disorder and comorbidity in early onset versus late-onset major depression. Am J Psychiatry 153:1308–1312, 1996

Fava M, Farabaugh AH, Sickinger AH, et al: Personality disorders and depression. Psychol Med 32:1049–1057, 2002

Frank E, Kupfer D: Axis II personality disorders and personality features in treatment-resistant and refractory depression, in Treatment Strategies for Refractory Depression. Edited by Roose SP, Glassman AH. Washington, DC, American Psychiatric Press 1990, pp 207–221

Gabbard GO: Psychodynamic psychotherapy of borderline personality disorder: a contemporary approach. Bull Menninger Clin 65:41–57, 2001

Ghaemi S, Ko J, Goodwin F: "Cade's disease" and beyond: misdiagnosis, antidepressant use, and a proposed definition for bipolar spectrum disorder. Can J Psychiatry 47:125–34, 2002

Greenberger D, Padesky C: Mind Over Mood: Change How You Feel By Changing the Way You Think. New York, Guilford, 1995

Greenspan S, Benderly B: Growth of the Mind: And the Endangered Origins of Intelligence. Cambridge, MA, Perseus Publishing, 1998

Hamilton M: A rating scale for depression. J Neurol Neurosurg Psychiatry 23:56–62, 1960

Hingley S: Psychodynamic theory and narcissistically related personality problems: support from case study research. Br J Med Psychol 74:57–72, 2001

Hirschfeld RM, Russell JM, Delgado PL, et al: Predictors of response to acute treatment of chronic and double depression with sertraline or imipramine. J Clin Psychiatry 59:669–675, 1998

Hollon S, De Rubeis R, Evans M, et al: Cognitive therapy and pharmacotherapy for depression: singly and in combination. Arch Gen Psychiatry 49:774–781, 1992

Ilardi S, Craighead W: Personality pathology and response to somatic treatments for major depression: a critical review. Depression 2:200–217, 1995

Keller MB, McCullough JP, Klein DN, et al: A comparison of nefazodone, the cognitive-behavioral analysis system of psychotherapy, and their combination for the treatment of chronic depression. N Engl J Med 342:1462–1470, 2000

Kennedy SH, Lam RW, Cohen NL, et al: Clinical guidelines for the treatment of depressive disorders, IV: medications and other biological treatments. Can J Psychiatry 46 (suppl 1):38S–58S, 2001

Kernberg O, Selzer M, Koenigsberg H, et al: Psychodynamic Psychotherapy of Borderline Patients. New York, Basic Books, 1989

Leahy R: Overcoming Resistance in Cognitive Therapy. New York, Guilford, 2001

Leichsenring F, Leibing E: The effectiveness of psychodynamic therapy and cognitive behavior therapy in the treatment of personality disorders: a meta-analysis. Am J Psychiatry 160:1223–1232, 2003

Levy J: The borderline patient: psychotherapeutic stalemates, in Handbook of Borderline Disorders. Edited by Silver D, Rosenbluth M. Madison, CT, International Universities Press, 1992, pp 307–334

Linehan M: Dialectical behavior therapy for borderline personality disorder: theory and method. Bull Menninger Clin 51:261–276, 1987

Linehan M: Cognitive-Behavioral Treatment of Borderline Personality Disorder. New York, Guilford, 1993

Linehan M, Armstrong H, Suarez, et al: Cognitive-behavioral treatment of chronically parasuicidal borderline patients. Arch Gen Psychiatry 48:1060–1064, 1991

Linehan M, Heard H, Armstrong H: Naturalistic follow-up of a behavioral treatment for chronically parasuicidal borderline patients. Arch Gen Psychiatry 50:971–974, 1993

Linehan MM, Tutek DA, Heard HL, et al: Interpersonal outcome in cognitive behavioral treatment for chronically suicidal borderline patients. Am J Psychiatry 151:1771–1776, 1994

Linehan MM, Schmidt H, Dimeff LA, et al: Dialectical behavior therapy for patients with borderline personality disorder and drug dependence. Am J Addict 8:279–292, 1999

Linehan M, Cochran B, Kehrer C: Dialectical behavior therapy for borderline personality disorder, in Clinical Handbook for Psychological Disorders. Edited by Barlow D. New York, Guilford, 2001, pp 470–522

MacQueen G, Young L: Bipolar II disorder: symptoms, course, and response to treatment. Psychiatr Serv 52:358–361, 2001

Masterson J: The Narcissistic and Borderline Disorders. New York, Brunner/Mazel, 1981

McCullough JP Jr: Treatment for Chronic Depression: Cognitive Behavioral Analysis System of Psychotherapy (CBASP). New York, Guilford, 2000

Michels R: The borderline patient: shifts in theoretical emphasis and implications for treatment, in Handbook of Borderline Disorders. Edited by Silver D, Rosenbluth M. Madison, CT, International Universities Press, 1992, pp 109–120

Mulder R: Personality pathology and treatment outcome in major depression: a review. Am J Psychiatry 159:359–371, 2002

Mullen LS, Blanco C, Vaughan SC, et al: Defense mechanisms and personality in depression. Depress Anxiety 10:168–174, 1999

Mundo E, Maina G, Uslenghi C: Multicentre, double-blind, comparison of fluvoxamine and clomipramine in the treatment of obsessive-compulsive disorder. Int Clin Psychopharmacol 15:69–76, 2000

Paris J: Borderline Personality Disorder: Etiology and Treatment. Washington, DC, American Psychiatric Association, 1992

Pepper CM, Klein DN, Anderson RL, et al: DSM-III-R axis II comorbidity in dysthymia and major depression. Am J Psychiatry 152:239–247, 1995

Perry J, Banon E, Ianni F: Effectiveness of psychotherapy for personality disorders. Am J Psychiatry 156:1312–1321, 1999

Safran J, Segal ZV: Interpersonal Aspects of Cognitive Therapy. New York, Basic Books, 1991

Shaver P, Mikulincer M: Attachment-related psychodynamics. Attach Hum Dev 4:133–161, 2002

Skodol AE, Stout RL, McGlashan TH, et al: Co-occurrence of mood and personality disorders: a report from the Collaborative Longitudinal Personality Disorders Study (CLPS). Depress Anxiety 10:175–182, 1999

Strupp H: Success and failure in time-limited psychotherapy. Arch Gen Psychiatry 37:595–603, 1980

Teasedale J, Segal Z, Williams J, et al: Prevention of relapse/recurrence in major depression by mindfulness-based cognitive therapy. J Consult Clin Psychology 68:615–623, 2000

Verheul R, Van den Bosch LM, Koeter MW, et al: Dialectical behaviour therapy for women with borderline personality disorder: 12 month, randomised clinical trial in the Netherlands. Br J Psychiatry 182:135–140, 2003

Vieta E, Colom F, Martinez-Aran A, et al: Bipolar II disorder and comorbidity. Compr Psychiatry 41:339–343, 2000

Weissman A, Beck A: Development and validation of the dysfunctional attitude scale: a preliminary investigation. Paper presented at the Annual Meeting of the Association for the Advancement of Behavior Therapy, Chicago, IL, May 12, 1978

Winston A, Laikin M, Pollack J, et al: Short-term psychotherapy of personality disorders. Am J Psychiatry 151:190–194, 1994

Young J, Klosko J: Reinventing Your Life: How to Break Free From Negative Life Patterns and Feel Good Again. New York, Dutton, 1994

Young J, Klosko J, Weishaar M: Schema Therapy: A Practitioner's Guide. New York, Guilford, 2003

Zanarini M, Frankenburg F, Hennen J, et al: The longitudinal course of borderline psychopathology: 6-year prospective follow-up of the phenomenology of borderline personality disorder. Am J Psychiatry 160:274–283, 2003

Zimmerman M, Mattia JI: Axis I diagnostic comorbidity and borderline personality disorder. Compr Psychiatry 40:245–252, 1999

Zimmerman M, Mattia J, Posternak M: Are subjects in pharmacological treatment trials of depression representative of patients in routine clinical practice? Am J Psychiatry 159:469–473, 2002

REFRACTORY AND CHRONIC DEPRESSION

The Role of Axis II Disorders in Assessment and Treatment

Robert H. Howland, M.D.

Michael E. Thase, M.D.

Despite the availability of a wide variety of antidepressant therapies, a substantial number of depressed patients have a chronic course of illness or have illness that is refractory to treatment (Howland 1993; Thase and Rush 1995). One approach to identify possible underlying causes of chronicity and treatment resistance in patients with depression is the study of personality disorders (Thase 1996; Thase and Howland 1994). Contemporary research on personality disorders has progressed beyond the historical interest in psychodynamic and intrapsychic principles (Hirschfeld and Shea 1992) to include investigations of cognitive and interpersonal processes (Beck et al. 1990; Kiesler 1996); the genetics and biology of personality traits and temperaments (Bond 2001; Bouchard and Loehlin 2001); interactions between genes and environment in the expression of behavioral traits and the development of psychiatric disorders (Kendler 2001; McGue and Bouchard 1998); and the pharmacological treatment of personality disorders (Aschauer and

Schlogelhofer 2003; Rivas-Vazquez and Blais 2002). As a result, under-standing the relationship between personality, depression, and treatment outcome is a very complex endeavor. In this chapter, we review the role of personality disorders in the assessment and treatment of refractory and chronic forms of depression.

Personality Disorders, Traits, and Temperaments

DSM-IV-TR (American Psychiatric Association 2000) organizes Axis II personality disorders into three descriptive clusters. Cluster A includes the personality types that share some clinical features with psychotic disorders: paranoid, schizoid, and schizotypal personality disorders. Antisocial, borderline, histrionic, and narcissistic personality disorders are grouped within Cluster B because of their common characteristics of emotional instability and dramatic, impulsive, or erratic behaviors. Cluster C consists of avoidant, dependent, and obsessive-compulsive personality disorders, which have features in common with anxiety disorders (see Table 7–1). Methods currently used to diagnose Axis II disorders include structured diagnostic interviews and self-report personality assessments (Klein et al. 2002; Rothschild and Zimmerman 2003).

TABLE 7–1.   DSM-IV-TR Axis II personality disorders

Cluster A	Paranoid, schizoid, schizotypal
Cluster B	Antisocial, borderline, histrionic, narcissistic
Cluster C	Avoidant, dependent, obsessive-compulsive

Source.   Reprinted from American Psychiatric Association: *Diagnostic and Statistical Manual of Mental Disorders,* 4th Edition, Text Revision. Washington, DC, American Psychiatric Association, 2000. Used with permission.

An alternative approach to the classification of personality is the assessment of traits and temperaments rather than specific categorical disorders (Aschauer and Schlogelhofer 2003; Klein et al. 2002). Personality traits and temperaments are dimensional characteristics that are heritable, manifest early in life, and involve biases in perceptual memory and habit formation. They underlie and/or influence cognitive processes, interpersonal and social function, emotional and affective states, and stress response systems (Buck 1999; Cloninger et al. 1993; Eley and Plomin 1997). Personality traits and temperaments span normal and psychopathological populations, differing only by a matter of degree or severity. There is developing evidence that the heritability and expression of personality traits also may be influenced by environmental factors (Kendler 2001; Ozkaragoz and Noble 2000). These findings suggest that the development of personality is dependent on not only genetic factors and environmental influences but also on complex interactions between genes and environment (Cloninger 1999).

Various personality traits and temperaments, such as neuroticism, extraversion, novelty seeking, harm avoidance, reward dependence, and persistence, have been studied in relation to depression and anxiety (Aschauer and Schlogelhofer 2003; Klein et al. 2002), although neuroticism has received the most attention in clinical and treatment studies (Petersen et al. 2002a). *Neuroticism* refers to a tendency to respond to distress in emotional, anxious, and somatic ways. The acute state of depression causes an increase in neuroticism scores, but high levels of neuroticism are also associated with an increased risk of developing depression (Hirschfeld et al. 1989) and with the development of chronicity (Scott et al. 1992; Tyrer et al. 1983). The cognitive concept of dysfunctional attitudes is closely related to neuroticism (Thase and Beck 1992). *Dysfunctional attitudes* are extreme and relatively rigid beliefs that guide thinking, emotional reactions, and behavior, and these beliefs concern two main areas: 1) attitudes about achievement and 2) attitudes related to interpersonal relationships. Acute depression increases the level of dysfunctional attitudes, but high levels are also associated with chronicity, risk of relapse, and poor treatment response (Miller et al. 1986; Peselow et al. 1990; Thase and Howland 1994). People with high levels of dysfunctional attitudes are more prone to developing depression in response to adverse life events (i.e., achievement events vs. interpersonal events) that "match" their particular personality vulnerabilities (i.e., sociotropy [interpersonal dependency] vs. autonomy [need for independence or control]) (Bagby et al. 2001; Robins et al. 1997). In addition, in these depressed patients, adverse interpersonal events are associated with a better antidepressant treatment outcome, and adverse achievement events are associated with a worse outcome (Mazure et al. 2000). Moreover, a better treatment outcome occurred in patients with higher levels of sociotropy who experienced negative interpersonal events and in patients with higher levels of autonomy who experienced negative achievement events (Mazure et al. 2000).

Most studies have found that patients with depression have increased rates of personality disorders and pathological personality traits compared with healthy control subjects (Rothschild and Zimmerman 2003). The relationship between depression and personality may

TABLE 7–2.   Relationship between depression and personality

- Personality and depression have common causes
- Personality is an early manifestation of depression
- Personality predisposes to developing depression
- Personality influences the expression or course of depression
- Personality features are the persistent effects after recovering from depression

Source.   Adapted from Klein et al. 2002.

be explained in several ways: personality and depression have common causes; personality is an early manifestation of depression; personality predisposes to developing depression; personality influences the expression or course of depression; and personality features are the persistent effects after recovering from depression (Klein et al. 2002) (see Table 7–2). The development or exaggeration of personality traits as a complication of depression or as a consequence of persistent or recurrent episodes of depression is relevant to the relationship between personality and chronicity or treatment resistance (Coryell et al. 1993; Friedman 1995; Thase and Howland 1994), especially in early-onset forms of depression (Parker et al. 2003; Sato et al. 1999a). In addition, depression and personality disorders are each associated with life stress. Many depressive episodes are triggered by stressful life events, and dysphoria amplifies the perception of stress (Brett et al. 1990). Adverse life events also do not happen randomly, and people with more chaotic and unstable lifestyles are at greater risk to suffer various stressors (Kendler 1995; Kendler et al. 1993). For example, adverse events that precipitate the onset of depression are shaped in part by a person's pathological personality traits, and the same personality traits may influence attempts to cope with these problems (Bender et al. 2001; Plomin 1994). Thus, depression and personality pathology have a reciprocal and interactive relationship with life stress, and people who are less well equipped to handle life stress are at increased risk to experience it (Kendler 2001; Rose 2001; Thase and Howland 1994).

The presence of depression may bias the perception or recollection of personal and interpersonal behavioral patterns and tendencies in a negative or distorted way, which affects the assessment of personality (Cohen et al. 1988; Farmer and Nelson-Gray 1990; Klein et al. 2002). Indeed, effective antidepressant treatment often leads to decreases in personality pathology in depressed patients (Aberg-Wistedt et al. 2000; Black and Sheline 1997; Corruble et al. 2002; Du et al. 2002; Hellerstein et al. 2000; Hirano et al. 2002), although antidepressant-induced changes in personality are not always associated with improvements in depression (Allgulander et al. 1998; Bagby et al. 1999; Tranter et al. 2002; Tse and Bond 2001). It is difficult to assess personality before onset of depression in people who have been depressed for many years and in persons with early-onset depression, which is often chronic or highly recurrent (Lewinsohn et al. 1997; Parker et al. 2003). Personality assessment may be deferred until after the person has recovered from depression, although this is obviously not helpful in evaluating the role of personality in people who are chronically depressed or are refractory to treatment. Using information from collateral sources, such as parents, friends, or spouses, can help to overcome this problem, although this information may also be biased or distorted in several ways. For example, because of the familial risks of depression and personality, as well as the process of assortative mating, it is possible that a collateral source also has depression or personality pathology (Bouchard and Loehlin 2001). In addition, a person's depression and/or personality may affect adversely the quality of life of a collateral source in a way that colors his or her perceptions and descriptions of the patient (Barnett and Gotlib 1988; Friedman 1995). Thus, investigating the relationship between personality disorders and treatment outcome is methodologically difficult, and the findings from clinical trials are not definitive (Thase 1996).

Personality Disorder and Antidepressant Response

A number of studies have investigated the relationship between personality disorders and antidepressant treatment response (Davidson et al. 1985; Reich and Green 1991; Reich and Vasile 1993; Rothschild and Zimmerman 2003). Many studies have found that patients with personality disorders have a less complete or delayed response to pharmacotherapy alone compared with depressed patients with no Axis II comorbidity (Bschor et al. 2001; Rothschild and Zimmerman 2003; Shea et al. 1990, 1992) or to pharmacotherapy and psychotherapy together (Frank and Kupfer 1990), although some studies have not supported this finding (Bagby et al. 2002; Mulder et al. 2003; Petersen et al. 2002b; Russell et al. 2003). Similarly, some studies of personality traits and temperaments, rather than specific disorders, have found that these dimensional variables may predict the response to antidepressant treatment, although there is no consistent finding regarding specific traits or specific antidepressant drugs (Bagby et al. 2002; Hirschfeld et al. 1998; Joyce et al. 1994; Nelson and Cloninger 1997; Sato et al. 1999b; Tome et al. 1997). Other studies have found no relationship between personality traits or temperaments and treatment outcome (Marijnissen et al. 2002; Newman et al. 2000; Petersen et al. 2002a).

In contrast to pharmacotherapy studies, very few studies have investigated the response to a depression-focused psychotherapy alone in depressed patients with personality disorders. Some studies (Ball et al. 2000; Merrill et al. 2003), but not all (Kuyken et al. 2001; Shea et al. 1990; Stuart et al. 1992), have found that depressed patients with personality disorders respond less well to cognitive-behavioral therapy (CBT) than do patients without personality disorders. One study found that comorbid personality pathology was associated with a delayed response to interpersonal psychotherapy (IPT) in depressed patients (Bearden et al. 1996). Two studies have suggested that IPT may be relatively less effective than CBT in depressed patients with comorbid personality disorders (Hardy et al. 1995; Shea et al. 1990). It would be clinically important and theoretically interesting to investigate prospectively whether the response to CBT and IPT generally differs in depressed patients with personality disorders, whether there are particular personality features that may predict patient response to CBT or IPT (Barber and Muenz 1996; Coombs et al. 2002; Sotsky et al. 1991), and whether modifications of these psychotherapies tailored to comorbid personality pathology are more effective (Jarrett et al. 1997; McCray and King 2003; Nelson-Gray et al. 1996; Weissman et al. 2000). Moreover, it would be especially interesting to compare treatment outcome with CBT or IPT in depressed patients according to adverse life events (i.e., achievement events vs. interpersonal events) and cognitive personality styles (i.e., sociotropy vs. autonomy) (Hammen et al. 1989; Mazure et al. 2000; Robins and Block 1989). Although depressed patients with personality disorders may respond less well to combination pharmacotherapy and psychotherapy than do patients without personality disorders (Frank and Kupfer 1990), there is some evidence that combination treatment may be more effective than pharmacotherapy alone in these patients (Hellerstein et al. 2001; Kool et al. 2003a, 2003b).

Personality disorders appear to be more prevalent among patients with various forms of chronic depression (Harkness et al. 2002; Keller et al. 2000; Kwon et al. 2000; Markowitz et al. 1992; Miller et al. 1986; Mulder et al. 2003; Russell et al. 2003; Sanderson et al. 1992). Rates of personality disorders are also greater in early-onset chronic depression than in late-onset chronic depression (Klein et al. 1999a, 1999b). Disentangling the early manifestations of personality traits from the early onset of mood symptoms, however, is difficult (Lewinsohn et al. 1997; Parker et al. 2003). Assessment of familial psychopathology (including personality disorders) may be helpful in early-onset depression and has been shown to predict a poorer outcome among patients with dysthymia (Durbin et al. 2000). The effect of personality pathology on treatment outcome in chronically depressed patients has not been as well studied. In a long-term follow-up study of dysthymia, patients with comorbid personality disorders were less likely to recover than those without personality disorders (Hayden and Klein 2001). In a study of patients with chronic major or double depression, depressive personality traits but not comorbid personality disorders were associated with a higher nonresponse to antidepressants (Hirschfeld et al. 1998; Russell et al. 2003). Chronic depression is generally associated with a 10%–20% reduction in antidepressant treatment response rates compared with nonchronic depression (Harrison and Stewart 1995; Howland 1991), but it is not clear to what extent comorbid personality pathology or other factors contributing to the persistence of depression also contribute to the relatively poorer treatment outcome (Lara and Klein 1999). As discussed previously, personality disorder diagnoses may be less valid when people have been continuously depressed for many years. Nevertheless, antidepressants and psychotherapy have been shown to improve some aspects of personality and psychosocial functioning in chronically depressed patients (Hellerstein et al. 2000; Hirschfeld et al. 2002; Kocsis et al. 1997, 2002; Miller et al. 1998).

How Can Personality Alter Antidepressant Effects?

Antidepressant treatments are generally more effective for people with moderately severe and circumscribed episodes of depression (Joyce and Paykel 1989; Thase and Rush 1995). In many ways, depression chronicity and antidepressant responsiveness are strongly correlated with various psychosocial factors (Lara and Klein 1999; Thase and Kupfer 1987). For example, patients with good social supports tend to respond better to treatment (Bagby et al. 2002), as do patients who are compliant with treatment (Sirey et al. 2001). An acute stress-related depression is more likely to have a shorter episode and better outcome, whereas chronic or intractable stresses are associated with more persistent and less treatment-responsive depressions. The presence of Axis I comorbidity, such as anxiety disorders and substance abuse, is also associated with chronicity and a poorer antidepressant response (see Table 7–3).

People with personality disorders may have a greater burden of factors that diminish the effectiveness of antidepressant treatments (Bender et al. 2001). Personality disorders begin early in life and are associated with many interpersonal difficulties and high rates of Axis I

TABLE 7–3.   Factors affecting treatment outcome for patients with depression

Positive	Negative
Good social supports and compliance	Chronic or intractable stresses
Acute stress-related depression—shorter episode and better outcome	Presence of Axis I comorbidity—chronicity

comorbidity, including anxiety disorders and substance abuse (Lewin-sohn et al. 1997; Parker et al. 2003). Their interpersonal difficulties and social skills deficits certainly affect social support systems, and they contribute to the development and persistence of stressful and adverse life events associated with family, social, and work environments. It is also likely that personality pathology is linked to a patient's antidepressant nonresponse through medication noncompliance (Ekselius et al. 2000; Sirey et al. 2001). Therefore, a number of predictors of antidepressant response overlap with the clinical and psychosocial features that characterize patients with personality disorders (Thase and Kupfer 1987; Thase and Rush 1995).

The relationship between personality and refractory depression may also be considered from the standpoint of recent work in psychiatric neurobiology and molecular genetics (Bond 2001; Lesch et al. 2002). For example, the serotonin transporter (5-HTT) gene is one of the most studied candidate genes in psychiatric genetics (Melke 2003). 5-HTT is best known as the site of action of the selective serotonin reuptake inhibitor (SSRI) antidepressants, which are widely used and generally effective in the treatment of depression, anxiety, and even some personality disorders (Aschauer and Schlogelhofer 2003; Rivas-Vazquez and Blais 2002). Certain polymorphisms of the gene that expresses the 5-HTT have been found to predict the response to SSRIs in some depression treatment studies (Melke 2003). Other studies have found that 5-HTT genetic polymorphisms are associated with some depression and anxiety-related personality traits (e.g., neuroticism and negative emotionality) (Melke 2003; Murphy et al. 2001) (see Table 7–4). Hence, it is conceivable that the attenuated antidepressant treatment response in a subgroup of depressed patients with personality disorders may be mediated by a common underlying neurobiological mechanism.

Another recent study found that people with short copies of the 5-HTT gene exhibited more depressive symptoms, diagnosable depres-

TABLE 7–4. Influence of serotonin transporter (5-HTT) polymorphisms on depression and its treatment

Symptom presentation (Caspi et al. 2003)	Short allele carriers have more depressive symptoms and suicidality in relation to stressful life events
Personality traits (Murphy et al. 2001)	Short allele is associated with patients' increased "neuroticism" and "negative emotionality"
Treatment response (Melke 2003)	Long allele predicts better patient response to selective serotonin reuptake inhibitors

sion, and suicidality in relation to stressful life events than people who had long copies of the gene (Caspi et al. 2003). In other words, a genetic polymorphism of the *5-HTT* was found to moderate the influence of environmental stress on depression rather than simply causing depression. This finding has several potentially important implications for understanding the role of personality in refractory and chronic depression. Stress responsiveness may be genetically determined in some people, which might represent a common underlying vulnerability in patients with comorbid depression and personality disorders (Eley and Plomin 1997). This genetic mechanism might also mediate the reciprocal and interactive relationship between depression, personality pathology, and life stress. For example, genes affect aspects of the social environment, such as exposure to stressful life events and levels of social support, which in turn feed back on the risk of depression (Kendler 2001; Rose 2001). What is observed clinically (that personality pathology is associated with chronicity of depressive symptoms or a poor antidepressant response) may represent the phenotypic expression of an underlying genetically determined heightened susceptibility to environmental stress and/or a neurobiologically attenuated response to antidepressant drugs. Moreover, this pathophysiological model does not trivialize the relevance of cognitive, interpersonal, and other psychosocial processes, which influence and are influenced by genetic and environmental factors (Denenberg 2000; Durbin et al. 2000; Kendler 2001; McGue and Bouchard 1998).

Integrative Treatment of Depression and Comorbid Personality

The initial approach to patients with refractory or chronic depression begins with a comprehensive assessment of Axis I psychiatric disorders, including information from the patient as well as collateral

TABLE 7–5. Integrative assessment of depression and comorbid personality

Assessment	Information to be gathered
1. Comprehensive assessment of Axis I disorders	Information from patient and collateral sources
2. Information regarding current psychosocial functioning and optimal functioning in past years	Personality traits as child, teenager, young adult
3. Pharmacotherapy history	Drug dose, duration, response, adverse effects, compliance, outcome
4. Psychotherapy history	Therapy modality, duration, response, compliance, outcome

sources. Unrecognized syndromal or subsyndromal psychiatric conditions (e.g., bipolar disorder, atypical depression, anxiety disorders, psychosis, substance abuse) may be found in some patients with chronic or treatment resistant depression, and the presence of any of these associated conditions has obvious implications for considering particular pharmacotherapy and/or psychotherapy treatment options (Thase 1996). Similarly, information (from the patient and collateral sources) about current psychosocial functioning; optimal functioning in past years; and "basic" personality traits as a child, teenager, and young adult, especially during times when the patient has not been depressed, is needed in the assessment of Axis II disorders. Finally, past medication and psychotherapy treatment history is essential, including quantitative and qualitative information about treatment type, duration, adequacy, tolerability, compliance, and outcome (see Table 7–5).

For patients with clear-cut Axis II comorbidity, it is helpful to provide a nonjudgmental and nonpejorative description of the clinical assessment to the patient, including education about the nature of personality disorders and their potential impact on the course and treatment of depression. The treatment plan should be guided by the case formulation and past treatment history and should include considerations of various medication alternatives (Howland and Thase 1997; Thase et al. 2002), medication combinations (Thase et al. 1998), and psychotherapies (Keller et al. 2000; Thase et al. 2001) (see Table 7–6).

Pharmacotherapy

The relationship between personality disorder clusters and Axis I disorders suggests particular medication strategies (Aschauer and

TABLE 7–6. Feedback for treatment of patients with depression

The clinician should provide...
- A nonpejorative, nonjudgmental description of the clinical assessment
- Psychoeducation regarding the nature of personality disorders and potential impact on the course and treatment of depression
- A treatment plan guided by case formulation and past treatment history
- Consideration of various medication alternatives, medication combinations, and psychotherapies

Schlogelhofer 2003; Thase 1996). Depressed patients with Cluster C anxiety-related personality disorders might benefit more from the use of serotonergic antidepressant drugs that have been found to be effective in the treatment of various anxiety disorders. The SSRIs (i.e., fluvoxamine, fluoxetine, paroxetine, sertraline, citalopram, or escitalopram) and venlafaxine are effective treatments for generalized and social anxiety symptoms. Venlafaxine also has been shown to be effective in treatment-resistant depression (Thase et al. 2000) and more effective than SSRIs in patients with nonrefractory depression (Thase 2003). The antidepressants nefazodone and mirtazapine also have beneficial effects on symptoms of anxiety among patients with depression, and these might be appropriate alternatives to the SSRIs or venlafaxine. The antianxiety drug buspirone may have antidepressant effects at higher doses and could be used alone or in combination with one of these antidepressant medications. Obsessive-compulsive symptoms respond preferentially to the SSRIs or to the tricyclic antidepressant (TCA) clomipramine. Depressed patients with Cluster C personality disorders who fail to respond to adequate trials of the newer generation antidepressants (e.g., two or more SSRIs, venlafaxine, nefazodone, and mirtazapine) might benefit from the older generation TCA or monoamine oxidase inhibitor (MAOI) antidepressant drugs (Thase and Rush 1995; Thase et al. 2002). In particular, the MAOI phenelzine and the TCA clomipramine have demonstrated efficacy in the treatment of anxiety disorders and have especially good track records in the treatment of refractory depression (Thase and Rush 1995). Atypical forms of depression also respond preferentially to MAOIs (Thase et al. 1995).

Subtle signs of bipolar disorder (e.g., mood instability and impulsive behaviors) in patients with Cluster B personality disorders provide a clinical rationale for trying different mood-stabilizing medications, such as lithium, anticonvulsant drugs, or atypical antipsychotic drugs, either alone or in combination with antidepressant drugs (Markovitz 2004), especially in patients with borderline personality disorder

(Grossman 2002; Soloff 2000). Despite potential concerns about toxicity among patients prone to impulsive overdoses, lithium has been found to reduce the risk of suicide attempts and suicide deaths in bipolar disorder (Goodwin et al. 2003) and to reduce anger and suicidal thoughts in borderline personality (Links et al. 1990). Lithium also is the best studied and most effective augmentation therapy for refractory depression. Anticonvulsant drugs (e.g., valproic acid, lamotrigine, carbamazepine, and oxcarbazepine) are now used relatively more often than lithium in clinical practice for the treatment of bipolar disorder. There is developing evidence that they also may be effective in the treatment of borderline personality (Grossman 2002; Pinto and Akiskal 1998; Townsend et al. 2001) and to have significant antidepressant effects in unipolar and bipolar depression, including refractory depression (Barbee and Jamhour 2002; Barbosa et al. 2003; Calabrese et al. 2003). However, anticonvulsants may be less effective than lithium in reducing suicide attempts and suicide deaths in patients with bipolar disorder (Goodwin et al. 2003), although these drugs have not been directly compared in the treatment of patients with borderline personality. Atypical antipsychotic drugs (e.g., risperidone, olanzapine, quetiapine, ziprasidone, and aripiprazole) are now being used with increased frequency, often in combination with antidepressants, for the treatment of patients with bipolar disorder (Thase 2002; Tohen et al. 2003), refractory depression (Barbee et al. 2004; Corya et al. 2003), and borderline personality (Markovitz 2004; Zanarini et al. 2004). A recent study found that olanzapine alone and in combination with fluoxetine was more effective than fluoxetine alone for treating depression and impulsive aggression in patients with borderline personality, although fluoxetine alone also led to a substantial reduction in depression and impulsive aggression (Zanarini et al. 2004). Bipolar depression, which is often chronic and refractory to treatment, may respond somewhat better to MAOIs (Thase et al. 1995), the novel antidepressant bupropion (Sachs et al. 1994), the anticonvulsant lamotrigine (Calabrese et al. 2003), or the combination of olanzapine and fluoxetine (Tohen et al. 2003). Because of pharmacological differences among drugs within the group of anticonvulsants and within the group of atypical antipsychotics, depressed patients with Cluster C personality disorders who fail to respond to an initial trial of a mood-stabilizing medication might benefit from switching to an alternative drug from the same class. However, after failing to respond to adequate trials of at least two drugs from the same group, consideration should be given to switching to an alternative class of medication.

Patients with Cluster A personality disorders show subtle psychotic symptoms (e.g., paranoia or odd thoughts and behaviors) that may support the use of antipsychotic drugs (Markovitz 2004). The antidepressant effects of atypical antipsychotics, especially when combined with antidepressants, provide further clinical justification for their use in refractory depression as well as in psychotic depression (Rothschild et al. 2004). Because of pharmacological differences among atypical antipsychotic drugs, depressed patients with Cluster A personality disorders who fail to respond to an initial adequate trial of one medication might benefit from switching to an alternative antipsychotic. The older tetracyclic antidepressant amoxapine has antipsychotic and antidepressant effects and has been found to be effective alone in the treatment of psychotic depression (Rothschild et al. 1993). Electroconvulsive therapy (ECT) is considered a viable alternative to medications for the treatment of psychotic depression and should not be overlooked in depressed patients with comorbid personality disorders, especially in the presence of severe levels of depression or treatment resistance (DeBattista and Mueller 2001). Some guidelines for the use of medications in treatment-refractory depression are listed in Table 7–7.

Psychotherapy

An active psychoeducational and skills-oriented approach to psychotherapy is generally most useful for refractory and chronic depression in patients with comorbid personality disorders (Thase 1996). This approach should emphasize practical interpersonal, cognitive, and behavioral interventions that are individually tailored to help the patient achieve well-defined goals (see Table 7–8). A specific and detailed problem list of psychosocial difficulties is needed for setting short- and long-term treatment goals. The therapist and patient must work together to establish an agreement about the problems, goals, and potential strategies to try in therapy, with a willingness to try alternative approaches when an initial strategy is ineffective. It should be emphasized that although problems generally have solutions, better ways of coping with problems may be available when solutions are not immediately possible. The use of an eclectic mix of psychosocial methods is designed to address comprehensively the myriad complicated problems encountered in these patients (Lara and Klein 1999; Thase and Howland 1994). Moreover, this approach uses various treatment strategies that have been specifically developed and/or used for these types of patients (Jarrett et al. 1997; Linehan 1993; McCullough 2000; Weissman et al. 2000).

CBT is the best studied form of psychotherapy for chronic and refractory depression (Howland 1996; Keitner and Cardemil 2003; Thase

---

TABLE 7–7.   Suggested guidelines for psychopharmacological intervention in patients with treatment-refractory depression

---

- The initial choice of antidepressant medication should be based on depression subtype, associated symptom features, comorbidity, desired and/or expected side-effect profile, and prior medication history.

- Each medication should be used at the maximum tolerated approved dose for at least 6–12 weeks. In select cases, doses higher than the manufacturer's recommended maximum can be used with appropriate clinical monitoring.

- The goal of treatment should be full remission of depressive symptoms and significant recovery of psychosocial functioning.

- For patients showing a significant partial improvement with a single antidepressant drug, augmentation with a second agent or combination with a second antidepressant is preferred over switching to an alternative antidepressant.

- Recommendations for antidepressant augmentation include lithium, atypical antipsychotic drugs, buspirone, thyroid hormone, lamotrigine, and stimulant drugs. Recommendations for antidepressant combinations include mirtazapine plus selective serotonin reuptake inhibitors (SSRIs) or venlafaxine, bupropion plus SSRIs or venlafaxine, and tricyclic antidepressants plus SSRIs or venlafaxine.

- For patients showing minimal or no improvement with a single antidepressant drug, switching to an alternative antidepressant is preferred over augmentation with a second agent.

- For patients failing an initial trial of an SSRI antidepressant, switching to an alternative SSRI is appropriate. Patients failing trials of two SSRI antidepressants should be switched to an alternative antidepressant from a different class.

- Lithium, anticonvulsant drugs, and atypical antipsychotic drugs can be used together with antidepressants to treat associated symptoms (e.g., anger, mood instability, impulsiveness, subtle psychosis) and may also augment the mood effects of antidepressants.

- For patients with chronic and refractory depression, an effective medication or combination of medications should be maintained indefinitely with periodic clinical assessments for safety and tolerability. Medications should be slowly tapered and discontinued only after a long period of full remission and recovery.

---

et al. 2001). Modifications of CBT also have been developed to address the treatment of anxiety disorders and personality disorders (Beck et al. 1990; Jarrett et al. 1997; Nelson-Gray et al. 1996). Homework assignments are used to monitor and record the particular problems, situations, negative or distorted thoughts, and behavioral responses that occur outside therapy, contribute to depression, and can be addressed

TABLE 7–8. Suggested guidelines for psychotherapeutic intervention in patients with treatment-refractory depression

- The therapy relationships should be collaborative and centered around the goal of teaching new skills to improve coping with a chronic illness. Pair core therapeutic skills (e.g., empathy and understanding) with the ability to provide appropriately specific, targeted interventions (e.g., relaxation training, activity scheduling, problem solving, or cognitive restructuring).
- Make judicious use of examples from other medical models in which rehabilitative interventions are used to enhance the outcome of a chronic disorder (e.g., poststroke rehabilitation, pain management, or orthopedic rehabilitation).
- Express cautious optimism that problems can be addressed with varying degrees of success. It is important, however, to understand the patient's pessimism and to elicit feedback about what has not worked well in the past.
- Establish stepwise, short-term goals that specifically address the patient's problems or symptoms. Use graded tasks or intermediate assignments to approach more daunting or potentially overwhelming problems.
- Meet frequently and, if necessary, shorten sessions to enhance learning and retention. Keep sessions active and avoid the "silent treatment." Obtain feedback at the beginning and the end of treatment sessions so that the patient's reactions to therapy can be monitored and properly addressed. Be vigilant concerning subtle affective and behavioral reactions within sessions as an in vivo source of feedback.
- Use homework assignments and in-session rehearsal to facilitate development of new coping skills. It is important to avoid implicit criticisms about difficulties in therapy, such as homework noncompliance. The therapist must address his or her own dysfunctional cognitions blaming the patient for "not wanting to get better."
- Involve spouse or significant others to provide psychoeducation and to enhance alliance with family members.
- Establish intermediate and long-term goals as symptomatic improvement and short-term goals are accomplished.
- Do not terminate treatment until the patient has achieved a remission and sustained it for at least 4–6 months.

Source. Reprinted from Thase ME: "The Role of Axis II Comorbidity in the Management of Patients With Treatment-Resistant Depression," *The Psychiatric Clinics of North America,* Vol. 19, No. 2, pp. 287–309, 1996, ©1996, with permission from Elsevier.

within therapy sessions. Refractory and chronically depressed patients are often predisposed to assume a more pessimistic, hopeless, and passive role in their lives, which reinforces the depressed state. In CBT, patients learn to approach problems one step at a time by breaking them down into more discrete and potentially solvable tasks. The important goal is task completion, however, and not necessarily a successful out-come. Patients are also encouraged to pursue various activities that can lead to feelings of pleasure and success and that can counter symptoms such as lack of motivation, isolation, and withdrawal. By way of exam-ple, a depressed person who has long been rigid, perfectionistic, overly preoccupied with details, indecisive, and excessively devoted to work may have a comorbid obsessive-compulsive personality disorder. Ther-apeutic techniques in CBT may be appropriate for addressing depres-sive symptoms as well as underlying obsessive-compulsive traits in such a patient.

Many depressed patients with personality disorders have difficul-ties with emotional dysregulation, and they may have significant prob-lems with irritability, anger, and controlling impulsive behaviors (Linehan 2000). Various cognitive and behavioral strategies, such as identification of cognitions associated with angry outbursts, distrac-tion, guided imagery, relaxation techniques, and skills training, have been used in anger management. For example, a comprehensive cogni-tive-behavioral treatment model known as dialectical behavior therapy (DBT) has been developed for patients with borderline personality dis-order (Linehan 1993). In DBT, patients learn greater awareness and ac-ceptance of their emotions, thinking, and patterns of behavior, and they develop alternative self-control skills that can be used to manage intol-erable emotional states and reduce maladaptive behaviors. Patients learn to identify the chain of thoughts and feelings that precede mal-adaptive behaviors, and they learn to implement alternative ways of coping. For example, a chronically depressed person who has a long-standing pattern of unstable interpersonal relationships, poor self-image, mood instability, and impulsive behaviors consistent with a comorbid borderline personality disorder would be a good candidate for DBT.

IPT is an effective treatment for depression, although it is not as well studied as CBT (Klerman et al. 1984; Weissman et al. 2000). Interper-sonal difficulties are an obvious problem in patients with personality disorders, and these problems are accentuated in the face of chronic or refractory depression. Some effort has been made to tailor IPT to these patients (Markowitz 1998, 2003; McCray and King 2003; Weissman et al. 2000). Much of the focus in IPT is on difficulties in the patient's current interpersonal relationships, including problems associated with grief, interpersonal role disputes, role transitions, and interpersonal deficits, although past interpersonal problems also are explored and are used to understand maladaptive patterns and to identify areas for change. Pa-tients are encouraged to examine how depression has affected their lives and how they can work to become well again. Techniques commonly used in IPT include facilitating affect (e.g., expressing repressed anger), encouraging activity and socialization, exploring different options for achieving life goals, examining communication problems, clarifying the patient's understanding of his or her interpersonal style, and using the therapy relationship to examine and work through interpersonal problems. For example, a chronically depressed person who is socially inept and inhibited avoids occupational activities that involve significant interpersonal contact and is inhibited in new interpersonal situations because of feelings of inadequacy may have an underlying avoidant personality disorder, and the use of IPT might be appropriate for targeting his or her depression and interpersonal difficulties. Marital discord also is associated with a poor antidepressant treatment outcome, and some patients may benefit from couple's therapy (Goering et al. 1992).

Social skills training (SST) is a particular behavioral approach that targets inadequate or dysfunctional interpersonal behaviors (Becker et al. 1987). Because important reinforcers for most adults occur in interpersonal activities, insufficient positive reinforcement of nondepressed behavior may contribute to the development or persistence of depression. Poor interpersonal function can be attributed to many factors, including inadequate or maladaptive social skills, a failure to recognize or accurately interpret social cues, a lack of assertiveness, and a belief that their skills will be ineffective in social situations. Chronically depressed patients, especially those with comorbid personality disorders, may be socially ineffective or may engage in interpersonally aversive behaviors that worsen their psychosocial problems (Gilbert and Connolly 1991). SST consists of evaluating the patient's social performance, practical social skills training, role playing and practice exercises to reinforce these skills, learning perceptual skills to use in interpersonal situations, and teaching patients to monitor their performance and to provide themselves with positive reinforcement. Thus, patients learn practical skills that will improve their relationships, increase their socialization, and enhance their self-esteem by their interpersonal success. SST has been shown to have a significant antidepressant effect and improve the psychosocial environment of depressed patients (Hersen et al. 1984). An SST treatment model has also been developed for use in the treatment of patients with personality disorders (Stanley et al. 2001). For example, a depressed person who has a pervasive pattern of social and interpersonal deficits because of odd beliefs, peculiar speech, and eccentric behaviors may have a comorbid schizotypal personality disorder. The use of SST may be helpful in the overall management of such a patient.

Cognitive-behavioral analysis system of psychotherapy (CBASP) is a psychotherapy model that was specifically developed for the treatment of chronic depression (McCullough 2000). CBASP is a highly structured therapy that combines important elements of CBT, IPT, and SST. The emphasis in CBASP is on teaching patients to associate their behavioral responses and faulty interpretations of events with interpersonal outcomes. Careful attention is paid to potential pitfalls in the therapeutic alliance that can derail therapy. An important goal of CBASP is for patients to learn to take a perspective that facilitates achieving their desired outcome in interpersonal situations and to take actions that lead more directly to their desired outcomes, with consequent improvements in social support systems. CBASP has been shown to be as effective as antidepressant medication in the treatment of chronic depression (Keller et al. 2000). Although CBASP has not yet been specifically applied to the treatment of personality disorders, the cognitive, interpersonal, and behavioral skills techniques that are used may be relevant to this patient population. For example, a chronically depressed person with a long-standing pattern of allowing others to make decisions, lacking initiative, having difficulty disagreeing with others, and feeling helpless when alone may have a comorbid dependent personality disorder, and CBASP might be very effective in targeting the patient's chronic depressive symptoms and associated personality traits. Of interest in this respect, CBASP alone was found to have significant effects on psychosocial function in chronically depressed patients, and this improvement was relatively independent of changes in depressive symptoms (Hirschfeld et al. 2002).

Combination Treatment

Most patients with refractory or chronic depression and comorbid personality disorders will benefit from some combination of pharmacotherapy and psychotherapy, which will often require coordination between a nonmedical psychotherapist and a pharmacotherapist (Chiles et al. 1991). Pharmacotherapy and psychotherapy can each be provided within a clearly focused and rigorous conceptual model of treatment (Howland and Thase 2003). Close collaboration will be needed, however, to avoid problems with treatment splitting that may undermine or contradict the efforts of each provider. Obviously, this problem is more likely to occur in the treatment of patients with comorbid personality disorders.

Although there are no formal controlled studies of combined treatment in refractory or chronic depression specifically addressing comorbid personality disorders, there is some evidence that combination treatment may be more effective than pharmacotherapy alone in these patients (Hellerstein et al. 2001; Kool et al. 2003a, 2003b). In addition, many studies have demonstrated the relative benefits of combining psychotherapy and pharmacotherapy in patients with chronic and refractory depression, who are more likely to suffer from comorbid personality pathology (Howland 1996, 2003; Keitner and Cardemil 2003; Thase et al. 2001).

A recent large randomized study comparing the antidepressant nefazodone alone, CBASP, and their combination in 681 patients with chronic major depression or double depression found that the treatment response rate to nefazodone or to CBASP alone was approximately 50% after 12 weeks (Keller et al. 2000). This response rate was impressive for a very chronically depressed group of patients (the average duration of their current episode of dysthymia was approximately 23 years and approximately 8 years for their current episode of major depression) but was significantly less than the astounding 70% response rate seen in the combined treatment group. Those patients receiving nefazodone (either alone or in combination) responded to treatment significantly earlier than the CPASP only group. Moreover, combination treatment resulted in relatively greater improvements in psychosocial functioning (Hirschfeld et al. 2002). An ongoing study is currently investigating the efficacy of adjunctive CBASP (compared with a supportive psychotherapy) in the treatment of patients with chronic depression who have not responded fully to antidepressant medication.

Conclusions

A significant proportion of patients with refractory and chronic depression have personality disorders. The relationship between personality, depression, and treatment outcome, however, is very complex. The development of chronicity or treatment resistance likely reflects the compounded effects of various psychosocial and neurobiological risk factors in these patients. Nevertheless, a variety of psychotherapeutic and pharmacological treatment options are available, and other promising therapies are currently being developed or are being investigated for these difficult-to-treat patients. Even among those patients who do not appear to benefit from any type of antidepressant therapy, ongoing therapeutic support should help patients to grieve the loss of their "healthy" self, to gain acceptance of their illness and its inherent limitations, and to rely on existing strengths and coping strategies to manage their lives. This is not unlike the approach to living with other chronic medical conditions. Moreover, it is important not to lose hope: long-term outcome studies have shown that there is a small cumulative chance of remission from chronic depression, even after having it for many years (Keller et al. 1992; Winokur and Morrison 1973).

References

Aberg-Wistedt A, Agren H, Ekselius L, et al: Sertraline versus paroxetine in major depression: clinical outcome after six months of continuous therapy. J Clin Psychopharmacol 20:645–652, 2000

Allgulander C, Cloninger CR, Przybeck TR, et al: Changes on the Temperament and Character Inventory after paroxetine treatment in volunteers with generalized anxiety disorder. Psychopharmacol Bull 34:165–166, 1998

American Psychiatric Association: Diagnostic and Statistical Manual of Mental Disorders, 4th Edition, Text Revision. Washington, DC, American Psychiatric Association, 2000

Aschauer HN, Schlogelhofer M: Anxiety, depression, and personality, in Handbook of Depression and Anxiety, 2nd Edition. Edited by Kasper S, den Boer JA, Ad Sitsen JM. New York, Marcel Dekker, 2003, pp 91–110

Bagby RM, Levitan RD, Kennedy SH, et al: Selective alteration of personality in response to noradrenergic and serotonergic antidepressant medication in depressed sample: evidence of nonspecificity. Psychiatry Res 86:211–216, 1999

Bagby RM, Gilchrist EJ, Rector NA, et al: The stability and validity of the sociotropy and autonomy personality dimensions as measured by the revised personal style inventory. Cognit Ther Res 21:765–779, 2001

Bagby RM, Ryder AG, Cristi C: Psychosocial and clinical predictors of response to pharmacotherapy for depression. J Psychiatry Neurosci 27:250–257, 2002

Ball J, Kearney B, Wilhelm K, et al: Cognitive behaviour therapy and assertion training groups for patients with depression and comorbid personality disorders. Behavioural and Cognitive Psychotherapy 28:71–85, 2000

Barbee JG, Jamhour NJ: Lamotrigine as an augmentation agent in treatment-resistant depression. J Clin Psychiatry 63:737–741, 2002

Barbee JG, Conrad EJ, Jamhour NJ: The effectiveness of olanzapine, risperidone, quetiapine, and ziprasidone as augmentation agents in treatment-resistant major depressive disorder. J Clin Psychiatry 65:975–981, 2004

Barber JP, Muenz LR: The role of avoidance and obsessiveness in matching patients to cognitive and interpersonal psychotherapy: empirical findings from the treatment for depression collaborative research program. J Consult Clin Psychology 64:951–958, 1996

Barbosa L, Berk M, Vorster M: A double-blind, randomized, placebo-controlled trial of augmentation with lamotrigine or placebo in patients concomitantly treated with fluoxetine for resistant major depressive episodes. J Clin Psychiatry 64:403–407, 2003

Barnett PA, Gotlib IH: Psychosocial functioning and depression: distinguishing among antecedents, concomitants, and consequences. Psychol Bull 104:97–126, 1988

Bearden C, Lavelle N, Buysse D, et al: Personality pathology and time to remission in depressed outpatients treated with interpersonal psychotherapy. J Pers Disorders 10:164–173, 1996

Beck A, Freeman A, Associates: Cognitive Therapy of Personality Disorders. New York, Guilford, 1990

Becker R, Heimberg R, Bellack A: Social Skills Training for Treatment for Depression. New York, Pergamon, 1987

Bender DS, Dolan RT, Skodol AE, et al: Treatment utilization by patients with personality disorders. Am J Psychiatry 158:295–302, 2001

Black KJ, Sheline YI: Personality disorder scores improve with effective pharmacotherapy of depression. J Affect Disord 43:11–18, 1997

Bond AJ: Neurotransmitters, temperament and social functioning. Eur Neuropsychopharmacol 11:261–264, 2001

Bouchard TJ, Loehlin JC: Genes, evolution, and personality. Behav Genet 31:243–273, 2001

Brett JF, Brief AP, Burke MJ, et al: Negative affectivity and the reporting of stressful life events. Health Psychol 9:57–68, 1990

Bschor T, Canata B, Muller-Oerlinghausen B, et al: Predictors of response to lithium augmentation in tricyclic antidepressant-resistant depression. J Affect Disord 64:261–265, 2001

Buck R: The biological affects: a typology. Psychol Rev 106:301–336, 1999

Calabrese JR, Bowden CL, Sachs G, et al: A placebo-controlled 18-month trial of lamotrigine and lithium maintenance treatment in recently depressed patients with bipolar I disorder. J Clin Psychiatry 64:1013–1024, 2003

Caspi A, Sugden K, Moffitt TE, et al: Influence of life stress on depression: moderation by a polymorphism in the 5-HTT gene. Science 301:386–389, 2003

Chiles JA, Carlin AS, Benjamin GAH, et al: A physician, a nonmedical psychotherapist, and a patient: the pharmacotherapist-psychotherapy triangle, in Integrating Pharmacotherapy and Psychotherapy. Edited by Beitman BD, Klerman GL. Washington, DC, American Psychiatric Press, 1991, pp 105–118

Cloninger CR: A new conceptual paradigm from genetics and psychobiology for the science of mental health. Aust N Z J Psychiatry 33:174–186, 1999

Cloninger CR, Svrakic DM, Przybeck TR: A psychobiological model of temperament and character. Arch Gen Psychiatry 50:975–990, 1993

Cohen LH, Towbes LC, Flocco R: Effects of induced mood on self-reported life events and perceived and received social support. J Pers Soc Psychol 55:669–674, 1988

Coombs MM, Coleman D, Jones EE: Working with feelings: the importance of emotion in both cognitive-behavioral and interpersonal therapy in the NIMH treatment of depression collaborative research program. Psychotherapy: Theory, Research, Practice, Training 39:233–244, 2002

Corruble E, Duret C, Pelissolo A, et al: Early and delayed personality changes associated with depression recovery? A one-year follow-up study. Psychiatry Res 109:17–25, 2002

Corya SA, Anderson SW, Detke HC, et al: Long-term antidepressant efficacy and safety of olanzapine/fluoxetine combination: a 76-week open-label study. J Clin Psychiatry 64:1349–1356, 2003

Coryell W, Scheftner W, Keller M, et al: The enduring psychosocial consequences of mania and depression. Am J Psychiatry 150:720–727, 1993

Davidson J, Miller R, Strickland R: Neuroticism and personality disorder in depression. J Affect Disord 8:177–182, 1985

DeBattista C, Mueller K: Is electroconvulsive therapy effective for the depressed patient with comorbid borderline personality disorder? J ECT 17:91–98, 2001

Denenberg VH: Evolution proposes and ontogeny disposes. Brain Lang 73:274–296, 2000

Du L, Bakish D, Ravindran AV, et al: Does fluoxetine influence major depression by modifying five-factor personality traits? J Affect Disord 71:235–241, 2002

Durbin CE, Klein DN, Schwartz JE: Predicting the 2 ½ year outcome of dysthymic disorder: the roles of childhood adversity and family history of psychopathology. J Consult Clin Psychol 68:57–63, 2000

Ekselius L, Bengtsson F, von Knorring L: Non-compliance with pharmacotherapy of depression is associated with a sensation seeking personality. Int Clin Psychopharmacol 15:273–278, 2000

Eley TC, Plomin R: Genetic analyses of emotionality. Curr Opin Neurobiol 7:279–284, 1997

Farmer R, Nelson-Gray R: Personality disorders in depression: hypothetical relations, empirical findings, and methodological considerations. Clin Psychol Rev 10:453–476, 1990

Frank E, Kupfer DJ: Axis II personality disorders and personality features in treatment-resistant and refractory depression, in Treatment Strategies for Refractory Depression. Edited by Roose SP, Glassman AH. Washington, DC, American Psychiatric Press, 1990, pp 207–221

Friedman RA: Social and occupational adjustment in chronic depression, in Diagnosis and Treatment of Chronic Depression. Edited by Kocsis JH, Klein DN. New York, Guilford Press, 1995, pp 89–102

Gilbert DG, Connolly JJ (eds): Personality, Social Skills, and Psychopathology: An Individual Differences Approach. New York, Plenum, 1991

Goering PN, Lancee WJ, Freeman SJJ: Marital support and recovery from depression. Br J Psychiatry 160:76–82, 1992

Goodwin FK, Fireman B, Simon GE, et al: Suicide risk in bipolar disorder during treatment with lithium and divalproex. JAMA 290:1467–1473, 2003

Grossman R: Psychopharmacologic treatment of patients with borderline personality disorder. Psychiatr Ann 32:357–370, 2002

Hammen C, Ellicott A, Gitlin M, et al: Sociotropy/autonomy and vulnerability to specific life events in patients with unipolar depression and bipolar disorders. J Abnorm Psychol 98:154–160, 1989

Hardy GE, Barkham M, Shapiro DA, et al: Impact of cluster C personality disorders on outcomes of contrasting brief psychotherapies for depression. J Consult Clin Psychol 63:997–1004, 1995

Harkness KL, Bagby RM, Joffe RT, et al: Major depression, chronic minor depression, and the five-factor model of personality. European Journal of Personality 16:271–281, 2002

Harrison WM, Stewart JW: Pharmacotherapy of dysthymic disorder, in Diagnosis and Treatment of Chronic Depression. Edited by Kocsis JH, Klein DN. New York, Guilford, 1995, pp 124–145

Hayden EP, Klein DN: Outcome of dysthymic disorder at 5-year follow-up: the effect of familial psychopathology, early adversity, personality, comorbidity, and chronic stress. Am J Psychiatry 158:1864–1870, 2001

Hellerstein DJ, Kocsis JH, Chapman D, et al: Double-blind comparison of sertraline, imipramine, and placebo in the treatment of dysthymia: effects on personality. Am J Psychiatry 157:1436–1444, 2000

Hellerstein DJ, Little SAS, Samstag LW, et al: Adding group psychotherapy to medication treatment in dysthymia: a randomized prospective pilot study. J Psychother Pract Res 10:93–103, 2001

Hersen M, Bellack AS, Himmelhoch JM, et al: Effects of social skill training, amitriptyline, and psychotherapy in unipolar depressed women. Behav Ther 15:21–40, 1984

Hirano S, Sato T, Narita T, et al: Evaluating the state dependency of the temperament and character inventory dimensions in patients with major depression: a methodological contribution. J Affect Disord 69:31–38, 2002

Hirschfeld RM, Shea MS: Personality, in Handbook of Affective Disorders, 2nd Edition. Edited by Paykel ES. New York, Guilford, 1992, pp 185–194

Hirschfeld RM, Klerman GL, Lavori P, et al: Premorbid personality assessment of first onset of major depression. Arch Gen Psychiatry 46:345–350, 1989

Hirschfeld RM, Russell JM, Delgado PL, et al: Predictors of response to acute treatment of chronic and double depression with sertraline or imipramine. J Clin Psychiatry 59:669–675, 1998

Hirschfeld RM, Dunner DL, Keitner G, et al: Does psychosocial functioning improve independent of depressive symptoms? A comparison of nefazodone, psychotherapy, and their combination. Biol Psychiatry 51:123–133, 2002

Howland RH: Pharmacotherapy of dysthymia. J Clin Psychopharmacol 11:83–92, 1991

Howland RH: Chronic depression. Hosp Community Psychiatry 44:633–639, 1993

Howland RH: Psychosocial therapies for dysthymia, in The Hatherleigh Guide to Managing Depression. Edited by Flach FF. New York, Hatherleigh Press, 1996, pp 225–241

Howland RH: Psychopharmacology of dysthymia, in Handbook of Chronic Depression. Edited by Alpert JE, Fava M. New York, Marcel Dekker, 2003, pp 139–158

Howland RH, Thase ME: Switching strategies for the treatment of unipolar major depression. Mod Probl Pharmacopsychiatry 25:56–65, 1997

Howland RH, Thase ME: Combining psychotherapy and pharmacotherapy for depression and anxiety, in Handbook of Depression and Anxiety, 2nd Edition. Edited by Kasper S, den Boer JA, Ad Sitsen JM. New York, Marcel Dekker, 2003, pp 151–163

Jarrett RB, Kraft D, Silver P: Cognitive therapy of mood disorders with comorbidity, in Treatment Strategies for Patients With Psychiatric Comorbidity. Edited by Wetzler S, Sanderson WC. New York, Wiley, 1997, pp 135–162

Joyce PR, Paykel ES: Predictors of drug response in depression. Arch Gen Psychiatry 46:89–99, 1989

Joyce PR, Mulder RT, Cloninger CR: Temperament predicts clomipramine and desipramine response in major depression. J Affect Disord 30:35–46, 1994

Keitner GI, Cardemil EV: Psychotherapy for chronic depressive disorders, in Handbook of Chronic Depression. Edited by Alpert JE, Fava M. New York, Marcel Dekker, 2003, pp 159–181

Keller MB, Lavori PW, Mueller TI, et al: Time to recovery, chronicity, and levels of psychopathology in major depression: a 5-year prospective follow-up of 431 subjects. Arch Gen Psychiatry 49:809–816, 1992

Keller MB, McCullough JP, Klein DN, et al: A comparison of nefazodone, the cognitive behavioral-analysis system of psychotherapy, and their combination for the treatment of chronic depression. N Engl J Med 342:1462–1470, 2000

Kendler KS: Adversity, stress, and psychopathology: a psychiatric genetic perspective. Int J Methods Psychiatr Res 5:163–170, 1995

Kendler KS: Twin studies of psychiatric illness: an update. Arch Gen Psychiatry 58:1005–1014, 2001

Kendler KS, Neale MC, Kesler RC, et al: A twin study of recent life events and difficulties. Arch Gen Psychiatry 50:589–596, 1993

Kiesler DJ: Contemporary Interpersonal Theory and Research: Personality, Psychopathology, and Psychotherapy. New York, Wiley, 1996

Klein DN, Schatzberg AF, McCullough JP, et al: Early- versus late-onset dysthymic disorder: comparison in outpatients with superimposed major depressive episodes. J Affect Disord 52:187–196, 1999a

Klein DN, Schatzberg AF, McCullough JP, et al: Age of onset in chronic major depression: relation to demographic and clinical variables, family history, and treatment response. J Affect Disord 55:149–157, 1999b

Klein DN, Durbin CE, Shankman SA, et al: Depression and personality, in Handbook of Depression and Its Treatment. Edited by Gotlib IH, Hammen CL. New York, Guilford, 2002, pp 115–140

Klerman GL, Weissman MM, Rounsaville BJ, et al: Interpersonal Psychotherapy of Depression. New York, Basic Books, 1984

Kocsis JH, Zisook S, Davidson J, et al: Double-blind comparison of sertraline, imipramine, and placebo in the treatment of dysthymia: psychosocial outcomes. Am J Psychiatry 154:390–395, 1997

Kocsis JH, Schatzberg AF, Rush AJ, et al: Psychosocial outcomes following long-term, double-blind treatment of chronic depression with sertraline vs placebo. Arch Gen Psychiatry 59:723–728, 2002

Kool S, Dekker J, Duijsens IJ, et al: Changes in personality pathology after pharmacotherapy and combined therapy for depressed patients. J Personal Disord 17:60–72, 2003a

Kool S, Dekker J, Duijsens IJ, et al: Efficacy of combined therapy and pharmacotherapy for depressed patients with or without personality disorders. Harv Rev Psychiatry 11:133–141, 2003b

Kuyken W, Kurzer N, DeRubeis RJ, et al: Response to cognitive therapy in depression: the role of maladaptive beliefs and personality disorders. J Consult Clin Psychol 69:560–566, 2001

Kwon JS, Kim YM, Chang CG, et al: Three-year follow-up of women with the sole diagnosis of depressive personality disorder: subsequent development of dysthymia and major depression. Am J Psychiatry 157:1966–1972, 2000

Lara ME, Klein DN: Psychosocial processes underlying the maintenance and persistence of depression: implications for understanding chronic depression. Clin Psychol Rev 19:553–570, 1999

Lesch KP, Greenberg BD, Higley JD, et al: Serotonin transporter, personality, and behavior: toward a dissection of gene-gene and gene-environment interaction, in Molecular Genetics and the Human Personality. Edited by Benjamin J, Ebstein RP. Washington, DC, American Psychiatric Publishing, 2002, pp 109–135

Lewinsohn PM, Rohde P, Seeley JR, et al: Axis II psychopathology as a function of axis I disorders in childhood and adolescence. J Am Acad Child Adolesc Psychiatry 36:1752–1759, 1997

Linehan MM: Cognitive-Behavioral Treatment of Borderline Personality Disorder. New York, Guilford, 1993

Linehan MM: Commentary on innovations in dialectical behavior therapy. Cogn Behav Ther 7:478–481, 2000

Links PS, Steiner M, Boiago I, et al: Lithium therapy for borderline patients: preliminary findings. J Personal Disord 4:173–181, 1990

Marijnissen G, Tuinier S, Sijben AES, et al: The temperament and character inventory in major depression. J Affect Disord 70:219–223, 2002

Markovitz PJ: Recent trends in the pharmacotherapy of personality disorders. J Personality Disord 18:99–101, 2004

Markowitz JC: Interpersonal Psychotherapy for Dysthymic Disorder. Washington, DC, American Psychiatric Press, 1998

Markowitz JC: Interpersonal psychotherapy for chronic depression. J Clin Psychology 59:847–858, 2003

Markowitz JC, Moran ME, Kocsis JH, et al: Prevalence and comorbidity of dysthymic disorders among psychiatric outpatients. J Affect Disord 24:63–71, 1992

Mazure CM, Bruce ML, Maciejewski PK, et al: Adverse life events and cognitive-personality characteristics in the prediction of major depression and antidepressant response. Am J Psychiatry 157:896–903, 2000

McCray JA, King AR: Personality disorder attributes as supplemental goals for change in interpersonal psychotherapy. Journal of Contemporary Psychotherapy 33:79–92, 2003

McCullough JP Jr: Treatment for Chronic Depression: Cognitive Behavioral Analysis System of Psychotherapy (CBASP). New York, Guilford, 2000

McGue M, Bouchard TJ: Genetic and environmental influences on human behavioral differences. Annu Rev Neurosci 21:1–24, 1998

Melke J: Serotonin transporter gene polymorphisms and mental health. Curr Opin Psychiatry 16:215–220, 2003

Merrill KA, Tolbert VE, Wade WA: Effectiveness of cognitive therapy for depression in a community mental health center: a benchmarking study. J Consult Clin Psychol 71:404–409, 2003

Miller IW, Norman W, Dow M: Psychosocial characteristics of "double depression." Am J Psychiatry 143:1042–1044, 1986

Miller IW, Keitner GI, Schatzberg AF, et al: The treatment of chronic depression, part 3: psychosocial functioning before and after treatment with sertraline or imipramine. J Clin Psychiatry 59:608–619, 1998

Mulder RT, Joyce PR, Luty SE: The relationship of personality disorders to treatment outcome in depressed outpatients. J Clin Psychiatry 64:259–264, 2003

Murphy DL, Li Q, Engel S, et al: Genetic perspectives on the serotonin transporter. Brain Res Bull 56:487–494, 2001

Nelson E, Cloninger CR: Exploring the TPQ as a possible predictor of antidepressant response to nefazodone in a large multi-site study. J Affect Disord 44:197–200, 1997

Nelson-Gray RO, Johnson D, Foyle LW, et al: The effectiveness of cognitive therapy tailored to depressives with personality disorders. J Pers Disord 10:132–152, 1996

Newman JR, Ewing SE, McColl RD, et al: Tridimensional personality questionnaire and treatment response in major depressive disorder: a negative study. J Affect Disord 57:241–247, 2000

Ozkaragoz T, Noble EP: Extraversion: interaction between D2 dopamine receptor polymorphisms and parental alcoholism. Alcohol 22:139–146, 2000

Parker G, Roy K, Hadzi-Pavlovic D, et al: Distinguishing early and late onset non-melancholic unipolar depression. J Affect Disord 74:131–138, 2003

Peselow ED, Robins C, Block P, et al: Dysfunctional attitudes in depressed patients before and after clinical treatment and in normal control subjects. Am J Psychiatry 147:439–444, 1990

Petersen T, Papakostas GI, Bottonari K, et al: NEO-FFI factor scores as predictors of clinical response to fluoxetine in depressed outpatients. Psychiatry Res 109:9–16, 2002a

Petersen T, Hughes M, Papakostas GI, et al: Treatment-resistant depression and axis II comorbidity. Psychother Psychosom 71:269–274, 2002b

Pinto OC, Akiskal HS: Lamotrigine as a promising approach to borderline personality: an open case series without concurrent DSM-IV major mood disorder. J Affect Disord 51:333–343, 1998

Plomin R: Genetics and Experience: The Interplay Between Nature and Nurture. Thousand Oaks, CA, Sage, 1994

Rivas-Vazquez RA, Blais MA: Pharmacologic treatment of personality disorders. Prof Psychol Res Pr 33:104–107, 2002

Reich JH, Green AI: Effect of personality disorders on outcome of treatment. J Nerv Ment Dis 179:74–82, 1991

Reich JH, Vasile RG: Effect of personality disorders on the treatment outcome of Axis I conditions: an update. J Nerv Ment Dis 181:475–484, 1993

Robins CJ, Block P: Cognitive theories of depression viewed from a diathesis-stress perspective: evaluations of the models of Beck and of Abramson, Seligman, and Teasdale. Cognit Ther Res 13:297–313, 1989

Robins CJ, Bagby RM, Rector NA, et al: Sociotropy, autonomy, and patterns of symptoms in patients with major depression: a comparison of dimensional and categorical approaches. Cognit Ther Res 21:285–300, 1997

Rose S: Moving on from old dichotomies: beyond nature-nurture towards a lifetime perspective. Br J Psychiatry 178 (suppl 40):S3–S7, 2001

Rothschild L, Zimmerman M: Interface between personality and depression, in Handbook of Chronic Depression. Edited by Alpert JE, Fava M. New York, Marcel Dekker, 2003, pp 19–48

Rothschild AJ, Samson JA, Bessette MP, et al: Efficacy of the combination of fluoxetine and perphenazine in the treatment of psychotic depression. J Clin Psychiatry 54:338–342, 1993

Rothschild AJ, Williamson DJ, Tohen MF, et al: A double-blind, randomized study of olanzapine and olanzapine/fluoxetine combination for major depression with psychotic features. J Clin Psychopharmacol 24:365–373, 2004

Russell JM, Kornstein SG, Shea MT, et al: Chronic depression and comorbid personality disorders: response to sertraline versus imipramine. J Clin Psychiatry 64:554–561, 2003

Sachs GS, Lafer B, Stoll AL, et al: A double-blind trial of bupropion versus desipramine for bipolar depression. J Clin Psychiatry 55:391–393, 1994

Sanderson WC, Wetzler S, Beck AT, et al: Prevalence of personality disorders in patients with major depression and dysthymia. Psychiatr Res 42:93–99, 1992

Sato T, Sakado K, Uehara T, et al: Personality disorder comorbidity in early onset versus late-onset major depression in Japan. J Nerv Ment Dis 187:237–242, 1999a

Sato T, Hirano S, Narita T, et al: Temperament and character inventory dimensions as a predictor of response to antidepressant treatment in major depression. J Affect Disord 56:153–161, 1999b

Scott J, Eccleston D, Boys R: Can we predict the persistence of depression? Br J Psychiatry 161:633–637, 1992

Shea MT, Pilkonis PA, Beckham E, et al: Personality disorders and treatment outcome in the NIMH treatment of depression collaborative research program. Am J Psychiatry 147:711–718, 1990

Shea MT, Widiger TA, Klein MH: Comorbidity of personality disorders and depression: implications for treatment. J Consult Clin Psychol 60:857–868, 1992

Sirey JA, Bruce ML, Alexopoulos GS, et al: Perceived stigma and patient-rated severity of illness as predictors of antidepressant drug adherence. Psychiatr Serv 52:1615–1620, 2001

Soloff PH: Psychopharmacology of borderline personality disorder. Psychiatr Clin North Am 23:169–192, 2000

Sotsky SM, Glass DR, Shea MT, et al: Patient predictors of response to psychotherapy and pharmacotherapy: findings in the NIMH treatment of depression collaborative research program. Am J Psychiatry 148:997–1008, 1991

Stanley B, Bundy E, Beberman R: Skills training as an adjunctive treatment for personality disorders. J Psychiatr Pract 7:324–335, 2001

Stuart S, Simons AD, Thase ME, et al: Are personality assessments valid in acute major depression? J Affect Disord 24:281–290, 1992

Thase ME: The role of axis II comorbidity in the management of patients with treatment-resistant depression. Psychiatr Clin North Am 19:287–309, 1996

Thase ME: What role do atypical antipsychotic drugs have in treatment-resistant depression? J Clin Psychiatry 63:95–103, 2002

Thase ME: Effectiveness of antidepressants: comparative remission rates. J Clin Psychiatry 64 (suppl 2):3–7, 2003

Thase ME, Beck AT: An overview of cognitive therapy, in Cognitive Therapy With Inpatients: Developing a Cognitive Milieu. Edited by Wright JH, Thase ME, Beck AT, et al. New York, Guilford, 1992, pp 3–34

Thase ME, Howland R: Refractory depression: relevance of psychosocial factors and therapies. Psychiatr Ann 24:232–240, 1994

Thase ME, Kupfer DJ: Characteristics of treatment-resistant depression, in Treating Resistant Depression. Edited by Zohar J, Belmaker RH. New York, PMA Publishing, 1987, pp 23–45

Thase ME, Rush AJ: Treatment-resistant depression, in Psychopharmacology: The Fourth Generation of Progress. Edited by Bloom FE, Kupfer DJ. New York, Raven, 1995, pp 1081–1097

Thase ME, Trivedi MH, Rush AJ: MAOIs in the contemporary treatment of depression. Neuropsychopharmacol 12:185–219, 1995

Thase ME, Howland RH, Friedman ES: Treating antidepressant nonresponders with augmentation strategies: an overview. J Clin Psychiatry 59 (suppl 5):5–15, 1998

Thase ME, Friedman ES, Howland RH: Venlafaxine and treatment-resistant depression. Depress Anxiety 12 (suppl 1):55–62, 2000

Thase ME, Friedman ES, Howland RH: Management of treatment-resistant depression: psychotherapeutic perspectives. J Clin Psychiatry 62 (suppl 18):18–24, 2001

Thase ME, Rush AJ, Howland RH, et al: Double-blind switch study of imipramine or sertraline treatment of antidepressant-resistant chronic depression. Arch Gen Psychiatry 59:233–239, 2002

Tohen M, Vieta E, Calabrese J, et al: Efficacy of olanzapine and olanzapine-fluoxetine combination in the treatment of bipolar I depression. Arch Gen Psychiatry 60:1079–1088, 2003

Tome MB, Cloninger CR, Watson JP, et al: Serotonergic autoreceptor blockade in the reduction of antidepressant latency: personality variables and response to paroxetine and pindolol. J Affect Disord 44:101–109, 1997

Townsend MH, Cambre KM, Barbee JG: Treatment of borderline personality disorder with mood instability with divalproex sodium: series of ten cases. J Clin Psychopharmacol 21:249–251, 2001

Tranter R, Healy H, Cattell D, et al: Functional effects of agents differentially selective to noradrenergic or serotonergic systems. Psychol Med 32:517–524, 2002

Tse WS, Bond AJ: Serotonergic involvement in the psychosocial dimensions of personality. J Psychopharmacol 15:195–198, 2001

Tyrer P, Casey P, Gall J: Relationships between neurosis and personality disorder. Br J Psychiatry 142:404–408, 1983

Weissman MM, Markowitz JC, Klerman GL: Comprehensive Guide to Interpersonal Psychotherapy. New York, Basic Books, 2000

Winokur G, Morrison J: The Iowa 500: follow-up of 225 depressives. Br J Psychiatry 123:543–548, 1973

Zanarini MC, Frankenburg FR, Parachini EA: A preliminary, randomized trial of fluoxetine, olanzapine, and the olanzapine-fluoxetine combination in women with borderline personality disorder. J Clin Psychiatry 65:903–907, 2004

CHAPTER 8

BIPOLAR DISORDER AND PERSONALITY

Constructs, Findings, and Challenges

Peter Bieling, Ph.D.

Glenda MacQueen, M.D., Ph.D.

The intersection between bipolar disorder and personality has intrigued the field of psychiatry for at least a century. Early psychiatric writers speculated about the extent to which temperament, traits, or character are precursors of the development of this mood disorder. In the last several decades, those observations and speculations have been tested in research paradigms that seek to specify the relation between personality, defined in myriad ways, and the development and expression of bipolar disorder. Work in this area often challenges conventional notions about what defines psychiatric "illness" and what is a manifestation of temperament, and such challenges have both scientific and sociocultural implications. The many theories of personality and personality development must also be considered to make sense of the relation between a cyclical, episodic, often chronic mood disorder and the presumably lifelong stable characteristics that make up personality and personality disorders. This relation may often provide clinicians with diagnostic and management dilemmas in the struggle to understand whether behaviors are manifestations of illness, character, or a complex interplay of both. These dilemmas pose equal challenges for our systems of diagnosis and the meanings that clinicians attach to personality versus mood disorders. In this chapter we review this work, focusing on five distinct areas that have emerged over time: 1) bipolar disorder and Axis II comorbidity, 2) the personality-bipolar disorder continuum, 3) the bipolar disorder and borderline personality disorder "spectrum," 4) temperament and trait markers of bipolar disorder, and 5) treatment implications for personality factors in bipolar disorder. For each area, we summarize available findings and also examine the methodological, conceptual, and clinical implications. We conclude with broader implications of these different areas for theory, research, and clinical work.

Bipolar Disorder and Axis II Comorbidity

A point of departure for many investigators has been to examine the relations between bipolar disorder and the personality disorders defined by the DSM-IV-TR (American Psychiatric Association 2000). This work tries to quantify the degree of overlap between this mood disorder and the serious and chronic personality dysfunctions described in DSM. Several important questions are addressed in this work. For example, what proportion of individuals with bipolar disorder has a personality disorder, and is the relation between these disorders more than incidental? What is the most common personality disorder associated with bipolar disorder? And do the relations between bipolar disorder and personality disorders have implications for underlying causes of these disorders?

Bipolar Disorder/Personality Disorder Comorbidity Research

Numerous researchers have examined the question of comorbidity of bipolar disorder and personality disorders defined by DSM-IV-TR. Typically, these studies focus on overall personality disorder rates and frequency of specific personality disorders in samples of patients with bipolar disorder seen in tertiary clinics or inpatient settings. Two early prevalence studies focusing on bipolar disorder and a variety of personality disorder assessment instruments were both based on a sample of 26 bipolar disorder and schizoaffective disorder, bipolar type, participants (Pica et al. 1990; Turley et al. 1992). The first study used a structured clinical interview (Structured Interview for DSM Personality

[SIDP]) and found that 62% of the sample had at least one personality disorder (Pica et al. 1990). Interestingly, the prevalence rate before interviewing informants was 20% lower. This study also included a comparison group of patients with schizophrenia and found that histrionic personality disorder, which was the most common personality disorder in the patients with bipolar disorder, was diagnosed more frequently in the group with bipolar disorder compared with subjects with schizophrenia.

A subsequent study (Turley et al. 1992) of this same data set examined a different assessment technology, the Millon Clinical Multiaxial Inventory-II (MCMI-II). Overall rates of personality disorder diagnosis across these two studies depended to a great extent on instrumentation, with the self-report MCMI-II concluding that 89% of the sample had at least one personality disorder and 58% had two or more (Turley et al. 1992). The MCMI-II self-report scale and the SIDP were seen to have poor agreement in this sample, with the interview resulting in a prevalence rate of 57% and little agreement within various personality disorder categories. However, at least according to the MCMI-II self-report scales, narcissistic personality disorder and antisocial personality disorder were the most prevalent disorders (Turley et al. 1992).

In a broader study of psychiatric inpatients using the DSM-III, Jackson and colleagues (1991) found that histrionic personality disorder was the most common disorder in a sample of 26 patients with recent-onset mania. Indeed, fully 50% of these patients who met criteria either for bipolar disorder or schizoaffective disorder, bipolar type, were found to have histrionic personality disorder based on structured interviews with both the patient and knowledgeable informants (Jackson et al. 1991). Moreover, relative to other diagnostic groups that included schizophrenia and unipolar depression, patients with bipolar disorder had fewer schizotypal, dependent, and avoidant diagnoses (Jackson et al. 1991).

Another early comorbidity study examined the ability of self-report instruments, in isolation, to diagnose personality disorder (O'Connell et al. 1991). Using the Personality Disorder Questionnaire–Revised (PDQ-R), the authors documented a 58% prevalence rate of at least one personality disorder in a sample of 50 patients with bipolar disorder. These authors also reported the number of diagnoses made in their sample (71) and the mean number of diagnoses per patient (1.42). The most common diagnoses were in Cluster B, with borderline personality disorder diagnosed 15 times and histrionic personality disorder diagnosed 10 times. The authors concluded that the PDQ-R has high sensitivity but moderate specificity, and that self-report should be supplemented with structured clinical interview in patients with bipolar disorder (O'Connell et al. 1991).

Carpenter and colleagues (1995), critical of previous studies that had not controlled for patients' state of illness at the time of personality disorder assessment, attempted to examine prevalence rates of personality disorder in patients with bipolar disorder, carefully separating out pathology caused by affective episodes. Various methodological and assessment-related maneuvers were attempted in 23 patients to establish a more accurate picture of character pathology, and the authors reported an overall personality disorder prevalence rate of 35%. Unfortunately, because of the small sample size and presence of several disorders in some individuals, data on specific personality disorders were difficult to establish reliably in that study.

In a study of 90 patients with bipolar disorder, Ucok and colleagues (1998) found that almost half (47.7%) of the sample had at least one personality disorder diagnosis. These researchers also included a control sample of patients without a history of mental illness from an orthopedic clinic, and this group had a much lower prevalence of personality disorder (15.5%). The two most common personality disorder diagnoses in the patients with bipolar disorder were obsessive-compulsive personality disorder (OCPD) and histrionic personality disorder, followed closely by paranoid and schizoid personality disorders. A diagnosis of at least one disorder from clusters A, B, and C was significantly more frequent in the bipolar disorder sample when compared with the nonpsychiatric control subjects.

Barbato and Hafner (1998) carefully screened 42 individuals with bipolar I disorder in Australia and found an overall personality disorder prevalence rate of 45.2%. Histrionic personality disorder was the most common diagnosis, but only in women, followed by borderline personality disorder and OCPD. Individuals with a personality disorder had spent more time in the hospital, rated themselves as more impaired, and had fewer periods of euthymia. Of note, the researchers examined clinical case notes and, based on that documentation, found a prevalence rate of just 7%. Only two of those patients had ever been informed that they had a diagnosis of personality disorder.

In a study of Axis II comorbidity in 61 bipolar I disorder patients, Kay and colleagues (1999) also focused on histories of alcohol use disorders. A total of 38% of their sample met criteria for at least one personality disorder, and those patients with a personality disorder were more than twice as likely to have abused alcohol as those patients who did not have a personality disorder (Kay et al. 1999). This study did not report prevalence for specific disorders but found that Cluster A (33%)

and C (33%) prevalence was more common than Cluster B (15%) prevalence among participants with alcohol use disorder comorbidity. In participants without an alcohol use disorder, the authors found that Cluster A disorders had the lowest prevalence (0%), followed by Cluster B (12%) and Cluster C (16%).

One personality disorder prevalence study focused on patients with bipolar II disorder to clarify rates in this specific variant of bipolar disorder (Vieta et al. 1999). In 40 patients, 13 (32.5%) had at least one personality disorder, and only one patient had two personality disorders. The most frequent diagnosis was borderline personality disorder (12.5%), followed by histrionic personality disorder (7.5%) and OCPD (7.5%). Patients with personality disorder had an earlier onset of illness and a higher rate of suicidal ideation (Vieta et al. 1999). In a follow-up study of this same sample, the patients with bipolar II disorder with comorbidity were found to be similar on a number of demographic and clinical course variables compared with patients with bipolar II disorder who had no comorbidity (Vieta et al. 2000).

Rossi and colleagues (2001) studied prevalence of Axis II conditions in both unipolar and bipolar disorder patients ($N=71$) in a psychiatric research unit in Italy. Using the Structured Clinical Interview for DSM (SCID) and SCID-II, the authors found that OCPD was the most frequent personality disorder (32.4%), followed by borderline (29.6%) and avoidant (19.7%) personality disorders. There were no differences in frequencies of personality disorder between the bipolar disorder and unipolar patients. Unfortunately, the authors of the study did not report an overall prevalence rate in their patients with bipolar disorder (Rossi et al. 2001).

One study attempted to integrate Axis II pathology and the five-factor model of personality in a sample of bipolar disorder patients ($n=60$) compared with unipolar patients ($n=117$) (Brieger et al. 2003). Overall, 38% of bipolar disorder patients and 51% of unipolar patients were found to have at least one personality disorder. Moreover, 13% of bipolar disorder patients had two or more personality disorders. The most frequently occurring personality disorder diagnoses in the bipolar disorder sample were OCPD (16.7%), narcissistic (8.3%), and borderline (6.7%). The five-factor model was associated with personality disorder, but the authors did not report specific relationships between this model and personality disorder within the bipolar sample.

Other studies have examined more specific questions of personality disorder comorbidity and bipolar disorder. Dunayevich and colleagues (1996) examined rates of personality disorder in patients with first versus multiple episodes of mania. This examination allowed for an initial exploration of the hypothesis that personality disorders may develop in response to repeated mood episodes. A total of 59 participants (33 in a first episode, 26 with multiple episodes) were compared using the SCID-II. Overall, 47% of the sample met criteria for at least one personality disorder, with avoidant personality disorder being the most common. However, the personality disorder rates were significantly different between first episode (33%) and multiple episode (65%) patients. Although the results were provocative and in line with the authors' hypotheses, the study did not follow individuals longitudinally; thus, it was not clear whether the higher prevalence rate in multiple episode patients was actually a result of experiencing multiple episodes.

The link between bipolar disorder and narcissistic personality disorder has also been investigated because of the conceptual and clinical links made between symptoms of inflated self-esteem and grandiosity common in both of these disorders (Stormberg et al. 1998). Because of the nature of the research question, patients in this study were assessed during an acute manic state, unless this state prevented them from participating in the diagnostic interviewing, and then again when they were euthymic. A total of 18 participants were able to complete all of the study, and they were compared with a control group of "other" psychiatric patients and patients with "pure" narcissistic personality disorder. The bipolar disorder patients, when manic, resembled patients with narcissistic personality disorder on structured interview; however, these similarities did not exist when these same bipolar disorder patients were euthymic. One interesting difference emerged between manic patients with bipolar disorder and "pure" narcissists. The latter group was much more preoccupied with need for admiration and having the envy of others, and the authors concluded that these symptoms are unique to narcissistic personality disorder (Stormberg et al. 1998).

Critique and Summary of Bipolar Disorder/ Personality Disorder Comorbidity

Despite the number of studies of personality disorder and bipolar disorder comorbidity, and apparent consistencies in findings, there are several methodological problems associated with this area. First, early studies in particular pay insufficient attention to the state of illness at the time of the personality disorder assessment. Even when researchers endeavor to assess individuals when they are not acutely ill, this is operationalized in a variety of ways. Some studies use clinical judgment of euthymia or stability, others specific cutoffs on symptom scales. Moreover, it is not yet clear to what extent variations in mood state actually affect diagnosis of personality disorder. Also, some studies include a variety of diagnostic categories, ranging from all types of bipolar disorder and schizoaffective disorder, bipolar type, to bipolar I or bipolar II disorder. Thus, overall conclusions about personality disorder prevalence rates in bipolar disorder may not generalize to specific bipolar disorder subtypes. Finally, because many studies have small sample sizes, the number of individuals diagnosed with any one disorder on Axis II can amount to no more than a single case or even no cases. In these studies, the number of individuals with a specific personality disorder typically is between 0 and 5, and this makes inferential statistics of any type difficult and unlikely to be reliable. Such small samples also lead to the appearance of large differences when reported as percentages of the total sample. Thus, many researchers are forced to draw conclusions on prevalence, and differences in prevalence rates, from a very small number of cases. More broadly, studies of bipolar disorder and personality disorder comorbidity are plagued by the more general problems associated with Axis II assessment and diagnosis, including reliability and validity of the disorders themselves and myriad diagnostic technologies with varying specificity and sensitivity.

Our review of this literature suggests that personality disorder comorbidity rates in bipolar disorder—defined broadly to include bipolar I disorder, bipolar II disorder, and schizoaffective disorder, bipolar type—are in the range of 30%–50%, with the most frequent personality disorder diagnoses being OCPD, histrionic personality disorder, and borderline personality disorder. At the level of individual disorders, Table 8–1 displays frequencies in the studies described here. Across studies, histrionic personality disorder had the highest rate of comorbidity (24.5%), followed by borderline personality disorder (17.7%) and narcissistic personality disorder and OCPD (12.7% and 12.6%, respectively). These observations are consistent with a similar pooled analysis of 7 studies described by Brieger and colleagues (2003) that resulted in a prevalence rate of 45.6% in data for 393 patients. OCPD, histrionic personality disorder, and borderline personality disorder each had a prevalence rate of approximately 15% in that pooled data (Brieger et al. 2003). The least likely personality disorder diagnoses associated with bipolar disorder appear to be schizotypal (3%), schizoid (4.9%), and dependent personality disorder (5.1%) in the studies we have reviewed here. Overall, comorbidity rates of personality disorder appear to be lower in patients with bipolar disorder when compared with those with unipolar depression. However, given the small number of studies that have used a unipolar depression control group, it is difficult to specify exactly which personality disorders occur at different frequencies in bipolar disorder and unipolar depression.

These data suggest that clinicians must be vigilant to the presence of comorbid personality disorder in patients with bipolar disorder as well as those with unipolar disorder. Certainly the presence of apparently refractory symptoms of illness should trigger a review for both Axis I and Axis II comorbidity that may be impeding treatment outcome. Some personality disorder symptoms may improve with pharmacological treatment of bipolar disorder, whereas others may be more amenable to psychotherapeutic intervention. Before initiation of complex polypharmacy with its inherent risks, it is important to clarify whether the refractory bipolar disorder or the symptoms of a comorbid illness are primarily contributing to the observed presentation of illness.

The Personality-Bipolar Disorder Continuum: From Disposition to Disorder

The notion of an underlying "bipolar" personality structure related directly to mania and hypomania alternating with depression has been evident in the psychiatric literature since the early twentieth century. This approach to the integration of personality factors and bipolar disorder is conceptually different from the approach of those who examine personality disorder and bipolar disorder comorbidity rates. In studies of bipolar disorder and Axis II comorbidity, personality disorders are seen as separate clinical entities with some amount of quantifiable, but not necessarily theoretically meaningful, overlap. Instead, in the work reviewed next, personality disposition is proposed as a precursor and crucible of the emergence of bipolar disorder or bipolar disorder–like illness. Although the notion of a "bipolar disposition" traces its roots to the work of Kraeplin and Kretschmer, more elaborated models were developed in the 1970s by von Zerssen and Akiskal. Building on the theory of a melancholic type that predisposes to unipolar depression, von Zerssen (1977, 2002) described a set of traits or temperament tantamount to a "mild chronic form of hypomania" (Hecht et al. 1998, p. 33) or as a manic type (von Zerssen 2002). These themes identified by von Zerssen are echoed by others who believe that bipolarity is not a discrete entity but a continuum ranging from a temperamental substrate that predisposes to cycling moods at one end to fully syndromal bipolar disorder at the other (Akiskal 1998; Akiskal et al. 1977). In this view bipolar disorders "arise from the soil of extraverted, cyclothymic, and related…temperamental disorders; a driven, work-oriented obsessoid quality" (Akiskal et al. 1983, p. 808). Akiskal's work has focused more

TABLE 8–1. Prevalence of Axis II personality disorders in populations with bipolar disorder (BD)

Study (method of personality disorder assessment)	BD population	N	Cluster A			Cluster B				Cluster C			Other/NOS	
			Prm	Scd	Szt	Ats	Bld	Hist	Nar	Oc	Avd	Dpd	Pag	Other[a]
Pica et al. 1990; Jackson et al. 1991 (SIDP)	BD-I, schizoaffective bipolar type	26	3.9	3.9	3.9	15.4	23.1	50	11.5	3.9	0	0	19.2	NA
O'Connell et al. 1991 (PDQ-R)	BD-NI	50	6	12	4	16	30	20	14	10	12	8	6	NA
Turley et al. 1992 (MCMI-II)	BD-NI, schizoaffective bipolar type	19	5.3	10.5	5.3	47.4	10.5	36.8	47.4	5.3	15.8	15.8	36.8	36.8
Turley et al. 1992 (SIDP)	BD-NI, schizoaffective bipolar type	19	0	5.3	5.3	21.1	21.1	52.6	10.5	5.3	0	0	21.1	15.8
Carpenter et al. 1995 (PDE)	BD-I	23						22					NA	NA
Dunayevich et al. 1996 (SCID-II)	BD-I	59		6.8				22			18.6		NA	NA
Barbato and Hafner 1998 (IPDE)	BD-I	42	7.9	2.6	0	10.5	15.8	21.1	2.6	15.8	13.2	2.6	NA	NA

TABLE 8–1. Prevalence of Axis II personality disorders in populations with bipolar disorder (BD) *(continued)*

Study (method of personality disorder assessment)	BD population	N	Cluster A			Cluster B				Cluster C			Other/NOS	
			Prm	Scd	Szt	Ats	Bld	Hist	Nar	Oc	Avd	Dpd	Pag	Other[a]
Stormberg et al. 1998 (DIN)	BD-I	18	NA	NA	NA	NA	NA	NA	11	NA	NA	NA	NA	NA
Ucok et al. 1998 (SCID-II)	BD-I	90	15.6	0	0	0	10	16.7	1.1	16.7	10	3.3	5.6	NA
Kay et al. 1999 (SCID-II)	BD-I	52		18				13.5			22		NA	NA
Kay et al. 1999 (PDQ-R)	BD-I	61		45			43	43			33		NA	NA
Vieta et al. 1999, 2000 (SCID-II)	BD-I	40	0	2.5	0	0	12.5	7.5	5	7.5	0	0	NA	NA
Rossi et al. 2001 (SCID-II)	BD-I	71	18.3	5.6	5.6	5.6	29.6	12.7	11.3	32.4	19.7	14.1	15.5	NA
Brieger et al. 2003 (SCID-II)	BD-I, BD-II	60	3.3	1.6	3.3	5	6.7	3.3	8.3	16.7	5	1.7	NA	3.3

Rates of personality disorders (%)

TABLE 8–1. Prevalence of Axis II personality disorders in populations with bipolar disorder (BD) *(continued)*

Study (method of personality disorder assessment)	BD population	N	Cluster A			Cluster B				Cluster C			Other/NOS	
			Prn	Scd	Szt	Ats	Bld	Hist	Nar	Oc	Avd	Dpd	Pag	Other[a]
Mean rate (%) across studies reporting individual PDs (number of studies)			9.0 (9)	3.8 (9)	2.6 (9)	8.7 (9)	17.4 (9)	18.7 (9)	9.6 (10)	15.8 (9)	9.7 (9)	5.3 (9)	12.7 (6)	12.2 (3)

Note. ATS=antisocial; AVD=avoidant; BD-I=bipolar I disorder; BD-II=bipolar II disorder; BD-NI=bipolar disorder, type not indicated; BLD=borderline; DIN=Diagnostic Interview for Narcissism; DPD=dependent; Hist=histrionic; IPDE=International Personality Disorder Examination; MCMI-II=Millon Clinical Multiaxial Inventory-II; NA=not assessed; NAR=narcissistic; NOS=not otherwise specified; Oc=obsessive-compulsive; PAG=passive-aggressive; PDE=Personality Disorder Examination; PDQ-R=Personality Diagnostic Questionnaire–Revised; PRN=paranoid; SCD=schizoid; SCID-II=Structured Clinical Interview for DSM-IV Axis II Personality Disorders; SIDP=Structured Interview for DSM Personality; SZT=schizotypal.

[a]Other includes negativistic, mixed, self-defeating, aggressive (sadistic).

on the spectrum of bipolar disorder illnesses, especially the middle of that spectrum, expansions of bipolar II disorder and so-called soft bipolar illnesses, whereas von Zerssen has focused more on the precursors of syndromal bipolar disorder.

Akiskal's perspective challenges current diagnostic schemes, as well as the traditional distinction between bipolar disorder and unipolar depression and personality disorder (Akiskal et al. 1983). Rather than seeing these as discrete entities, or in the case of personality disorder being on a different classificatory axis, Akiskal has advanced the position that these conditions are often intertwined and therefore part of the same spectrum. Thus, Akiskal's approach truly fuses the concepts of personality and Axis I mental disorders, at least for those disturbances related to affective dysregulation. In Akiskal's continuum model the construct of borderline personality disorder is also seen to be part of the bipolar disorder spectrum, a contention we examine in a subsequent section of this chapter.

Research on the Bipolar Disorder Spectrum

The spectrum approach is supported by three distinct lines of empirical evidence. First, expansion of the classic definition of bipolarity appears to result in the inclusion of many individuals with clear impairment related to mood cycling. Thus, some have argued that the boundary between unipolar and bipolar forms of illness is not as clear as suggested by DSM. Second, numerous studies suggest that the presence of a "bipolar temperament" affects expression of disorder and clinical course. Third, treatments, including mood stabilizers, useful in bipolar disorder are also hypothesized to be effective in broader spectrum conditions. Next we provide a summary of these lines of research.

Several studies suggest that there is a significant subset of individuals who have chronic cycling depression/dysthymia and also mild hypomania or mood elevations, both of which interfere with normal functioning and yet fall just outside the classification of bipolar disorder (Perugi and Akiskal 2002). Examination of this group of individuals suggests that affective dysregulation and other negative affective states, including anxiety, irritability, and possibly binge eating, are facets of the bipolar disorder spectrum (Perugi and Akiskal 2002). A study of the clinical epidemiology of mania in a multisite study involving 104 manic patients found support for the notion of a "spectrum of mixity" and a distinct form of mania that includes some depressive symptoms (Akiskal et al. 1998). Similarly when the course of illness of unipolar patients is examined closely, as many as 30% of individuals actually show evidence of significant mood cycling (Cassano et al. 2002). Moreover, when the course of their illness is examined carefully, depressed patients in whom antidepressants trigger mania or hypomania appear also to belong on the bipolar disorder spectrum (Akiskal et al. 2000). High rates of bipolar II disorder and cyclothymic temperament have also been noted in patients with HIV, and it has been suggested that the impulsivity and risk taking associated with the bipolar disorder spectrum may lead to risky behavior and thus increase the probability of infection with HIV (Perretta et al. 1998).

There has been little research to examine the notion of the bipolar disorder spectrum from a population perspective, in part because the concept is novel and controversial. Klein and colleagues (1996) studied hypomanic personality features in a representative sample of over 1,700 adolescents and found that adolescents with hypomanic traits were more likely to have a history of unipolar depression, disruptive behavior disorders, and substance problems but not a history of bipolar disorder. Hypomanic traits were associated with more social dysfunction and problems in functioning, and they predicted more severe levels of depression (Klein et al. 1996). Taken together, studies that carefully examine bipolar disorder spectrum symptoms in already diagnosed patients, as well as at least one population-based study, support the notions that bipolarity can be broadly expressed and that mania can express itself in "temperament" forms. Interestingly, when using a more spectrum-based perspective on bipolar disorder, prevalence in the population is closer to 5% as compared with 1% for bipolar disorder as currently defined in DSM-IV-TR (Angst 1998).

The second line of evidence supporting a spectrum approach is that presence versus absence of an underlying bipolar disorder temperament appears to affect the expression of disorder. For example, in a study of 196 patients with bipolar II disorder, Akiskal and colleagues (2003) found that the presence of a cyclothymic temperament was associated with greater mood instability and younger age at onset. These "cyclothymic depressions" are also associated with family history of bipolar disorder and therefore should be considered bipolar spectrum illnesses rather than personality disorders (Akiskal et al. 2003). Perugi and colleagues (2001) used a factor-analytic approach to mania subtyping in 153 patients with bipolar disorder. Five factors were identified: depressive, irritable-agitated, euphoric-grandiose, accelerated-sleepless, and paranoid-anxious. Those patients with hyperthymic temperament scored higher on the euphoric-grandiose, paranoid-anxious, and accelerated-sleepless factors. In contrast, the bipolar disorder patients with depressive temperaments had more depressive symptoms. A third group that had both a depressive and hyperthymic temperament scored highest on irritable-agitated when hospitalized for mania. The authors suggest that these findings support the notion that underlying temperament impacts expression of bipolar disorder illness.

The third argument for this spectrum perspective is that treatments, specifically mood stabilizers, that are beneficial for bipolar I disorder are also effective in individuals with more broadly defined bipolar disorder features. Indeed, some have advanced the position that appropriate mood stabilizer treatment is likely to be withheld when patients are inappropriately diagnosed with personality-based, rather than bipolar disorder spectrum–based, illnesses (Perugi and Akiskal 2002). Data on this topic are difficult to ascertain, however, because most medication trials are carried out in carefully screened bipolar I and bipolar II disorder patients, and this would systematically exclude the subgroups that are described in the spectrum model (Cassano et al. 2002). Thus this line of argument must await broader studies of mood stabilizers in these spectrum illnesses.

There are other important issues that have been studied from the perspective of a bipolar spectrum. Some writers have suggested that factors including stigma against bipolarity, relegation of mood fluctuations as caused by personality factors or seasonality, and the presentation of patients with soft bipolar illnesses as "highly verbal and opinionated" (Cassano et al. 1999, p. 321) as reasons that bipolar spectrum illnesses are under-recognized. The notion of a bipolar disorder spectrum has also led some to propose the addition of several new categories of bipolarity (for a review, see Hirschfeld 2001). Some schemes advocate for as many as seven categories of bipolar illness to fully express the range of this putative continuum (Akiskal and Pinto 1999). Such schemes have not gone without criticism, and some argue that treating characterological factors as episodic illness is unlikely to produce positive outcomes because it may obscure aspects of illness that are best treated with medications and that are more amenable to psychotherapy (Hutto 2001).

Another approach to the general notion of "bipolar personality" has been described over some three decades by von Zerssen and his group. With this approach, they emphasize the premorbid characteristics of bipolar disorder patients and have developed several unique methods and instruments to assess this vulnerability to bipolar disorder. These approaches probe for long-term and pre-illness patterns of behavior and affectivity. Several studies do suggest that bipolar disorder patients with more mania and hypomania do display a more manic personality type before illness onset (Hecht et al. 1998; von Zerssen 2002). In one study of 122 patients with affective disorders, there was a significant trend for melancholic personality type to be less prominent in individuals with more depression and fewer episodes of mania. In contrast, there was evidence of linear increases in the manic personality type for patients who had more mania and hypomania in their course of illness (Hecht et al. 1998). However, these results were not consistent across instruments, and in some cases the bipolar patients in particular were not distinguishable from control subjects. von Zerssen (2002) reviewed numerous studies that included questionnaire and biographical methods that supported a link between a manic type predisposition and bipolar disorder, and consistent differences in temperament markers between unipolar and bipolar patients (von Zerssen and Possl 1990; von Zerssen et al. 1994). There is also evidence of significant familial correlations for hypomanic personality features. Meyer and Hautzinger (2001) found parent-offspring correlations of 0.15 in a sample of 717 index participants and family members.

Summary and Critique of Spectrum Research

Validation of the existence of a bipolar disorder spectrum will require evidence from basic descriptive and longitudinal research as well as studies examining mood stabilizers and other forms of treatment in carefully assessed samples. Instruments to assess bipolar spectrum illnesses have been developed, and validation of these will be an important step in attempting to validate the spectrum notion (Cassano et al. 1999). However, because this approach seeks to combine temperament and disorder, operational definitions of dependent and independent variables are not as clear as they should be. By denying a clear distinction between temperament and illness, a host of definitional problems can be encountered. For example, is mood lability in childhood best defined as a temperament marker, subclinical indicator of future illness, or an emerging bipolar disorder symptom? This area will require clearer concepts and hypotheses that can be both supported and refuted based on carefully developed a priori definitions. Also, advanced psychometric tools, including statistical methods for discriminating taxons from continuous constructs, will be required to validate the notion of a bipolar disorder spectrum. The availability of such tools is critical because the last several years have witnessed an explosion of interest in childhood- and adolescent-onset bipolar disorder. Identifying those who have not exhibited typical symptoms of mania or hypomania and yet fall within the bipolar spectrum will be a necessary first step in identifying the best treatment interventions, either pharmacological or psychotherapeutic, for these individuals. Similarly, we must be vigilant that, in our attempts to improve the course of bipolar disorder with early intervention, we do not misidentify a group of individuals whose temperamental characteristics do not warrant aggressive intervention with pharmacological agents whose safety has often not been established for each developmental period.

The Bipolar Disorder and Borderline Personality Disorder Spectrum

The following case example illustrates the difficulty involved in sorting out symptoms secondary to bipolar disorder versus those symptoms secondary to borderline personality disorder. The case highlights the benefit of longitudinal information on the patient's course of illness, information about the effectiveness of various treatment strategies that have been attempted, and the fact that targeted treatment of symptoms, independent of formal diagnosis, may be necessary in many instances.

Case Example

Ms. Z was a 26-year-old married woman who was not working outside her home when she was first assessed in our mood disorders program. She asserted that a previous psychiatrist had given her a diagnosis of bipolar disorder with rapid cycling that was refractory to lithium and valproate, medications she disliked because of weight gain. She described rapidly fluctuating moods, with "highs" consisting of irritability, hypersexuality, and poor judgment exemplified by excessive, although not extreme, shopping. Her "lows" tended to be more prolonged, with periods of a week or two when she would spend most of her time in bed and have suicidal thoughts. Ms. Z was morbidly obese and usually poorly groomed; she often dressed inappropriately, wearing sandals over dirty, bare feet in winter or layers of ripped, revealing clothing in summer, dying her hair green or shaving it into unusual cuts. She described a chaotic childhood with a physically abusive, substance-abusing father; a passive, possibly depressed mother; and a brother with conduct disorder about whom she felt very protective. Apart from being close to her brother, she was estranged from her family, including from a sister who was married with children. She resented her sister, "the good one," for having children and disclosed that she did not have regular menses and despaired over never becoming pregnant, which she desperately wanted. Although she was frequently verbally disparaging of her husband, the marriage was fundamentally stable. Her husband, who had a secure job and supportive family, would often accompany her to appointments to advocate quietly for her. She was remarkably sensitive to perceived slights, had a strong dislike for her past psychiatrist with no well-articulated reason for this, and quickly idealized the tertiary care program to which she had been referred.

Although she did meet criteria for bipolar II disorder, rapid cycling, on a structured clinical interview, she also scored very high on structured interviews for borderline personality disorder and was initially formulated as having bipolar disorder comorbid with borderline personality disorder. When she first entered treatment, she forcefully attributed her impulsive and sometimes chaotic behavior to the bipolar illness only; she was ambivalent about medication but refused to discuss psychotherapy of any sort. She consented, with much discussion, to a low dose of an atypical antipsychotic. She tolerated it well and agreed that it "took the edge off her cycling"; in other words, the medication made her less irritable and less impulsive, and it improved her sleep. During the first winter of treatment she experienced a sustained low mood. Psychotherapeutic decisions were limited by what she was willing to add to the low dose of atypical antipsychotic. A serotonin reuptake inhibitor was negotiated and Ms. Z did well, with an improvement in symptoms and no evidence of increased mood instability. She was behaviorally managed with explicit limits on contact with the clinic and descriptions of acceptable behavior, and she was generally respectful of these limits, with only sporadic crisis calls and no emergency room visits as long as a regular appointment schedule was maintained. She was an intelligent woman, and when her physical appearance, often profane language, and occasional threats of harm to self or others failed to alienate her treating physician, she and the treating physician developed a mutual respect.

Over time it became apparent that most periods of fluctuating mood and inappropriate behavior were preceded by pathological interactions with her family, by whom she felt criticized, belittled, and helpless to respond. She began to work at using cognitive strategies to prevent extreme emotional responses to such situations with reasonable results. She also began to see fertility experts and to explore options regarding childbearing. Her struggle to modulate her emotional response to perceived criticism was ongoing. However, for example, a straightforward suggestion by a physician that weight loss might improve her physical health was met with hostility and an immediate disinterest in returning to that physician.

With several years of psychiatric treatment and no observed instances of mania or hypomania, Ms. Z's medications were gradually weaned until she was prescribed only low doses of zopiclone for sleep, which she took intermittently. As she became more willing to understand the origins of her emotions and behaviors outside the context of a bipolar illness, she was referred for dialectical behavior therapy (DBT), to which she was adherent. DBT, pioneered by Marsha Linehan and colleagues (Linehan 1993), was constructed to help patients with borderline personality disorder better manage their affective dysregulation using a variety of behavioral strategies. Ms. Z was able to incorporate a number of the skills she learned into her daily routine and normal coping methods during treatment and maintained a number of skills after this treatment ended. Thus, after approximately 6 years of psychiatric treatment, which diminished in intensity significantly over time, Ms. Z was discharged from care. No definitive manic or hypomanic episodes had ever been observed, and she had not had a depressive episode in over 2 years. She was happy with her marriage, resigned to the issues in her family of origin, and applying to be evaluated for in vitro fertilization.

Patients such as Ms. Z are common in mood disorder specialty clinics, and indeed the interface between mood and borderline personality disorder has generated a large volume of research and caused considerable controversy. The research work in this area combines, to a great extent, a simple "comorbidity-rate" perspective with aspects of the bipolar disorder spectrum approach. At one level, borderline personality disorder and bipolar disorder would appear to be a particularly difficult combination of disorders to diagnose accurately; these two disorders have a number of shared symptom features that in clinical practice are clearly hard to differentiate. However, some see this diagnostic and management conundrum as evidence that the two disorders, rather than being two categories with some amount of intersection, really represent different manifestations of a single pathophysiological continuum (Akiskal et al. 1985; Perugi and Akiskal 2002). This represents an important dilemma and debate both for researchers and clinicians. Borderline personality disorder is one of most chronic and impairing psychiatric conditions and is a significant challenge for treating clinicians, as it was in the preceding case example. Moreover, there is no doubt that affective instability is a shared feature of both types of disorder, and this instability can lead to significant diagnostic dilemmas, especially when the patient is new to the presenting clinician (Bolton and Gunderson 1996). The outcome of this debate will also have important consequences for making and communicating diagnosis and treatment in affected individuals, the critical issue being the extent to which individuals with borderline personality disorder/bipolar disorder comorbidity (or, alternatively, a bipolar disorder spectrum illness) are treated mainly with pharamacologic or some combination of medication and psychosocial interventions (Bolton and Gunderson 1996; Feiner 1997).

Relevant areas of inquiry on this topic include studies that address comorbidity of bipolar disorder with Axis II conditions but also the reverse perspective—that is, studies of comorbidity associated with borderline personality disorder. Also, various studies have been conducted to better understand the nature of the relationship between bipolar disorder and borderline personality disorder. Typically such studies focus on individuals with both bipolar disorder and borderline personality disorder and patients in whom bipolar disorder (defined either in DSM or in soft bipolar terms) or borderline personality disorder is present in isolation. Some studies focus strictly on the overlap between bipolar disorder and borderline personality disorder from a spectrum perspective; others attempt to determine differences between these separate disorders. Next we review the comorbidity rates for bipolar disorder and borderline personality disorder, followed by an examination of the evidence that these two disorders exist on a continuum of affective dysregulation disorders.

Research on the Bipolar Disorder/Borderline Personality Disorder Distinction

The issue of comorbidity of Axis I conditions with borderline personality disorder has been pressing for several reasons. First, patients with borderline personality disorder are often found to have accompanying Axis I conditions. Second, the nature of Axis I complaints in patients with borderline personality disorder is typically not isolated to a single type of disorder, and indeed the nature of these Axis I conditions appears to change over time. Most relevant for this chapter, if bipolar disorder and borderline personality disorder exist on a spectrum, one would expect substantial rates of overlap between bipolar disorder and borderline personality disorder. Table 8–2 provides a summary of studies examining rates of bipolar disorder in samples of individuals with BPD. Zanarini and colleagues (1998) reviewed 15 studies of Axis I comorbidity in patients with borderline personality disorder and identified major depression and substance abuse as the most common comorbid conditions. Their own sophisticated study of 520 patients suggested that 96% of patients with borderline personality disorder had a mood disorder compared with 72% of patients with other personality disorders (Zanarini et al. 1998). Of the 379 patients with borderline personality disorder, 9.5% had bipolar disorder, whereas 83% had major depression. Interestingly, 88% of the sample with borderline personality disorder had at least one anxiety disorder, and anxiety disorders better discriminated the borderline personality disorder group from the other personality disorder group.

In a study of borderline personality disorder recognition and treatment in primary care settings with a relatively small sample size, the most common Axis I conditions were anxiety disorder (57%), major depression (36%), and bipolar disorder (21%) (Gross et al. 2002). In that study no cases of bipolar disorder were present in the psychiatric control group, and the authors concluded that comorbidity between borderline personality disorder and bipolar disorder is likely to be higher than chance and higher than the comorbidity rates of between 0.3% and 14% identified in other studies. One limitation of these comorbidity studies, which suggest a modest but significant bipolar disorder/borderline personality disorder co-occurrence rate, is that they define bipolar disorder rigorously using DSM criteria. Researchers more focused on the spectrum approach have also used broader criteria to better gauge the degree of overlap between borderline personality disorder and soft bipolarity.

Deltito and colleagues (2001) used a novel approach to the question of overlap between bipolar disorder and borderline personality disorder by applying different criteria of bipolarity. Although the sample size ($N=16$) was small, patients in the study were carefully diagnosed with borderline personality disorder. Presence of bipolarity was then assessed in depth, with varying levels of evidence used to determine whether a bipolar spectrum illness was also present. The range of levels of evidence and associated comorbidity rates included history of spontaneous mania (12.5%), spontaneous mania or hypomania (31.5%), spontaneous mania or hypomania or bipolar temperament (43.75%), spontaneous mania or hypomania or bipolar temperament or pharmacological response pattern (68.78%), and spontaneous mania or hypomania or bipolar temperament or pharmacological response pattern or family history of bipolar disorders (81.25%). Moreover, there was a pattern, not tested with inferential statistics, of better response to mood stabilizers compared with antidepressants (Deltito et al. 2001). Findings in this study were consistent with an earlier but considerably larger study of 60 patients that focused on the connection between borderline personality disorder and cyclothymia (Levitt et al. 1990). In that study, 41% of borderline personality disorder patients were found to have cyclothymia, whereas in the control group of other personality disorders there were no cases of cyclothymia. Perugi and colleagues (2003) studied 107 patients with atypical depression, and 45 (42%) of these patients were found to have a cyclothymic temperament. In that subsample of atypical patients, a diagnosis of borderline personality disorder was more common (62%) than in the noncyclothymic group (29%). The cyclothymic group also had a greater frequency of personality disorder diagnoses in a number of categories.

Together these studies suggest that as the definition of bipolarity is broadened, the intersection between bipolar disorder conditions and borderline personality disorder rises substantially. Table 8–3 displays the comorbidity rates of borderline personality disorder/bipolarity

TABLE 8–2. Rates of bipolar disorder in samples with borderline personality disorder (BPD)

Study	Sample	Definition of bipolarity	Bipolar disorder/ BPD comorbidity rate (%)
Levitt et al. 1990	60 BPD subjects	Spectrum	41
Zanarini et al. 1998	379 BPD subjects	Strict	9.5
Deltito et al. 2001	16 BPD subjects	Strict	31.5
Deltito et al. 2001	16 BPD subjects	Spectrum	68.8
Gross et al. 2002	14 BPD subjects	Strict	21.4
Perugi et al. 2003	45 cyclothymic subjects	Spectrum	62.2

across these six studies and suggests that a broader definition of bipolarity as much as triples the rate of overlap (20.8% overlap with bipolarity strictly defined and 57.3% when bipolarity is broadly defined). Nonetheless, the degree to which borderline personality disorder and bipolar disorder represent different points on a continuum cannot be answered definitively by comorbidity studies alone.

Other research focuses less on the degree of overlap between bipolar disorder illnesses and borderline personality disorder and examines the extent to which these two constructs share common, underlying features. There is relatively less work in this area, but such an approach is important in determining to what extent these entities have similar or different underlying substrates. Henry and colleagues (2001) examined two specific, potentially temperament-based factors in both bipolar II disorder and borderline personality disorder: affective instability and impulsivity. These researchers divided their sample of 148 into groups of "pure" borderline personality disorder, "pure" bipolar II disorder, borderline personality disorder and bipolar II disorder, and other personality disorder, no bipolar disorder. Although affective lability was present in both the borderline personality disorder and bipolar disorder groups, the nature of this lability was significantly different. In patients with borderline personality disorder, affect shifts from euthymia to anxiety and anger were more common, whereas affect shifts from euthymia to depression and from depression to elation were more common in patients with bipolar disorder (Henry et al. 2001). Also, in this sample only the patients with borderline personality disorder had elevations on impulsiveness and aggressiveness. The authors suggest that these differences do not support a simple spectrum model and that the differences identified are borne out

TABLE 8–3. Comorbidity of bipolar disorder (BD) and borderline personality disorder (BPD)

Author	Sample	Findings
Zanarini et al. 1998	Reviewed 15 studies of Axis I comorbidity in BPD patients	Most commonly occurring comorbid conditions: Major depression Substance abuse
Zanarini et al. 1998	520 patients	Comorbid mood disorder; 96% of BPD patients had mood disorder compared with 72% with other personality disorders
Zanarini et al. 1998	379 BPD patients	9.5% with BD 83% with major depressive disorder
Gross et al. 2002	Small sample (size not given); BPD recognition and treatment in primary care settings	57% with anxiety disorder 36% with major depressive disorder 21% with BD Conclusion: comorbidity between BPD and BD likely higher than chance

in the different clinical presentations associated with borderline personality disorder, specifically self-harm and anger control problems, that are not commonly associated with bipolar disorder.

Another study employed Cloninger's personality model, hypothesizing that if bipolar disorder and borderline personality disorder are on the same spectrum, underlying personality traits in these individuals should be very similar (Atre-Vaidya and Hussain 1999). Although the sample in this study was small ($N=23$), there were significant differences on harm avoidance, self-directedness, and cooperativeness. The authors suggest that because differences in these traits are mediated by different neurobiological pathways, bipolar disorder and borderline personality disorder are best considered distinct types of disorders.

Summary and Critique of Bipolar Disorder/ Borderline Personality Disorder Distinction

The area of bipolar disorder/borderline personality disorder distinction presents enormous conceptual and methodological challenges to researchers. As a result of these challenges, the nature of the evidence is such that a vigorous debate about bipolar disorder and borderline personality disorder continues. For example, some investigators interpret comorbidity rates of bipolar disorder and borderline personality disorder that are higher than chance as evidence of an underlying continuum. However, others see the same comorbidity rates and descriptive psychopathology studies and conclude that the two disorders are discrete taxons with some amount of overlap. These two positions have important clinical but also sociopolitical implications. Those who see borderline personality disorder as a form of mood disorder believe that patients are being misdiagnosed by a system that is deeply flawed and that such patients will be medically undertreated and made to needlessly suffer the stigmatizing effects of being labeled with a disorder of "character." Those who believe that borderline personality disorder is a valid clinical entity believe that considering this constellation of symptoms as a mood disorder will lead to undertreatment with psychosocial interventions and will prevent a necessary focus on emotion regulation skills, acceptance, and recovery.

This debate, with its political overtones and long entrenched advocates on both sides, may not be settled by scientific data alone. What is clear from the data is that there is a link in the phenomenology of bipolar disorder and borderline personality disorder symptoms, and a rate of comorbidity between the two "conditions" that rises well above chance, especially when a broader definition of bipolar disorder is employed. At the same time there are differences in presentations and underlying traits in the two disorders that would seem to argue for a clear distinction. Moreover, even if these disorders are on the same continuum, not all of the symptoms seen in borderline personality disorder necessarily overlap with bipolar disorder (e.g., chronic self-harming behaviors, disturbed sense of self, chronic interpersonal problems, difficulty controlling anger). Therefore, to accurately communicate the nature of illness, it will still be necessary to use different sets of terms for bipolar disorder– and borderline personality disorder–like illnesses. Nonetheless, this area does call attention to difficulties with distinguishing Axis I and Axis II disorders and questions the use of categorical ways of viewing clinical problems that may have considerable overlap.

Temperament and Trait Markers of Bipolar Disorder

Another group of researchers have examined trait markers that are associated with development of bipolar disorder, independent of the notion of a bipolar temperament or bipolar spectrum. These markers tend to be drawn from the literature on "normal" personality characteristics or individual difference variables relevant to the population. What is unique about this area is that the personality factors of focus are not usually related to mood or affective regulation characteristics per se. This research may be particularly important for prevention because, theoretically, temperament markers are likely to predate the onset of mood disorder symptoms. However, to date most research in this area is cross sectional and focuses on associations between traits and expression of illness rather than testing the germane predictive hypotheses.

Interestingly, the majority of early studies of temperament variables found few differences between euthymic bipolar disorder patients and healthy control subjects (for a review, see Solomon et al. 1996). The exceptions to these were characteristics such as emotional instability, aggression, and impulsiveness, which may also have been markers of illness or at least spectrum conditions (Solomon et al. 1996). Also, these early researchers tended to focus on personality constructs that were themselves imprecise, often based on flawed and now outmoded theories of personality development, and measured with inadequate tools such as projective tests. Better measurement of personality variables has helped renew interest in this area.

Two comprehensive measurement systems for personality traits have evolved in the psychology and psychiatric literatures, respectively: Costa and McCrae's five-factor model (FFM) and Cloninger's psychobiological model. The FFM was originally derived from a lexical analysis of human trait adjectives and includes 1) neuroticism, 2) extraversion, 3) agreeableness, 4) conscientiousness, and 5) openness. The second frequently used approach to personality/temperament measurement is Cloninger's psychobiological model, operationalized by the Tridimensional Personality Questionnaire (TPQ) (Cloninger et al. 1993). The instrument assesses four dimensions of personality putatively related to underlying neurotransmitter systems: 1) novelty seeking, 2) harm avoidance, 3) reward dependence, and 4) persistence.

On the basis of Cloninger's system, Osher and colleagues (1996) compared 50 euthymic patients with bipolar disorder to U.S. norms on the TPQ and found that the bipolar disorder sample had lower than average scores on persistence and higher scores on harm avoidance and reward dependence. Subsequently, Osher and colleagues (1999) compared 25 euthymic patients with bipolar disorder with 25 normal healthy subjects on the TPQ and found that novelty seeking and persistence were both significantly lower in the bipolar disorder sample (Osher et al. 1999). The findings in the second study replicated the earlier results pointing to persistence as problematic in patients with bipolar disorder, and the authors described mechanisms by which low persistence could mediate the link between stress and disorder.

Results using Cloninger's TPQ have not always been consistent, however. Others have found that novelty seeking is actually higher in patients with bipolar disorder than in recovered unipolar patients, whereas harm avoidance is elevated in both bipolar disorder and unipolar patients compared with healthy control subjects (Young et al. 1995). In a study of clinical outcomes, novelty seeking was associated with a worse functional outcome 6 months after discharge from the hospital (Strakowski et al. 1993). Finally, Blairy and colleagues (2000) focused on a potential genetic connection between the harm avoidance trait and bipolar disorder. In 40 patients with bipolar disorder compared with 89 healthy control subjects, they did find elevations on harm avoidance in bipolar disorder but no contribution of the serotonin 2A receptor gene polymorphism to either bipolar disorder or harm avoidance.

Several studies using a variety of comparison groups and data analytic strategies, including prediction of clinical course, have been completed using the FFM approach. Bagby and colleagues (1996) compared 34 euthymic patients with bipolar disorder with 74 unipolar depressed patients and found that extraversion, specifically the positive emotions facet, was elevated in bipolar disorder versus unipolar patients. There was a trend for patients with bipolar disorder also to be higher on overall openness and for significant differences on two specific facets of openness (Bagby et al. 1996). In a study using a comparison group of patients with seasonal affective disorder ($n=24$), patients with bipolar disorder ($n=13$) were found to have higher neuroticism scores and lower scores on extraversion, openness, and conscientiousness (Jain et al. 1999). Carpenter and colleagues compared the FFM profiles of patients with bipolar disorder ($N=33$) to published norms and found that although profiles had considerable variability, aggregate personality scores in the patients with bipolar disorder did not deviate substantially from healthy control subjects (Carpenter et al. 1999). However, over the course of 1 year, higher levels of neuroticism levels did predict a negative clinical course. Similarly, a study by Lozano and Johnson (2001) sought to predict changes in depression and mania symptoms from the FFM in a sample of 39 patients with bipolar disorder. Participants were assessed when relatively stable, and FFM scores were used to predict symptoms at 6-month follow-up. Neuroticism scores predicted more depression symptoms, whereas conscientiousness, particularly achievement striving, predicted presence of mania symptoms. Finally, in one study comparing bipolar disorder patients with mixed episodes as opposed to pure mania, none of the FFM variables distinguished between these two presentations of bipolar disorder (Brieger et al. 2002).

Beyond the FFM and Cloninger's model, several other similar studies of personality traits are available. For example, Solomon and colleagues (1996) conducted a broad survey of personality features in patients with bipolar disorder ($n=30$) and compared this group to a sample of healthy control subjects ($n=974$). These researchers used 17 scales that assessed four broad factors: 1) emotional strength—somewhat akin to neuroticism and emotional dependency, 2) need for contact and approval, 3) extraversion, and 4) a miscellaneous category. The patients with bipolar disorder had less emotional strength on a number of scales and lower levels of extraversion including less ego control. Benazzi (2000) found a higher rate of interpersonal rejection sensitivity in patients with bipolar disorder as opposed to unipolar patients. Stable, euthymic patients with bipolar disorder were found to have higher perfectionism, need for approval, and dependency scores compared with healthy control subjects in a study of vulnerability to psychopathology (Scott et al. 2000). Bipolar disorder also appears to be related to trait-based impulsivity that goes beyond the confines of discrete mood episodes (Moeller et al. 2001).

The connection between bipolar disorder and creativity, potentially a traitlike variable, has also been investigated. Critically, given the base rate of bipolar disorder and a sufficient sample of time, it is a given that a certain number of artists will also happen to have bipolar disorder. Moreover, it is difficult to ascertain to what extent bipolar disorder, and particularly mania, are causal agents in the creative process (Rothenberg 2001). To date few studies examining these ideas are available that could be seen to be strong tests of these hypotheses (for a review, see Rothenberg 2001). Case studies and biographical surveys often support the view that bipolar disorder rates are elevated in creative individuals; those studies that use more population-based methods and larger samples typically find no relations.

Taken in sum, several significant, although not always consistent, differences have emerged in cross-sectional studies that compare patients with bipolar disorder to control groups. Through use of the Cloninger approach, elevations in harm avoidance and novelty seeking appear to be the most consistent findings and to be associated with significant clinical outcomes. Based on the FFM, elevated neuroticism and decreased extraversion scores emerge as the most consistent finding across different studies. However, the overall number of studies in the area is still relatively small, and there are a number of conceptual issues to be resolved. These include the selection of an appropriate control group; some studies compare patients with bipolar disorder to norms or healthy control subjects, and others compare patients with bipolar disorder to unipolar patients. Also, cross-sectional studies are unlikely to be the strongest possible tests of personality markers because there is no way to ensure that personality differences predated the emergence of the mood illness. A more persuasive examination of personality markers would involve a longitudinal study either in a large population or in a sample of high-risk participants. This would allow not only for a comparison of personality scores between individuals with and without bipolar disorder but also for statistical examination of the predictive potential (e.g., sensitivity and specificity) of such markers for identifying who will develop bipolar disorder. In addition to such important practical and clinical questions, this area provides an interesting intersection of basic personality and applied psychopathology research that may ultimately influence both fields.

Treatment Implications of Personality Factors in Bipolar Disorder

There are very few studies that have systematically examined the impact of personality disorders or personality traits on outcome in bipolar disorder. Most studies that have examined the effect of a comorbid personality disorder on outcome in bipolar disorder suggest that the presence of the personality disorder exerts a negative impact. These studies are summarized in Table 8–4. Dunayevich and colleagues (1996, 2000) assessed 56 patients who were hospitalized with a diagnosis of mania or mixed state using the SCID-II to obtain diagnoses of personality disorder. Patients were interviewed on the SCID-II shortly before discharge, and the investigators specifically noted that patients were judged sufficiently recovered from an affective episode that they were able to answer questions using their premorbid function as the standard reference. Using this method, 48% of patients received a diagnosis of personality disorder, with the most common diagnoses being avoidant (14.3%), passive-aggressive (8.9%), and self-defeating personality disorder (8.9%). There was no difference in age, sex distribution, education or employment status, substance use disorder, or mania or depression rating scale scores of the patients with or without personality disorder, but patients with a personality disorder diagnosis were five times more likely to have had a past hospitalization than those with no personality disorder diagnosis. Following the index episode, the presence of a personality disorder was associated with a lack of symptomatic recovery, with only 35% of patients with personality disorder attaining symptomatic recovery compared with 69% of patients without a personality disorder. Similarly, only 12% of patients with a personality disorder achieved symptomatic recovery, whereas 38% of patients without a personality disorder achieved symptomatic recovery. Finally, only 10% of patients with personality disorder achieved full functional recovery over the 1 year of follow-up compared with 31% of patients without a personality disorder. The authors note several features that may have contributed to the poor outcome in the patients with comorbid personality disorder, including compliance as a mediating factor and the fact that more patients with personality disorder had multiple past episodes of illness.

Dunayevich and colleagues (2000) raised the possibility that treatment compliance is a variable mediating between personality disorder and outcome in bipolar disorder. The association between pharmacological treatment compliance and personality disorder in bipolar disorder was studied in more detail by Colom and colleagues (2000). They assessed 144 patients with bipolar I disorder and 56 patients with bipolar II disorder who were enrolled in a 2-year naturalistic follow-up study at the University Hospital in Barcelona, Spain. All patients received the Spanish version of the SCID-II to assess rate and type of personality disorder, and in this sample histrionic (8%) and borderline personality disorder (5.5%) were described most frequently. Patients were divided into those with good compliance ($n=121$) and those with poor compliance ($n=79$). A higher proportion of patients in the poor compliance group (39.2%) had Axis II comorbidity than in the good compliance group (17.4%), and the presence of personality disorder was more predictive of poor compliance than substance abuse, socioeconomic status, marital status, education level, or specific medications prescribed (Colom et al. 2000). This association between personality disorder diagnosis and poor compliance has been observed previously (Keck et al. 1997).

In contrast to studies that focused on syndromic outcome in bipolar disorder, Hammen and colleagues (2000) studied 52 patients with bipolar I disorder ascertained from an outpatient sample and focused on work adjustment as a marker of outcome in bipolar disorder. This group completed the Eysenck Personality Questionnaire, the Interpersonal Dependency Inventory, and the PDQ-R when in remission. The focus of this study was predictors of work adjustment, using regression analyses to examine the impact of both clinical and psychosocial factors on work adjustment in patients with bipolar I disorder. Psychosocial variables overall were found to be significant in hierarchical regression analyses, whereas a variety of clinical variables such as past hospitalizations, chronicity, and severity of relapse did not account for work functioning. Unfortunately scores on the PDQ-R were combined with other psychosocial variables for the analysis, so the contribution of specific aspects of personality function or dysfunction was not determined independent of other variables such as relationship quality ratings.

One study used a different marker of outcome—suicide attempts in bipolar disorder—and examined factors associated with this negative outcome (Leverich et al. 2003). In 648 outpatients with bipolar disorder followed through the Stanley Foundation Bipolar Network, 34% of patients had a history of suicide attempts. In a hierarchical cluster analysis, Cluster B personality disorders were a significant predictor of a serious suicide attempt in addition to history of sexual abuse, lack of a confidant before illness, hospitalizations for depression, and suicidal thoughts when depressed.

Finally, Bieling and colleagues (2003) used a "life-charting" approach in which 87 bipolar I and II disorder patients were followed regularly and treated according to published guidelines. Patients were assessed by use of the SCID-II and were then followed for an average of 3.4 years. Better outcomes on symptom severity and functioning were noted for patients with lower scores on 7 out of 10 personality disorder categories, and Cluster A personality disorder symptoms best distinguished euthymic and symptomatic patients (Bieling et al. 2003). Thus, presence of personality symptoms predicted negative outcome over this relatively long-term follow-up.

There are a few studies that have examined normal personality traits and outcome in bipolar disorder. One study of 44 adolescents with a DSM-III-R–based diagnosis of bipolar disorder examined spectrum personality traits by very broad definitions such as "leadership potential" or "good peer relationships" (Quackenbush et al. 1996). This study found very high rates of functioning in these adolescents before the onset of bipolar disorder, which then appeared to decline dramatically following illness onset. For example, 33% of the sample was described as possessing leadership qualities before illness onset, whereas after illness onset, the estimate of the proportion possessing leadership qualities dropped to 0. Other investigators have also noted low rates of personality psychopathology before onset of bipolar disorder (Werry et al. 1991), which leads to an understudied question regarding the extent to which mood instability in years that are critical for formation of stable personality structure can result in the observed high rates of personality problems in adults with established bipolar disorder.

Another study examined temperament in bipolar disorder and its impact on prognosis (Henry et al. 1999). A total of 72 patients with a diagnosis of bipolar I disorder based on the French version of the Diagnostic Interview for Genetic Studies were assessed using the depressive temperament (DT) and hyperthymic temperament (HT) scales developed by Akiskal and Mallya (1987) when patients were remitted. After controlling for age, sex, and educational attainment, there was a positive association with DT scores and outcome as assessed by total number of past manic or depressive episodes. There was a negative correlation between DT score and percentage of manic episodes but a positive correlation between HT score and percentage of manic episodes. Dell'Osso and colleagues (1991) have shown that the incidence of mixed states is predicted by depressive temperament, and Akiskal (1992) has suggested that such mixed states arise when the temperament and episode are of opposite polarity.

A recent study of cognitive therapy for bipolar disorder relapse prevention identified that patients who were highly driven with extreme goal attainment beliefs were vulnerable to poor outcome (Lam et al. 2003). The study noted that "a vigorous attempt to challenge these beliefs was warranted but not necessarily successful" (p. 152).

One study of self-esteem in patients with bipolar disorder suggested that remitted patients did not differ from control subjects on self-esteem scores (Daskalopoulou et al. 2002) but that there was an association between low self-esteem and suicidality during depression in this group. Another study examined stigma and self-esteem in 186 patients with bipolar disorder who completed the Self-Esteem and Stigma Questionnaire but reported that only self-esteem varied as a function of mood state without directly assessing whether low self-esteem appeared to lead to low mood states (Hayward et al. 2002).

Summary and Critique of Bipolar Disorder/Personality Disorders and Traits Outcome Research

In summary, the available data, summarized in Table 8–4, suggest that the presence of a personality disorder exerts a negative effect on outcome in bipolar disorder, regardless of the definition of outcome employed. At least one study has suggested that personality disorders contribute to poor treatment adherence as a mediating variable in outcome (Colom et al. 2000). Others have speculated that the co-occurring personality disorder is the hallmark of a severe or persistent mood disorder, and that it is therefore not surprising that presence of a personality disorder is a negative prognostic indicator (Akiskal et al. 1983). Unfortunately, relatively few treatment trials have systematically examined the effect of comorbid personality disorder on treatment responsiveness in patients with bipolar disorder, and there is, therefore, little information that allows us to determine whether certain pharmacological or nonpharmacological treatments are particularly indicated in the presence of co-occurring personality disorder and bipolar disorder. There is a literature beyond the scope of this chapter suggesting that mood stabilizers such as valproate (Frankenburg and Zanarini 2002; Hollander et al. 2001), carbamazepine (Cowdry and Gardner 1988), and lamotrigine (Pinto and Akiskal 1998; Preston et al. 2004) may be useful in treating borderline personality disorder with or without bipolar disorder, but these studies have largely focused on treating symptoms of the personality disorder and have not examined how to optimally treat bipolar disorder in the presence of comorbid personality disorder. Given the poor long-term outcome that is often associated with bipolar disorder, it is important to recognize the presence of personality disorder and assess its effect on the course and outcome of bipolar disorder, with intervention targeted at minimizing the dysfunction associated with the personality disorder as a possible strategy to improve patients' overall outcome.

Conclusions and Future Direction

The interface of bipolar disorder and personality poses significant challenges conceptually, methodologically, and practically during the course of assessment and treatment of bipolar disorder. Overall, research has only begun to deal with those challenges. By comparison, work on personality factors in unipolar depression offers an illustrative example. In that field, well-articulated models have been advanced to describe how personality interacts with the onset and experience of depression. Those models, termed *predisposition, pathoplasty, complication,* and *spectrum,* seek to explain the relations between personality and depression (Clark et al. 1994). Briefly, the predisposition model postulates that personality plays its most important role by serving as a vulnerability to a depressive episode. The pathoplasty model predicts that personality factors modify the expression and course of the depressive episode but do not have a causal effect. The complication (or "scar") model predicts that the experience of depression negatively affects personality in a more or less permanent manner. Finally, the spectrum model predicts that depression and personality have similar causes

TABLE 8–4. The effect of personality disorders (PDs) on outcome in bipolar disorder (BD)

Author	Sample	Measure	Comment
Dunayevich et al. 1996, 2000	56 BD-I hospitalized for mania or mixed state	SCID-II before discharge	Patients with PD were 5 times more likely to have had past hospitalizations; 35% of patients with PD attained syndromic recovery compared to 69% without PD
Henry et al. 1999	72 BD-I	Depressive and hyperthymic temperament scales	Positive association between depressive temperament scores and outcome
Colom et al. 2000	144 BD-I 56 BD-II	SCID-II	Patients with PD were over 2 times more likely to be poorly compliant
Hammen et al. 2000	52 BD-I	Eysenck Personality Questionnaire; Interpersonal Dependency Inventory; Personality Disorders Questionnaire	Personality scores combined with other psychosocial variables predicted poor work adjustment
Bieling et al. 2003	87 BD-I and BD-II	SCID-II	High scores on PD scales distinguished symptomatic from euthymic patients in long-term follow-up
Leverich et al. 2003	648 BD-I and BD-II	PDQ-4+	Cluster B PD predictor of past serious suicide attempt

Note. BD-I=bipolar I disorder; BD-II=bipolar II disorder; PDQ-4+ =Personality Diagnostic Questionnaire—4+; SCID-II =Structured Clinical Interview for DSM-IV Axis II Personality Disorders.

(similar to the bipolar disorder spectrum approach) and argues that major depressive illness is essentially an extreme manifestation of "normal" personality traits.

These models have considerable value as organizing heuristics and ways to describe research in the area of unipolar depression. But perhaps more importantly, they allow for a priori theoretical predictions rather than exploratory hypotheses or simple comparative analyses; such models can lead to the construction of specific hypotheses and different kinds of predictions that can be tested against one another with data. Research on bipolar disorder and personality factors now needs to move in that direction, going beyond simple exploratory comparisons between bipolar disorder patients and control subjects or cross-sectional correlational analyses. Instead, future research needs to develop a clear conceptual argument based on comprehensive models or theories and to make specific, refutable hypotheses.

More sophisticated conceptual models of the role of personality in bipolar disorder could be developed, perhaps with the approaches used in unipolar depression as a springboard. Clearly, the spectrum model is already well represented, but a predisposition and complication model could also evolve. The number of significant findings reviewed here clearly suggests that the relation between bipolar disorder, temperament and traits, and personality disorders is important phenomenologically and that personality has an impact on clinical outcome.

Aside from moving toward explicit theories, methodological advances will also be necessary. Because personality theory and assessment is itself fraught with challenges, researchers need to carefully operationalize constructs and use gold-standard measures. Also, exploring the relations between personality features and a chronic mood illness such as bipolar disorder requires longitudinal methods to understand the development of symptoms and personality, and the predictive ability of temperament variables. Further, the best approach would be to assess temperament/personality variables before the emergence of illness and then follow individuals through episodes of mania/hypomania and depression. The importance of large, longitudinal studies of patients with bipolar disorder has been recently recognized with a number of large-scale, longitudinal studies of bipolar disorder (Stanley Foundation Bipolar Network, Systematic Treatment Enhancement Program for Bipolar Disorder [STEP-BD]). These may provide the power to detect and evaluate relations between bipolar disorder and personality disorder and advance our understanding of the interrelatedness of these conditions and their impact on patient outcome.

Finally, clinicians who treat bipolar disorder must be comfortable with assessing and managing personality disorders because these occur frequently in patients with mood disorders. The presence of maladaptive personality features may significantly influence many aspects of treatment, including the development of a therapeutic alliance, adherence to treatment, and type and efficacy of psychotherapy and pharmacotherapy. These factors can obviously, then, influence overall outcome of illness. Patients with personality disorders bring unique and challenging treatment issues that should not be minimized or ignored in the face of the Axis I disorders but rather encompassed as part of the overall assessment and treatment plan.

The following case example describes a woman with both bipolar disorder and a number of prominent Axis II features who was treated over a span of 12 years. This particular case illustrates many of the principles and challenges described in this chapter, including 1) difficulties with accurate diagnosis and separating bipolar disorder from long standing personality features, especially during the acute phase of bipolar disorder; 2) optimization of pharmacotherapy and balancing of other psychosocial approaches, especially in patients whose personality features can make treatment alliances difficult; and 3) a focus on maximizing functioning and stability even when some amount of mood variability as well as problematic personality traits are likely to persist chronically.

Case Illustration

Ms. B was 29 years old, married with three children, and had just completed her bar exams when she was first diagnosed with bipolar I disorder, with rapid cycling, during a manic episode that cost her a job. She had a classic presentation of mania, with grandiosity, sleeplessness, hypersexuality, poor insight, rapid speech and thoughts, and increased energy. She was initially treated with valproic acid because of her recent history of rapid cycling. The mania settled and she was discharged from the hospital, but she felt sedated and gained weight on the valproic acid and after a trial of several months refused to take the medication any longer. Lithium was tried but again she did not tolerate the side effects, and it was also withdrawn after a trial of several months. During this time she began to use clonazepam liberally in doses greater than that prescribed. She was then tried on a controlled-release preparation of carbamazepine. She tolerated the carbamazepine well, and this formed the mainstay of her treatment regimen for many years. She has never again required hospitalization. She periodically required carefully monitored quantities of benzodiazepine to regulate sleep when she became mildly hypomanic, which occurred at a greater frequency than the depressed periods early in her illness. More recently she began to experience an increase in cycling with prolongation of the depressive phases associated with high anxiety. Several agents were added in sequence to the carbamazepine, including gabapentin, an atypical antipsychotic, and finally lamotrigine, which she tolerated at low doses with appreciable stabilization in her mood, although not her anxiety. Antidepressants have been avoided because of the ongoing tendency to cycle.

From a psychosocial perspective, Ms. B was unable to return to work and her marriage ended in divorce during the years in which her illness resulted in rapid cycling. Also, because of the frank bipolar disorder symptoms and the uncertainty this causes for strong conclusions about underlying personality issues, the diagnostic formulation did not yet contain personality-related features. During that initial phase of her illness she had been offered a group cognitive-behavioral therapy (CBT) approach for bipolar disorder. Unfortunately, Ms. B did not find the group very helpful, began to attend sporadically, and was noncompliant with a number of therapy tasks. Her case was reviewed after her bipolar disorder had settled, and the CBT had been considered unsuccessful. This psychodiagnostic assessment, as well as clinical judgment by several clinicians involved in her care over years at the clinic, led to a more formal description of pervasive features of narcissism, grandiosity, and dependency. Before her illness, these traits had manifested in almost a positive manner; the narcissism and grandiosity were actually somewhat useful in her role as an attorney. However, after the onset of her bipolar disorder, these personality features seemed to have been exacerbated and were interfering with her recovery. In retrospect, her strong narcissistic traits were probably a negative indicator for participation in a group treatment, and indeed she reported that the group was too simplistic and did not take into her account the "special" nature of her illness and her needs, for example the "fall from grace" of having been an attorney who was ultimately hospitalized for a psychiatric illness. She did not present these concerns in the group so that these thoughts and feelings could be processed or discussed in that context. Instead, Ms. B sought out one of the group leaders as an individual therapist for more long-term psychotherapy. This therapy continued for at least 2 years, sometimes with more frequent meetings because of crises; other times sessions occurred only on a monthly basis. As might be expected with her high degree of dependency, Ms. B had difficulty contemplating termination, but at the same time there was little substantive progress from the therapy. Even though she had much less frank mania and limited dysphoria with the combination of medications and support, she struggled to reclaim any ground on functioning. She had doubts about her abilities as a mother to her children and was profoundly hurt when they chose to spend time with their father. Similarly, she found herself at loose ends occupationally, but thoughts about her work as an attorney were painful reminders of her loss of identity and more difficult times in her life.

Ms. B was subsequently referred for therapy that focused on behavioral activation, values, and problem solving rather than insight or unconditional positive regard. Despite having this new form of treatment offered, Ms. B struggled with the decision to end treatment with her other clinician. She had a strong tendency to "test" therapists' credentials, reputations, and intelligence so that they earned her respect. The new therapist tolerated this period of ambivalence, responding nondefensively to several challenges, and eventually Ms. B committed herself, in writing, to the new therapeutic approach. The therapeutic alliance was, at the beginning, somewhat tenuous especially because of the new emphasis on action and responsibility taking on Ms. B's part. In early sessions, the therapist did not challenge Ms. B's claims of "specialness" and instead focused on her understanding that the tasks of therapy were in her own best interests, even when this was not immediately apparent. Over time, this allowed the therapist to place Ms. B and her current difficulties in the here and now, rather than her history of cycling and the "fall from grace," at the center of the therapy work. Ms. B began to see the merit in redirecting her own behavior to try to increase her functional capacities, taking responsibility for changing her life in a positive direction, and learning to accept the losses of her past as well as acknowledging the limitations imposed by bipolar disorder. There were noted improvements in her ability to tolerate frustrations with parenting, and through several exercises related to values Ms. B began to consider how to change her life in light of her illness. She identified mental health advocacy and interest in the law, devoid of the shame of losing her career, as areas of interest. With the additional services of a vocational rehabilitation specialist, Ms. B found a volunteer position in which she represented mentally ill individuals in certain quasilegal contexts. This activity, and a number of individuals she met through the activity, considerably expanded her social circle and allowed her to form attachments beyond her therapists. Eventually, the therapist was able to "wean" Ms. B from therapy by spacing sessions at longer intervals while also leaving open the possibility of sessions during a crisis.

Ms. B's case emphasizes the complex interplay between the Axis I mood disorder and the Axis II personality features. It highlights the dissociation between symptom control and functional recovery, and the role that Axis II traits may have in limiting both while demonstrating that with adequate pharmacological treatment as a background the personality issues can be successfully addressed with appropriate psychotherapeutic formulation. Finally, Ms. B's long course toward functional improvement emphasizes not only the chronicity of this illness but also the possibility that significant gains may be accrued even after many years of seemingly "partial illness responsiveness."

References

Akiskal HS: Delineating irritable and hyperthymic variants of the cyclothymic temperament. J Personal Disord 6:326–342, 1992

Akiskal HS: The childhood roots of bipolar disorder. J Affect Disord 51:75–76, 1998

Akiskal HS, Mallya G: Criteria for the "soft" bipolar spectrum: treatment implications. Psychopharmacol Bull 23:68–73, 1987

Akiskal HS, Pinto O: The evolving bipolar spectrum: prototypes I, II, III, and IV. Psychiatr Clin North Am 22:517–534, 1999

Akiskal HS, Djenderedjian AM, Rosenthal RH, et al: Cyclothymic disorder: validating criteria for inclusion in the bipolar affective group. Am J Psychiatry 134:1227–1233, 1977

Akiskal HS, Hirschfeld RM, Yerevanian BI: The relationship of personality to affective disorders. Arch Gen Psychiatry 40:801–810, 1983

Akiskal HS, Chen SE, Davis GC, et al: Borderline: an adjective in search of a noun. J Clin Psychiatry 46:41–48, 1985

Akiskal HS, Hantouche EG, Bourgeois ML, et al: Gender, temperament, and the clinical picture in dysphoric mixed mania: findings from a French national study (EPIMAN). J Affect Disord 50:175–186, 1998

Akiskal HS, Bourgeois ML, Angst J, et al: Re-evaluating the prevalence of and diagnostic composition within the broad clinical spectrum of bipolar disorders. J Affect Disord 59 (suppl 1):S5–S30, 2000

Akiskal HS, Hantouche EG, Allilaire JF: Bipolar II with and without cyclothymic temperament: "dark" and "sunny" expressions of soft bipolarity. J Affect Disord 73:49–57, 2003

American Psychiatric Association: Diagnostic and Statistical Manual of Mental Disorders, 4th Edition, Text Revision. Washington, DC, American Psychiatric Association, 2000

Angst J: The emerging epidemiology of hypomania and bipolar II disorder. J Affect Disord 50:143–151, 1998

Atre-Vaidya N, Hussain SM: Borderline personality disorder and bipolar mood disorder: two distinct disorders or a continuum? J Nerv Ment Dis 187:313–315, 1999

Bagby RM, Young LT, Schuller DR, et al: Bipolar disorder, unipolar depression and the five-factor model of personality. J Affect Disord 41:25–32, 1996

Barbato N, Hafner RJ: Comorbidity of bipolar and personality disorder. Aust N Z J Psychiatry 32:276–280, 1998

Benazzi F: Exploring aspects of DSM-IV interpersonal sensitivity in bipolar II. J Affect Disord 60:43–46, 2000

Bieling PJ, MacQueen GM, Marriot MJ, et al: Longitudinal outcome in patients with bipolar disorder assessed by life-charting is influenced by DSM-IV personality disorder symptoms. Bipolar Disord 5:14–21, 2003

Blairy S, Massat I, Staner L, et al: 5-HT$_{2A}$ receptor polymorphism gene in bipolar disorder and harm avoidance personality trait. Am J Med Genet 96:360–364, 2000

Bolton S, Gunderson JG: Distinguishing borderline personality disorder from bipolar disorder: differential diagnosis and implications. Am J Psychiatry 153:1202–1207, 1996

Brieger P, Ehrt U, Roettig S, et al: Personality features of patients with mixed and pure manic episodes. Acta Psychiatr Scand 106:179–182, 2002

Brieger P, Ehrt U, Marneros A: Frequency of comorbid personality disorders in bipolar and unipolar affective disorders. Compr Psychiatry 44:28–34, 2003

Carpenter D, Clarkin JF, Glick ID, et al: Personality pathology among married adults with bipolar disorder. J Affect Disord 34:269–274, 1995

Carpenter D, Clarkin JF, Isman L, et al: The impact of neuroticism upon married bipolar patients. J Personal Disord 13:60–66, 1999

Cassano GB, Dell'Osso L, Frank E, et al: The bipolar spectrum: a clinical reality in search of diagnostic criteria and an assessment methodology. J Affect Disord 54:319–328, 1999

Cassano G, Frank E, Miniati M, et al: Conceptual underpinnings and empirical support for the mood spectrum. Psychiatr Clin North Am 25:699–712, 2002

Clark LA, Watson D, Mineka S: Temperament, personality, and the mood and anxiety disorders. J Abnorm Psychol 103:103–116, 1994

Cloninger CR, Svrakic DM, Przybeck TR: A psychobiological model of temperament and character. Arch Gen Psychiatry 50:975–990, 1993

Colom F, Vieta E, Martinez-Aran A, et al: Clinical factors associated with treatment noncompliance in euthymic bipolar patients. J Clin Psychiatry 61:549–555, 2000

Cowdry RW, Gardner DL: Pharmacotherapy of borderline personality disorder: alprazolam, carbamazepine, trifluoperazine, and tranylcypromine. Arch Gen Psychiatry 45:111–119, 1988

Daskalopoulou EG, Dikeos DG, Papadimitriou GN, et al: Self-esteem, social adjustment and suicidality in affective disorders. Eur Psychiatry 17:265–271, 2002

Dell'Osso L, Placidi GF, Nassi R, et al: The manic-depressive mixed state: familial, temperamental and psychopathologic characteristics in 108 female inpatients. Eur Arch Psychiatry Clin Neurosci 240:234–239, 1991

Deltito J, Martin L, Riefkohl J, et al: Do patients with borderline personality disorder belong to the bipolar spectrum? J Affect Disord 67:221–228, 2001

Dunayevich E, Strakowski SM, Sax KW, et al: Personality disorders in first- and multiple-episode mania. Psychiatry Res 64:69–75, 1996

Dunayevich E, Sax KW, Keck PE, et al: Twelve-month outcome in bipolar patients with and without personality disorders. J Clin Psychiatry 61:134–139, 2000

Feiner NF: Borderline personality and bipolar disorder. Am J Psychiatry 154:1175–1176, 1997

Frankenburg FR, Zanarini MC: Divalproex sodium treatment of women with borderline personality disorder and bipolar II disorder: a double-blind placebo-controlled pilot study. J Clin Psychiatry 63:442–446, 2002

Gross R, Olfson M, Gameroff M, et al: Borderline personality disorder in primary care. Arch Intern Med 162:53–60, 2002

Hammen C, Gitlin M, Altshuler L: Predictors of work adjustment in bipolar I patients: a naturalistic longitudinal follow-up. J Consult Clin Psychol 68:220–225, 2000

Hayward P, Wong G, Bright JA, et al: Stigma and self-esteem in manic depression: an exploratory study. J Affect Disord 69:61–67, 2002

Hecht H, van Calker D, Berger M, et al: Personality in patients with affective disorders and their relatives. J Affect Disord 51:33–43, 1998

Henry C, Lacoste J, Bellivier F, et al: Temperament in bipolar illness: impact on prognosis. J Affect Disord 56:103–108, 1999

Henry C, Mitropoulou V, New AS, et al: Affective instability and impulsivity in borderline personality and bipolar II disorders: similarities and differences. J Psychiatr Res 35:307–312, 2001

Hirschfeld RM: Bipolar spectrum disorder: improving its recognition and diagnosis. J Clin Psychiatry 62 (suppl 14):5–9, 2001

Hollander E, Allen A, Lopez RP, et al: A preliminary double-blind, placebo-controlled trial of divalproex sodium in borderline personality disorder. J Clin Psychiatry 62:199–203, 2001

Hutto B: Potential overdiagnosis of bipolar disorder. Psychiatr Serv 52:687–688, 2001

Jackson HJ, Whiteside HL, Bates GW, et al: Diagnosing personality disorders in psychiatric inpatients. Acta Psychiatr Scand 83:206–213, 1991

Jain U, Blais MA, Otto MW, et al: Five-factor personality traits in patients with seasonal depression: treatment effects and comparisons with bipolar patients. J Affect Disord 55:51–54, 1999

Kay JH, Altshuler LL, Ventura J, et al: Prevalence of axis II comorbidity in bipolar patients with and without alcohol use disorders. Ann Clin Psychiatry 11:187–195, 1999

Keck PE Jr, McElroy SL, Strakowski SM, et al: Compliance with maintenance treatment in bipolar disorder. Psychopharmacol Bull 33:87–91, 1997

Klein DN, Lewinsohn PM, Seeley JR: Hypomanic personality traits in a community sample of adolescents. J Affect Disord 38:135–143, 1996

Lam DH, Watkins ER, Hayward P, et al: A randomized controlled study of cognitive therapy for relapse prevention for bipolar affective disorder: outcome of the first year. Arch Gen Psychiatry 60:145–152, 2003

Leverich GS, Altshuler LL, Frye MA, et al: Factors associated with suicide attempts in 648 patients with bipolar disorder in the Stanley Foundation Bipolar Network. J Clin Psychiatry 64:506–515, 2003

Levitt AJ, Joffe RT, Ennis J, et al: The prevalence of cyclothymia in borderline personality disorder. J Clin Psychiatry 51:335–339, 1990

Linehan M: Cognitive-Behavioral Treatment of Borderline Personality Disorder. New York, Guilford, 1993

Lozano BE, Johnson SL: Can personality traits predict increases in manic and depressive symptoms? J Affect Disord 63:103–111, 2001

Meyer TD, Hautzinger M: Hypomanic personality, social anhedonia and impulsive nonconformity: evidence for familial aggregation? J Personal Disord 15:281–299, 2001

Moeller FG, Barratt ES, Dougherty DM, et al: Psychiatric aspects of impulsivity. Am J Psychiatry 158:1783–1793, 2001

O'Connell RA, Mayo JA, Sciutto MS: PDQ-R personality disorders in bipolar patients. J Affect Disord 23:217–221, 1991

Osher Y, Cloninger CR, Belmaker RH: TPQ in euthymic manic-depressive patients. J Psychiatr Res 30:353–357, 1996

Osher Y, Lefkifker E, Kotler M: Low persistence in euthymic manic-depressive patients: a replication. J Affect Disord 53:87–90, 1999

Perretta P, Akiskal HS, Nisita C, et al: The high prevalence of bipolar II and associated cyclothymic and hyperthymic temperaments in HIV-patients. J Affect Disord 50:215–224, 1998

Perugi G, Akiskal HS: The soft bipolar spectrum redefined: focus on the cyclothymic, anxious-sensitive, impulse-dyscontrol, and binge-eating connection in bipolar II and related conditions. Psychiatr Clin North Am 25:713–737, 2002

Perugi G, Maremmani I, Toni C, et al: The contrasting influence of depressive and hyperthymic temperaments on psychometrically derived manic subtypes. Psychiatry Res 101:249–258, 2001

Perugi G, Toni C, Travierso MC, et al: The role of cyclothymia in atypical depression: toward a data-based reconceptualization of the borderline-bipolar II connection. J Affect Disord 73:87–98, 2003

Pica S, Edwards J, Jackson HJ, et al: Personality disorders in recent-onset bipolar disorder. Compr Psychiatry 31:499–510, 1990

Pinto OC, Akiskal HS: Lamotrigine as a promising approach to borderline personality: an open case series without concurrent DSM-IV major mood disorder. J Affect Disord 51:333–343, 1998

Preston GA, Marchant BK, Reimherr FW, et al: Borderline personality disorder in patients wth bipolar disorder and response to lamotrigine. J Affect Disord 79:297–303, 2004

Quackenbush D, Kutcher S, Robertson HA, et al: Premorbid and postmorbid school functioning in bipolar adolescents: description and suggested academic interventions. Can J Psychiatry 41:16–22, 1996

Rossi A, Marinangeli MG, Butti G, et al: Personality disorders in bipolar and depressive disorders. J Affect Disord 65:3–8, 2001

Rothenberg A: Bipolar illness, creativity, and treatment. Psychiatr Q 72:131–147, 2001

Scott J, Stanton B, Garland A, et al: Cognitive vulnerability in patients with bipolar disorder. Psychol Med 30:467–472, 2000

Solomon DA, Shea MT, Leon AC, et al: Personality traits in subjects with bipolar I disorder in remission. J Affect Disord 40:41–48, 1996

Stormberg D, Ronningstam E, Gunderson J, et al: Brief communication: pathological narcissism in bipolar disorder patients. J Personal Disord 12:179–185, 1998

Strakowski SM, Stoll AL, Tohen M, et al: The Tridimensional Personality Questionnaire as a predictor of six-month outcome in first episode mania. Psychiatry Res 48:1–8, 1993

Turley B, Bates GW, Edwards J, et al: MCMI-II personality disorders in recent-onset bipolar disorders. J Clin Psychol 48:320–329, 1992

Ucok A, Karaveli D, Kundakci T, et al: Comorbidity of personality disorders with bipolar mood disorders. Compr Psychiatry 39:72–74, 1998

Vieta E, Colom F, Martinez-Aran A, et al: Personality disorders in bipolar II patients. J Nerv Ment Dis 187:245–248, 1999

Vieta E, Colom F, Martinez-Aran A, et al: Bipolar II disorder and comorbidity. Compr Psychiatry 41:339–343, 2000

von Zerssen D: Premorbid personality and affective psychoses, in Handbook of Studies on Depression. Edited by Burrows GD. Amsterdam, The Netherlands, Excerpta Medica, 1977, pp 79–103

von Zerssen D: Development of an integrated model of personality, personality disorders and severe axis I disorders, with special reference to major affective disorders. J Affect Disord 68:143–158, 2002 von Zerssen D, Possl J: The premorbid personality of patients with different subtypes of an affective illness: statistical analysis of blind assignment of case history data to clinical diagnoses. J Affect Disord 18:39–50, 1990

von Zerssen D, Tauscher R, Possl J: The relationship of premorbid personality to subtypes of an affective illness: a replication study by means of an operationalized procedure for the diagnosis of personality structures. J Affect Disord 32:61–72, 1994

Werry JS, McClellan JM, Chard L: Childhood and adolescent schizophrenic, bipolar, and schizoaffective disorders: a clinical and outcome study. J Am Acad Child Adolesc Psychiatry 30:457–465, 1991

Young LT, Bagby RM, Cooke RG, et al: A comparison of Tridimensional Personality Questionnaire dimensions in bipolar disorder and unipolar depression. Psychiatry Res 58:139–143, 1995

Zanarini MC, Frankenburg FR, Dubo ED, et al: Axis I comorbidity of borderline personality disorder. Am J Psychiatry 155:1733–1739, 1998

EVALUATING THE CONTRIBUTION OF PERSONALITY FACTORS TO DEPRESSED MOOD IN ADOLESCENTS

Conceptual and Clinical Issues

Darcy A. Santor, Ph.D.
Michael Rosenbluth, M.D.

Determining the clinical significance of maladaptive personality traits and characteristics is one of the main challenges clinicians face in working with youth who are being treated for depression or depressed mood. Maladaptive traits, characteristics, and styles, internal to the person, may either precipitate or exacerbate both the severity of symptoms defining the illness and the interpersonal and achievement difficulties frequently associated with those conditions.

Research has identified a number of personality characteristics and vulnerability factors that may increase the risk for developing mood problems in adolescence, ranging from temperamental differences identified early in development to differences in self-esteem and coping styles that may change over the course of adolescence. Assessing the contribution of personality traits and characteristics to the onset and maintenance of mood symptoms requires an understanding of how such factors can constitute a vulnerability for mood difficulties, as well as a set of tools and strategies for assessing the severity or degree of that vulnerability.

In the first section of this chapter, we highlight many of the theoretical issues concerning the definition of personality and vulnerability and the manner in which vulnerability factors might be related to depressed mood. In the second section, we review some of the key vulnerability factors that have been associated with mood difficulties in adolescents. In the third section, we illustrate how vulnerability factors can and should be assessed in clinical practice by reviewing a clinical case involving a 14-year-old adolescent dealing with depression. In the final section, we review general clinical issues and challenges.

Theoretical Issues in Defining Personality and Vulnerability

Defining Personality

Whether any personality trait or characteristic constitutes a vulnerability factor depends on how personality and vulnerability are defined. Numerous attempts have been made to provide a comprehensive and general definition of personality. Consider the following general definition of personality from Maddi (1980):

> Personality is a stable set of characteristics and tendencies that determine those commonalities and differences in the psychological behaviour (thoughts, feelings and actions) of people that have continuity in time and which cannot be explained by current social and biological events. *Tendencies* are the processes that determine directionality in thoughts, feelings and actions and are in the service of goals or functions. *Characteristics* are static or structural entities usually implied by tendencies that are used to explain content of goals. (p.10)

This definition highlights many of the key features of personality traits. The definition includes both *characteristics* and *tendencies*. Characteristics are the structural components of personality and would include characteristics such as dependency and self-criticism, which for theorists such as Blatt (1974) emerge when basic developmental processes are disrupted. Tendencies, in contrast, are the processes that determine the direction that thoughts, feelings, and actions take. They are the different strategies that dependent and self-critical individuals take in adapting to or coping with threats to self-worth and interpersonal relatedness (see Santor 2003).

The definition provided by Maddi (1980) emphasizes that personality is both stable and continuous over time. Stability implies that how individuals feel, think, and act will generalize (to a degree) across a number of situations and contexts. Individuals who need reassurance and attempt to elicit reassurance from others by expressing their own distress are expected to require reassurance from most people who are important to them and will adopt similar strategies with those individuals. Continuity implies that these traits and strategies are expected to persist over time and not merely be the concomitant of a mood disorder or a temporary response to a novel (social) situation.

Defining Vulnerability

Whether any personality trait, characteristic, or style counts as a vulnerability factor for depressed mood depends also on the manner in which vulnerability and clinical sequelae are defined. Personality traits such as shyness may be problematic at face value but do not necessarily confer a heightened risk for depressive moods or illness. Historically, the term *vulnerability* has been used in a number of ways, referring to a diverse group of conditions and individual dispositions that have been hypothesized either alone or in connection with other factors to explain the onset of mood problems. Early formulations of vulnerability referred to a diathesis defined as a "constitutional disposition, or predisposition, to some anomalous or morbid condition, which no longer belongs within the confines of normal variability, but already begins to represent a potential disease condition" (Campbell 1989, p. 202). This view of vulnerability dates to the humoral theory of temperament and disease articulated by the early Greeks and by Galen in the second century. However, over the past few decades the use of the term has been expanded to include both broad and specific traits, characteristics, and styles and has been used to designate whether individuals are vulnerable or at risk for a broad array of outcomes, ranging from sad and depressed moods to full episodes of depression (see Figure 9–1).

Some theorists have argued that *risk* and *vulnerability* are conceptually distinct. Ingram and Price (2001) characterize risk factors as exogenous and descriptive, whereas vulnerability factors are viewed as endogenous and causal. For Ingram and Price, risk should be used to refer to any factor that is empirically associated with an increased likelihood of experiencing a disorder. They cite poverty and stress related to social injustice as examples of risk factors, which are exogenous, but view negative thinking styles as vulnerability factors, which are endogenous and therefore believed to be capable of accounting for or explaining why an onset of difficulty has occurred. This distinction implies that

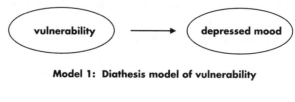

Model 1: Diathesis model of vulnerability

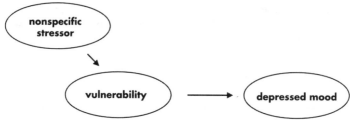

Model 2: Diathesis-stress model of vulnerability

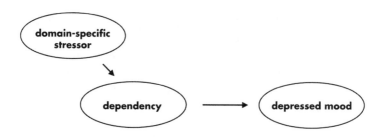

Model 3: Congruency model of vulnerability

FIGURE 9–1.   Three models of vulnerability.

identifying an exogenous risk factor (e.g., poverty) may not necessarily explain the mechanism of onset of disorder but that the identification of the endogenous factor could. Indeed, without a predisposition to negative thinking (the endogenous vulnerability factor), the stress associated with poverty alone (the exogenous risk factor) would not likely lead to the onset of an episode. Risk and vulnerability factors may be difficult to distinguish and are likely to act in conjunction, which is the heart of most contemporary stress diatheses models (see Munroe and Simons 1991).

Distinguishing risk and vulnerability factors in this manner may be arbitrary. Indeed, assigning any person factor the status of causal mechanism should be considered carefully, particularly given the importance of biological factors (Dahl and Ryan 1996; Kendler et al. 1993b), familial environment (Hammen et al. 1991), and childhood adverse events (Kessler 1994), which can increase the risk for developing clinical difficulties. In some instances the vulnerability factor may only be a sufficient (and not a necessary) cause of onset. Indeed, a high level of stress may precipitate, on its own, the onset of illness in most individuals, irrespective of the underlying vulnerabilities. In other instances, the status of the risk or vulnerability factor may not be clear. For example, a family history of mood disorder increases the risk for mood disorders in offspring. However, in any given offspring of a depressed parent, the risk for onset may be either the family environment or the genetic disposition passed from parent to offspring, some combination of both, or neither.

Whether any personality factor should be viewed as a vulnerability or risk factor also depends on the relationship between that factor and the clinical endpoint. For example, self-esteem is a characteristic that is generally stable across time and context and that has been associated with depressed mood (Schmitz et al. 2003). Although related to depressed mood at any given time, whether self-esteem should be considered a vulnerability factor for the onset of clinical episode of depression depends on 1) the magnitude of the (relative) risk for developing a future clinical depression given low self-esteem relative to the magnitude of the risk for developing a future clinical depression given high self-esteem, and 2) the extent to which cases of clinical depression can be attributed (attributable risk) to low self-esteem. The evidence for self-esteem in terms of either relative or attributable risk is weaker than other factors such as subthreshold symptoms of depression, which have far stronger associations with depressive episodes both in terms of relative and attributable risk (Horwarth et al. 1992).

Defining the clinical endpoint more liberally, say as just a mood disturbance, may reveal a stronger association between self-esteem and depressed mood. However, this raises the question of the clinical significance of mood disturbances; they do not meet the criteria of a disorder, which by definition requires that there be a degree of impairment in functioning. The majority of research conducted to date has examined depressed mood rather than cases of depression, which has been evaluated through the use of psychometric scales. There has been considerable debate about the value of studying depressed mood, defined on the basis of high scores on measures of severity rather than the onset of diagnosable cases of depression. Research has shown that high scores on a number of measures of depressed mood tend not to be good proxies of a clinical disorder. However, other research has shown that elevated scores on measures of depressed mood (Lewinsohn et al. 2000) and subthreshold levels of depressive symptoms (Johnson 1995) do predict the onset of depression.

Stability of Personality in Young Adults

There are a number of additional issues to consider in understanding the contribution of personality and vulnerability to the onset and maintenance of clinical difficulties in adolescence. Identifying what characteristics in adolescence will become enduring traits and vulnerability factors may be difficult given that adolescence is by definition a period of development in which those traits and styles are consolidated within a person. Moreover, how a young person thinks, feels, and acts (i.e., tendencies), or the degree to which a young person either is shy, dominant, or self-critical (i.e., characteristics), can and will change in response to the various familial, social, individual pressures and needs a young person experiences. The extent to which personality and vulnerability can contribute to the onset of difficulties, rather than be viewed as the outcome of difficulties, will depend on the degree of stability and consistency that can be achieved during this period of development.

One of the most important criteria for viewing any individual characteristic or trait as a personality or vulnerability factor is that these traits are stable across time and situations. Some characteristics of the individual such as attachment style and temperament should show relatively more permanence over time. Evidence is beginning to emerge for some degree of stability in personality over adolescence. In one of the few studies conducted to date, McCrae and colleagues (2002) showed that the broad dimensions of personality, as measured by the five-factor model (*neuroticism, extraversion, agreeableness, conscientiousness,* and *openness*) of personality (Digman 1990), were evident throughout adolescence, with different degrees of stability. Levels of neuroticism were shown to increase in girls, openness was found to increase in both boys and girls, but levels of extraversion, agreeableness, and conscientiousness remained stable. Other research has shown that stability in self-esteem is generally comparable to stability in personality traits (Trzesniewski et al. 2003), remaining low in childhood but increasing during adolescence and young adulthood.

Results of research conducted to date suggest that stability in personality factors should be considered carefully on a trait-by-trait basis. However, this consideration does not preclude the possibility of stability either across (some) situations or over (short) periods of time. Vulnerability theorists, such as Blatt (Blatt 1974; Blatt and Homann 1992; Blatt and Shichman 1983), acknowledge that depressive vulnerability factors such as dependency and self-criticism emerge during childhood and adolescence and are malleable. Even though the degree of vulnerability may not be immutable, vulnerability is nonetheless considered to be relatively stable across contexts and (shorter) periods of time, which longitudinal studies confirm (Kuperminc et al. 1997). On balance, the evidence to date favors viewing traits and vulnerability factors such as dependency and self-criticism as stable albeit over short periods of time.

Vulnerability Factors Emerging During Adolescence: Interpersonal Rejection and Peer Pressure

Many of the depressive vulnerability factors studied to date, such as attributional style, dependency, self-criticism, and reassurance thinking have been extrapolated from research and theorizing in adults and then adapted and validated in adolescent populations (Blatt et al. 1992). Although theorists such as Blatt (Blatt 1974; Blatt and Homann 1992; Blatt and Shichman 1983) have formulated vulnerability factors within a developmental perspective, many of the depressive vulnerability factors extrapolated from adults to adolescents are not necessarily characteristic of adolescence.

In contrast, peer pressure and peer rejection first emerge during adolescence. Because of their importance to the development of personality and interpersonal relationships at this time, they may exert greater influence on mood during adolescence then at other times over the life span. In this regard, personality characteristics such as a susceptibility to peer pressure and interpersonal rejection deserve special attention given that they have been shown to be related to depressed mood (Boivin et al. 1995; Bond et al. 2001; Santor et al. 2000). It is, however, unclear to what extent susceptibility to peer rejection and peer pressure contributes directly to mood problems or is related to other depressive vulnerability factors such as dependency and self-criticism.

Situating Vulnerability Factors Within a Developmental Framework

One other challenge facing clinicians assessing personality and vulnerability in adolescence is how to decide which of the numerous vulnerability factors that have been empirically related to depression should be assessed in the clinic. Developing a framework that articulates the manner in which various vulnerability and risk factors might be related is central to this task. Indeed, many of the personality and vulnerability factors highlighted in this chapter are likely to be related in important ways. For example, temperamental differences observed in infancy are likely to affect the ways in which children learn to manage emotional experiences with caregivers, who are likely to affect the extent to which individuals become self-critical or dependent during adolescence.

At present, few programs of research have attempted to explicate the manner in which various individual difference and vulnerability factors are related either theoretically or empirically in adolescent populations, although some general frameworks (Cicchetti and Toth 1995) and empirical investigations (Fichman et al. 1994) have appeared. Developmental psychopathology constitutes one of the few attempts to integrate and conceptualize the emergence of different forms of psychopathology during adolescence (Cicchetti and Rogosch 2002; Cicchetti and Toth 1995). The key elements of a developmental psychopathology framework include 1) that individuals play a role in directing the course of development; 2) that there is an ongoing transaction between different development domains (biological, emotional, cognitive, interpersonal) and the environment (familial, social, community); and 3) that developmental pathways be conceptualized in terms of two broad principles, namely *multifinality* and *equifinality* (von Bertalanffy 1968) (see Figure 9–2).

Multifinality specifies that diverse outcomes can emerge from a single starting point. For example, being the child of a depressed parent increases the risk for a range of difficulties, including depression, in addition to a number of other clinical, academic, and psychosocial difficulties that may or may not be accompanied by depressed mood, and still most children of depressed parents will not develop a clinical depression by adulthood. This illustrates the notion that individuals with similar risk factors can have different outcomes.

In contrast, equifinality specifies that a common outcome may develop over time from different starting points. For example, adolescents who develop depression may do so for different reasons. Some may have a genetic predisposition to depression, whereas others may have experienced the loss of a parent or some other negative life event. For example, a growing body of research shows that there may be two very different specific pathways to depression for boys and girls (see Block et al. 1991).

The principles of multifinality and equifinality also have a number of important implications for the assessment of risk and vulnerability. The principle of multifinality emphasizes the importance of assessing young people for a variety of outcomes even though they may be at

1: Principle of multifinality

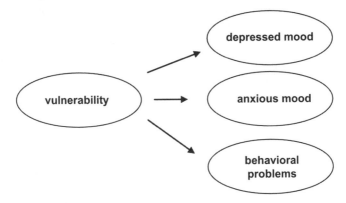

2: Principle of equifinality

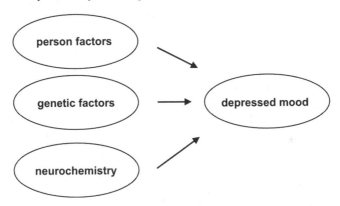

FIGURE 9–2. Principles of multifinality and equifinality of outcomes.

greatest risk for depressed mood, which can complicate how measures are chosen and what vulnerability factors get assessed. However, the principle of equifinality acknowledges that despite the extremely large number of different vulnerability factors examined to date, many of these vulnerability factors are likely to reflect a common underlying vulnerability that is expressed in different ways and at different periods of development, which despite any differences may confer the same degree of risk or vulnerability. Accordingly, it is recommended that clinicians select vulnerability factors that assess either broad dimensions of personality, such as neuroticism or introversion (McCrae et al. 2002), or select more specific measures of vulnerability, such as dependency, self-criticism, or temperament (Blatt 1974; Thomas et al. 1963), which can be mapped on to broader dimensions of personality that confer a vulnerability to depression, such as neuroticism or introversion (Zuroff 1994). However, it is also recommended that choosing a broad approach to assessing vulnerability should be done with care. Even though specific vulnerability factors such as dependency and self-criticism may all be related to broader common underlying vulnerability, such as neuroticism, differences in temperament, attributional style, and level of self-criticism and dependency may indicate different points of therapeutic intervention than the broader dimension.

Mechanisms of Onset: How Are Vulnerability Factors Related to Depressed Mood?

Understanding the precise relation between personality and depression is both complex and controversial. Adolescence is also a period of time during which some clinical difficulties, such as mood disorders, become prevalent. Epidemiological studies show that the occurrence of mood disorders in childhood is relatively rare but that their prevalence increases dramatically during adolescence—between 3- and 10-fold (Flemming et al. 1989; Poznanski and Mokros 1994)—which may affect the development of personality. Several models examining the relationship between personality and depression have been proposed (see L.A. Clark et al. 1994; D.N. Klein et al. 2002; and M.H. Klein et al. 1993 for reviews). One group of models suggests that personality traits can influence the onset or maintenance of depression in some way. These include 1) that personality factors predispose individuals to depressive episodes (vulnerability model), 2) that personality can influence the course and expression of a depressive episode (pathoplasty and exacerbation models), or 3) that personality interacts with vulnerability-congruent events (congruency model). A second group of models suggests that personality is largely incidental to the onset or course of depression. These include 4) that personality is an early manifestation (precursor model) of a mood disorder, 5) that personality is either a complication (or scar) of a depressive episode (complication model), 6) that personality is the result of a third factor also responsible for the onset of a depressive episode (common cause model), or 7) that personality is contingent on the mood disturbance (state dependence model). In the first group of models, personality can modify the onset, course, or expression of depression, whereas in the second group of models, personality does not. These models are not exhaustive nor are they mutually exclusive (see L.A. Clark et al. 1994; M.H. Klein et al. 1993).

Critics of personality and vulnerability models of depression have argued that there is little evidence in support of a stable vulnerability to depression. Elevated levels on personality traits such as neuroticism may reflect the severity of depressive symptoms but do not exist independently of depressive symptoms (Barnett and Gotlib 1988; Coyne and Gotlib 1983). Support for this view comes from a large number of studies, generally in adults, showing that scores on personality scales are either no different in remitted depressed patients than in nondepressed control subjects or are significantly lower in depressed patients tested in remission (see Barnett and Gotlib 1988; Segal and Ingram 1995, for reviews). Some studies have shown that personality factors do predict the onset of depressive symptoms (Block et al. 1991) and depressive episodes (Kendler et al. 1993a), but many studies have not (see Barnett and Gotlib 1988 for a review). Because scores generally decrease after treatment interventions, critics have concluded that personality and vulnerability factors believed to constitute a vulnerability to depression are not stable, depend on levels of depressive severity, and cannot be used as markers of risk or vulnerability for depressive states (Haynes 1992). However, research directly examining the relationship between changes in personality and depression has shown that one cannot be attributed directly to the other (Santor et al. 1997).

Proximal Versus Distal Effects of Vulnerability

Theoretical models of mental illness increasingly have emphasized the reciprocal effects of risk factors and the importance of developing transactional or dynamic models, wherein events and diatheses exert reciprocal influences on one another (Bandura 1977; Cicchetti and Tucker 1994; Folkman and Lazarus 1985; Neufeld 1999). Understanding the dynamic nature of proximal and distal risk factors and their sequelae is not only theoretically important for understanding the onset and evolution of mood difficulties, it is also important for developing appropriate prevention and treatment models for the management of the disorder.

Examining the influence of risk factors in a dynamic model implies that risk factors can exert different effects during different phases of the illness. There is good reason to believe that the influence of many risk factors identified in previous research is not static but rather changes dynamically with the development of the illness and onset of symptoms. Research examining the impact of stressors has shown that depressive episodes alter the degree of vulnerability for subsequent disorder (Post 1992). A number of studies have now shown that more psychosocial stressors are typically involved in the onset of the first episode than in subsequent episodes and that psychosocial stressors have less impact on subsequent episodes than in early episodes (Kendler et al. 2000; Lewinsohn et al. 1999; Post 1992). Research has also suggested that many negative life events may actually be a consequence of the individual's depression rather than a cause, the majority of the events being interpersonal (Hammen 1991), and that vulnerability to severe depressive states is influenced by patterns of information processing that occur during mild states of dysphoria, which are believed to be required to activate negatively biased interpretations of events (Hankin and Abramson 2001; Teasdale 1983, 1988).

Although the development and expansion of vulnerability research has been considerable, the vulnerability literature remains conceptualized largely in terms of a cognitive-affect stress-diathesis model (e.g., D. A. Clark et al. 1999). Studies, examining personality character as vulnerabilities for depressed mood have focused primarily on the content of personality, rather than on the tendencies, processes, or behavioral strategies that personality theorists such as Maddi (1980) view as integral components of personality.

Continued progress in understanding the link between vulnerability factors and mood depends on a fuller understanding of depressive vulnerability factors themselves. Viewing vulnerability factors more broadly in terms of their effects on both mood and behavior may be central to understanding the role of vulnerability factors in the premorbid phase of the illness as well as the kindling and stress-generation effects observed by Post (1992) and Hammen and colleagues (1991). Results of experimental work examining the proximal effects of vulnerability factors on behavior have shown that depressive vulnerability factors can contribute to stressful environments in a number of ways, for example 1) by moderating the manner in which individuals exert control over a shared, limited resource (Santor and Zuroff 1998); 2) by influencing whether individuals adopt strategies that ameliorate or aggravate the quality of interpersonal relations (Santor and Zuroff 1997, 1998; Santor et al. 2001); 3) by affecting the manner in which negative interpersonal events are recalled (Santor and Zuroff 1998) and characterized (Santor and Zuroff 1997); 4) by moderating the degree to which vulnerable individuals persist in making unfavorable comparisons with others (D. A. Santor, A. Yazbek: "Soliciting Unfavorable Social Comparisons: Effects of Self-Criticism." Unpublished manuscript, 2001); and 5) by the extent to which vulnerability factors are related to sustained, subthreshold mood disturbances (Santor and Patterson 2004).

Distinguishing the proximal versus distal effects of vulnerability factors also carries important implications for clinical assessment and practice, namely that the impact of vulnerability factors such as dependency and self-criticism should be considered not only with respect to their direct effects on mood but also with respect to other domains of functioning such as peer, familial, and romantic relationships, which have also been shown to adversely affect mood and functioning.

Assessing Depressive Vulnerability Factors in Young Persons

The breadth and number of personality factors studied in association with depressive moods and symptoms is enormous, ranging from specific individual difference factors such as self-esteem (Schmitz et al. 2003) and helplessness (Nolen-Hoeksema et al. 1986) to broad, higher order personality dimensions, such as neuroticism and extraversion (Jorm et al. 2000), onto which the majority of specific personality dimensions can be mapped. However, the most frequently studied and well-understood person factors associated with depressive moods include cognitive and interpersonal factors such as explanatory style and reassurance seeking, which are well situated within existing theories of depression. In this section, we review a number of central domains of vulnerability (see Table 9–1).

Cognitive Personality Factors

The cognitive vulnerability factors most frequently studied as vulnerability factors for depression include both attributional and explanatory style and personality factors, which characterize the extent to which individuals emphasize achievement and self-worth over maintaining interpersonal relatedness.

Attributional Style

Attributional or *explanatory* style refers to individual difference in how people explain the occurrence of bad events (Alloy et al. 1984). Indeed, negative events can be explained in different ways. Studies have shown that how young people tend to explain the occurrence of negative life events is related both concurrently and prospectively to depressed mood. That is, young people who attribute the cause of negative life events to themselves (internal) view these events as a result of circumstances that are unlikely to change (stable), and those who believe that failure is likely to occur in other situations (global) are more likely to experience sad mood. For example, the attribution "I failed a course because I am stupid" is internal (i.e., it is not because of the instructor or course work),

---

TABLE 9–1.   Domains of vulnerability

Broad personality dimensions

   Neuroticism

   Extraversion

Specific personality traits

   Self-esteem

   Helplessness

   Attributional style

   Dependency

   Self-criticism

Neurocognitive factors

   Attention

   Executive functioning

Attachment

   Temperament

   Reassurance seeking

   Insecure attachment styles

Developmental factors

   Interpersonal rejection

   Peer pressure

---

stable (i.e., having a low IQ is unlikely to change), and global (i.e., having a low IQ is likely to bring about failure in other areas as well).

Research on attributional style in children and adolescents has been substantial (Joiner and Wagner 1995). Meta-analyses of some 27 studies in children and adolescents support the association between attributional style and depressed mood both concurrently and to a degree prospectively. Support is mixed for the view that attributional style was associated with depressed mood only in the presence of negative life events but not their absence. However, research has shown that attributional styles predict increases in depressive symptoms 12 months prospectively irrespective of the occurrence of negative life events, even after accounting for baseline depressive severity (Spence et al. 2002).

Dispositions Emphasizing the Importance of Self and Others

Cognitive models of depression propose that individuals possess elaborate and complex schemata that contain predisposing attitudes, dysfunctional beliefs, or modes of thinking that constitute a diathesis or vulnerability for depressive symptoms. Situations and events congruent with one's schema or personality style are believed to activate dysfunctional beliefs, threaten self-worth, and precipitate depressive symptoms. Two broad domains of vulnerability have been defined and studied by cognitive and psychodynamic theorists such as Beck (1963, 1967) and Blatt (1974). Although the formulation of sociotropy/autonomy and dependency/self-criticism differ somewhat (Zuroff 1994), these and related constructs have generally distinguished two broad domains of vulnerability. One domain involves a vulnerability to interpersonal loss or rejection (dependency); the other domain involves a vulnerability to failure (self-criticism).

In Beck's cognitive model of depression, *sociotropy* defines a personality style characteristic of individuals who value "positive interchange with others, focusing on acceptance, intimacy, support and guidance" (Beck et al. 1983, p. 3), whereas *autonomy* defines a second personality style characteristic of individuals who value "independent functioning, mobility, choice, achievement, and integrity of one's domain" (p. 3). In Blatt's model of depression, *dependent* individuals are motivated to "establish and maintain good interpersonal relationships" and "rely on others to provide and maintain a sense of well-being" (Blatt and Zuroff 1992, p. 528). Highly dependent individuals may have difficulty expressing dissatisfaction or negative emotion because they fear losing the support and satisfaction gained from someone they are close to. As a result, they may attempt "to minimize overt conflict by conforming to and placating others" (p. 528). *Self-critical* individuals are preoccupied with issues of self-definition and self-worth. They strive for "excessive achievement and perfection and are often highly competitive" (p. 528). They desire respect and admiration but fear disapproval and recrimination. Consequently, they may be ambivalent about interpersonal relationships and "can be critical and attacking of others as well as themselves" (p. 528).

Research has shown that sociotropy and autonomy (Baron and Peixoto 1991) as well as dependency and self-criticism (Fichman et al. 1994; Kuperminc et al. 1997; Little 2000; Luthar and Blatt 1993, 1995) are positively associated with higher levels of depressed mood in adolescents. Prospective studies have also shown that self-criticism in young adults also predicts the number of prospective major depressive episodes (Spasojevic and Alloy 2001).

Temperament, Attention, and Executive Functioning

Temperament is comprised of two main components, namely reactivity and self-regulation, as observed in the domains of emotionality, motor activity, and attention (Rothbart et al. 2002). *Reactivity* refers to the manner in which individuals respond to changes in the environment; *self-regulation* refers to the various and cognitive processes that moderate this response. Both components may be assessed and conceptualized in terms of behavioral activity levels, including *easy, difficult, intermediate,* and *slow-to-warm-up* (Thomas et al. 1963) as well as their underlying neural substrates, including behavioral activation and inhibition systems (Gray 1979, 1982). Temperament may be linked to various forms of psychopathology, including depression (see Rothbart et al. 2002 for a review). For example, Block and colleagues (1991) showed that depressive mood in 18-year-old girls was predicted from higher preschool intelligence scores and from oversocialized and overcontrolling behavior at age 7 years, and that depressive mood in 18-year-old boys was predicted from higher aggressive and undercontrolled behavior at age 7 years. Others have shown that peer rejection may be the central mediating factor on the level of depressed mood. That is, undercontrolled behavior has been shown to precipitate peer rejection, which in turn is related to depressed mood (Patterson and Capaldi 1990).

Recent neuropsychological research also suggests that mood disorders may be associated with a variety of performance deficits on tests associated with inhibitory control (for a review, see Veiel 1997), which may account for risk taking and poor frustration tolerance associated with the disorder and which have been associated with increases in verbal (Santor et al. 2003) and physical (Giancola 1995; Giancola and Zeichner 1994, 1995; Lau and Pihl 1994) aggression in nonclinical samples.

Reassurance Seeking and Attachment

Interpersonal models of depression challenge a number of components of cognitive models of depression. Proponents of interpersonal models of depression view depression "as a response to the disruption of social space in which the person obtains support and validation for his experience" (Coyne 1976, p. 33). How the social environment of the depressed individual becomes disrupted and maintains an individual's depressive symptoms is a complex process, involving the depressed person's demand and need for approval and support as well as the ability of individuals within the depressed person's environment to provide genuine, nonambiguous support and validation. Depressed individuals use symptoms to elicit reassurance from others and to test both the "nature of [their] acceptance and the security of [their] relationship[s]" (p. 34). However, depressive symptoms are believed to be aversive to persons in the depressed individual's environment. Individuals in the social environment may feel both irritated and obliged to assure depressed individuals of their acceptance. Consequently, support and validation may be withdrawn or be disingenuous.

It follows that a strong disposition toward seeking reassurance from others should therefore moderate the onset and maintenance of depressive symptoms, particularly in individuals with poor self-esteem, for whom reassurance may be more important, valued, or needed. Support for the utility of viewing reassurance seeking as a personality or vulnerability factor was discovered by Joiner and colleagues (1992), who showed that depression was most strongly associated with rejection from college roommates in individuals with a strong need for reassurance. Research with adolescents has been generally sparse but supportive of this model (Joiner 1999).

Although an individual is motivated from different theoretical frameworks, the degree to which he or she is likely to seek reassurance, in particular following instances of rejection, will be influenced by attachment styles. Attachment theory proposes that caregiving experiences from infancy on influence the development of individuals and their capacity to adapt to disturbances in close relationships (Bowlby 1973). All individuals are believed to develop internal working models of themselves and attachment figures from their emotional experiences with caregivers, which then govern their future attachment behavior and adaptation to situations that give rise to negative emotions (Bowlby 1980; Bretherton and Munholland 1999; Zimmerman 1999). Research shows that attachment styles are relatively stable from infancy to childhood (Grossmann et al. 1999; Solomon and George 1999) as well as over middle to late adolescence (Zimmerman and Becker-Stoll 2002). Emerging evidence shows that nonsecure attachment styles place individuals at risk for a variety of clinical difficulties, including depression during early adolescence (Sund and Wichstrom 2002) and throughout the life span (see Cicchetti and Toth 1995, for a review).

Assessing the Severity of Vulnerability

One other main challenge in assessing personality and vulnerability factors is to locate problematic traits, characteristics, or styles along a continuum severity that may range from periodic obstacles associated with a specific trait or characteristic (e.g., dependency) to chronically severe difficulties associated with a level of severity and impairment that may constitute an emerging personality disorder itself (e.g., dependent personality disorder). Assessing this continuum of severity will be further complicated given the practical constraints of clinical practice that will limit how much can be assessed during an evaluation, in addition to the more theoretical difficulty of evaluating personality disorders during a period of development in which personality itself is still developing. Standardized tools can help guide decisions about the nature and severity of vulnerability. However, at present few of these psychometric instruments provide clear cutoff scores to facilitate decisions about risk or the focus of treatment. In the absence of clear cutoff scores, what constitutes a "high" score on a vulnerability measure is open to some degree of interpretation but can still inform clinical judgment.

The definition of *personality disorders* is, however, a useful starting point for assessing the severity of vulnerability irrespective of the particular personality characteristic or disorder. DSM-IV-TR (American Psychiatric Association 2000) defines a *personality disorder* as "an enduring pattern of inner experience and behavior that deviates markedly from the expectations of the individual's culture, is pervasive and inflexible, has an onset in adolescence or early adulthood, is stable over time, and leads to distress or impairment" (p. 685). This formulation of a personality disorder reflects both the key features of both personality and vulnerability, namely that 1) the characteristic in question is stable and enduring, 2) that it is excessive or extreme, and 3) that it results or is likely to result in some degree of distress or impairment. It is important to note that the definition also acknowledges that there may be some fluctuation over time: "[T]he features must have been present for a least 1 year…[and] may be exacerbated following the loss of a significant supporting persons (e.g., spouse) or previously stabilizing social situations (e.g., job)" (p. 687).

In the past few years, there has been a gradual acceptance that personality disorders can be assessed reliably in adolescence (Petti and Vela 1990), although the validity of such a diagnosis required ongoing validation. Efforts to adopt a more dimensional framework for personality disorders are important for a number of psychometric and substantive reasons (Trull et al. 2003), but perhaps most importantly they offer an opportunity to bring the extensive amount of clinical research on vulnerability factors such as dependency and self-criticism into routine clinical practice.

Accordingly, it is recommended that in the absence of clear cutoff scores with which individuals can be designated as at risk or vulnerable, that scores on well-validated measures of personality (McCrae et al. 2002), temperament (Windle and Lerner 1986), and depressive vulnerability measures (Blatt et al. 1992; D.A. Clark and Beck 1991) be interpreted with caution but may still inform clinical judgment.

Case Example and Treatment Implications

Personality and vulnerability factors may have a number of treatment implications for any individual in treatment with respect to 1) the identification of the underlying problems or difficulties, 2) specifying the various treatment goals, or 3) influencing the nature of the therapeutic process and the degree of therapeutic gain. Viewing personality factors as the tendencies or dispositions that determine thought, feeling, and action that are in the service of specific goals or needs (Maddi 1980, p. 10) can provide important insights into the source of the individuals' difficulties or at least the driving motivations for the personality styles that clinicians may observe at intake. There is now good evidence documenting the various problematic behavioral strategies and coping styles that are typically observed in individuals who show high levels of dependency and self-criticism (see previous section), which may become a specific or necessary treatment goal in their own right. For illustrative purposes, consider the following example.

Case Example

S is a 14-year-old female with a predisposition toward dependency and who currently meets criteria for a major depressive episode. As with many depressed adolescents, S feels that many of her friends, as well as her parents in particular, do not understand her. Her parents' admonitions about letting school work suffer and their frustration at not being able to help her feel better have intensified S's feelings of loneliness and isolation. Before the onset of her depression, S was able to fulfill most of her dependency needs through friends and family, preferring to spend her free time with others rather than alone. However, with the onset of the depressive symptoms and associated irritability with other people, friends and family members who once filled her dependency needs became increasingly distant and less satisfying, which subsequently intensified her need to feel loved and supported by others. To address this absence of support, S adopted increasingly extreme strategies to elicit the support from others, first by demanding reassurances from others that they still wanted to be friends with her and later by demonstrating the direness of her situation by harming herself and openly telling friends and family about her cutting. Therapeutically, S initially made some improvements in treatment, but her progress soon stalled and then waned. Only after identifying her maladaptive strategies at eliciting support from others and finding new ways to express her need for closeness was she able to achieve and maintain an adequate level of functioning.

The case was selected because it illustrates how a preexisting vulnerability factor can influence the behavioral strategies that an individual adopts in dealing with circumstances and events that threaten basic (interpersonal) needs. The case also illustrates how vulnerability factors and their associated behavioral strategies can influence the course of symptoms while not necessarily determining the onset of symptoms or the course of treatment. Further, knowing that an individual is more likely to be self-critical than dependent can serve as an important cue with respect to the domain or class of stressors that may initially trigger or intensify dysphoric moods or alert the clinician to the different types of interpersonal strategies that a patient may adopt in managing his or her own distress or interacting with others.

Some research has begun to articulate the specific goals, underlying needs, and behavioral strategies that are likely to be associated with dependency and self-criticism (Santor 2003), and some recent work has also demonstrated how vulnerability factors such as perfectionism can influence both the therapeutic process and treatment outcome. Blatt and colleagues (1998) and Zuroff and colleagues (Stuart 2000; Zuroff et al. 2000); have shown in some recent reanalyses of the National Institute of Mental Health Treatment of Depression Collaborative Research Program that 1) patients high on perfectionism showed smaller increases in their therapeutic alliance over the course of treatment, 2) patients high on perfectionism made small gains in treatment, and 3) the negative relationship between perfectionism and treatment outcome was explained (i.e., mediated) by perfectionistic patients' failure to develop stronger therapeutic alliances in treatment.

Strategies for Assessing Personality and Vulnerability Factors

Assessing the contribution of vulnerability or personality factors to a young person's current mood difficulties is certainly complex, particularly in the context of a depressive episode, and potentially intractable following the recent occurrence of negative life events or in the context of various types of social or economic adversity. Individuals with major depressive disorder are likely to be more negative or pessimistic in assessing the relative importance of various situational factors such as friends, family, and partners. Any assessment that relies on the depressed person's self-report is likely to be influenced by both the young person's personality as well as that person's current depressive symptoms. Indeed, there is good evidence to show that depressed people tend to be able to estimate certain negative events, such as the likelihood of failing a test, more accurately than nondepressed people, which has been termed *depressive realism* (Alloy and Abramson 1988). Indeed, depressed people are not only more likely to view themselves as ineffective, weak, ugly, unintelligent, or unlovable, they are also more likely to admit to such characteristics and are more likely to seek out information and evidence that supports their negative self-view (Swann and Read 1981; Swann et al. 1992). In addition, depressed people are more likely to view their significant others in more extreme terms, as either unloving or demanding (Barnett and Gotlib 1988), and are more likely to recall past memories and experiences in a negative way (Cohen et al. 1988). However, there is good evidence to suggest that memory biases associated with psychopathology have been exaggerated and that steps can be taken to overcome the limitations of retrospective reports to enhance reliability (Brewin 1996; Brewin et al. 1993).

In addition to the biases associated with the recollection of past negative events, considerable evidence has also shown that scores on measures of personality inventories tend to be inflated during a depressive episode (Barnett and Gotlib 1988; Coyne and Gotlib 1983; Segal and Ingram 1995). This has traditionally been taken as evidence of the instability and unreliability of vulnerability factors and personality traits; however, this is not necessarily incompatible with the nature of vulnerability factors (Santor 2003). Indeed, it may be reasonable to expect that levels of dependency and self-criticism increase during a depressive episode, and if this increase is associated with an exacerbation of problematic behavioral strategies that may influence the course or recovery from depression, then this "inflation" should not be discounted but rather accommodated in a case formulation and treatment plan. Research by Santor and colleagues (1997) has shown that changes in vulnerability scores experienced in the context of a depressive episode are not entirely attributable to changes in depressive severity and that despite changes in mean scores vulnerability scores still demonstrate high levels of relative stability over time (Santor et al. 1997). This finding argues for a more complex view of personality and depression that accommodates changes in vulnerability factors without viewing them merely as a concomitant of depressed mood (see Santor 2003).

In addition to the effects of depressive illness on vulnerability and personality factors, it is equally important to consider the effects of situational events and circumstances that may influence vulnerability factors for circumscribed periods of time. This is particularly important during adolescence, when some negative events, such as peer rejection and teasing, are common and where romantic dissolution may be more frequent than during adulthood. Similarly, contextual factors such as social and economic adversity or disruptive family dynamics may represent ongoing factors, which either perpetuate a temporarily heightened vulnerability within an individual, or which have influenced the emergence and development of a stable and likely sustained vulnerability in a young person. Differentiating the contribution of time-limited situational factors such as relationship dissolution from ongoing contextual factors such as social adversity is central to developing an appropriate case formulation and treatment plan.

There are a number of strategies that may be used to attempt to delineate the contribution of both individual vulnerability factors from situational or contextual factors, both of which typically require assessment while in the midst of a depressive episode but which will be complicated given the cognitive biases and inflated vulnerability levels associated with the depressive episode (Thase 1996) (see Table 9–2). First, personality assessment may be deferred until after the person has recovered from his or her depression or until after the effects of situational factors have subsided. This approach solves the problem of situational or state-dependent "inflation" of pathological traits and vulnerabilities as well as minimizing the effect of cognitive biases associated with the depressive episode. However, deferring the assessment of personality traits and their associated behavioral strategies until after symptoms have remitted or the effects of some negative event have subsided may not be possible, given that a complete remission of symptoms is unlikely because they are being sustained by the effects of vulnerability factors or negative events themselves. Moreover, deferring the assessment of vulnerability may offer little practical help to the clinician. Even though the level of vulnerability experienced by a young person may in some instance be the direct result of the depressive mood, if a vulnerability factor such as dependency or self-criticism has an effect on therapeutic rapport, patient compliance, or treatment outcome (see Blatt et al. 1998; Zuroff et al. 2000), then its assessment and management are crucial.

TABLE 9–2.   Strategies to assess personality factors

- Defer assessment of personality until depressive episode has remitted to minimize the impact of depressive mood.
- Assess person factors before the onset of illness or return of symptoms, particularly in individuals at high risk for onset or relapse.
- Assess person factors using standardized measures designed to minimize biases. Integrate information from multiple sources (patient, family, peers), contexts (home and school), and multiple domains (mood, thought, and behavior).

A second approach involves asking patients to rate their personality before the onset of the depressive illness. This approach deals with the issue of both recall biases and the inflation of vulnerability scores by establishing a baseline before the emergence of symptoms or the occurrence of some negative event. However, there are a number of practical problems associated with achieving this goal in a clinical setting given that most individuals will only be seen during the acute episode. Given the high rates of relapse already in individuals with even just one episode of depression and the high rates of onset in some groups (i.e., the children of depressed parents), the assessment of personality and vulnerability factors may still be conducted strategically, either during periods of remission among individuals likely to experience relapse or just among individuals at higher risk for a first episode during a premorbid phase of illness.

A third approach involves the integration of data from collateral sources such as parents, siblings, or even peers. This approach attempts to reduce the impact of the patient's distorted thinking on the assessment by balancing the information gathered from the young person with information gathered from others. The viability of this approach does, however, depend on balancing the degree of bias introduced as a result of the young person's illness against any biases introduced by the parents, siblings, or peers. Although helpful, particularly in judging the degree of dysfunction or the type of problematic behavioral strategies adopted by young people, reliance on judgments made by parents *may* still be problematic for a number of reasons, which stands to undermine both the reliability and validity of the information provided (Christensen et al. 1983; Forehand et al. 1982; Rickard et al. 1981; Velting et al. 1998; Webster-Straton 1988). Potential obstacles to obtaining accurate data from parents and others include the presence of pathology among the informant as well as the inherent difficulty of making complex judgments about psychopathology in others.

Cantwell and colleagues (1997) examined the correspondence of parent-adolescent reports for major psychiatric disorders. Results of this study question the validity of information gathered from parents. Kappa values for parent-adolescent agreement ranged from 0.19 for alcohol abuse/dependence to 0.79 for conduct disorder, with a mean kappa value of 0.42. In addition, results showed that information provided by the young person corresponded extremely well ($\kappa=0.74$ across all disorders) with consensus judgments made by clinicians, whereas information provided by parents did not corresponded well ($\kappa=0.50$ across all disorders) with clinician judgments. On the basis of this research, Cantwell and colleagues concluded that greater reliance on the adolescent will result in the detection of more diagnosed cases.

In summary, although there are a number of approaches to assessing vulnerability factors in the context of depressive episode, each approach and hypothesis about how vulnerability factors are related to and contribute to depressive illness must be evaluated carefully. Moving from nomothetic theories about personality and vulnerability and their influence on the onset, maintenance, and treatment of depression in groups of individuals, to idiographic predictions about single patients or clients is difficult and very often erroneous. Blatt and colleagues (1998) showed that perfectionism can begin to impede therapeutic gains in approximately two-thirds of the sample in the latter half of treatment. This study suggests that more perfectionistic patients may be affected adversely when anticipating an arbitrary, externally imposed termination date. These findings are useful in explaining not only why perfectionistic individuals do poorly in treatment but also offers a clear suggestion on how to circumvent those difficulties—namely by making treatment more open ended. Although these difficulties were observed in some two-thirds of patients, one-third did not show any related difficulties—which underscores the need for careful assessment and ongoing evaluation of progress for each and every patient.

General Treatment Considerations

Before concluding this chapter, we will highlight several issues regarding the treatment of affective disorder and personality disorder in adolescents.

Clinically, the issue of personality disorder in adolescence is complicated. The DSM-IV-TR cautions against routine diagnosis of personality disorders in adolescents, but there is a growing body of research over the last decade that has suggested that personality syndromes are recognizable in adolescents (Westen et al. 2003).

Becker and colleagues (2002) note that the borderline personality disorder construct in young patients has been a topic of debate. Their epidemiological and follow-up studies have suggested that personality disorders in adolescents can be reliably diagnosed, occurs frequently, and has concurrent validity (i.e., they are valid indicators of distress and dysfunction). However, they believe that they have only modest predictive validity and are relatively unstable over time. They conclude that symptoms of personality disorder in adolescents may accurately reflect current distress but may not represent coherent differentiable syndromes with stability over time. They observe that borderline personality disorders encompass a more diffuse range of psychopathology in adolescents than in adults.

Kasen and colleagues (2001) note that in adolescents the probability of personality disorder substantially increases for those who have a prior diagnosis of major depressive disorder. In an interesting conceptualization, they suggest that personality disorders may represent alternative pathways of continuity from major depressive disorder and other Axis I disorders across the child/adult transition. These findings relate to the discussion of the stability of personality in young adults earlier in this chapter.

Fava and colleagues (1996) have shown that early-onset depressive illness (before age 18 years) is distinguished from late-onset depressive illness (18 or later) by more frequent association with persistent disturbances in behaviors and attitudes. Patients with early-onset major depressive disorder had a significantly higher prevalence of personality disorders (including avoidant, histrionic, narcissistic, and borderline personality disorders) according to SCID-II. This finding suggests again the importance of not overlooking an Axis I diagnosis in the adolescent population.

Whereas these observations are conceptually interesting, the clinical point is to be sure to identify all Axis I diagnoses and provide robust treatments with both psychotherapy and pharmacotherapy to ensure that Axis I amplification of personality traits is not occurring. It is important to ensure that the patient has received a robust treatment trial so that apparent personality disorder is not an expression of the impact of Axis I disorder on the patient's personality.

In adults, it is very important to obtain a longitudinal picture of functioning to make a diagnosis of personality disorder. In Chapter 10 of this book, the authors point out that in the geriatric patient with affective disorder and personality disorder, a longitudinal decade-by-decade review of behaviors is called for to clarify if current behavior is of long-standing origin (Axis II) or related to Axis I or organic brain changes. When working with adolescents, although a longitudinal review instead of a decade-to-decade review is certainly advocated to ensure that behavioral problems are not "just" current Axis I expressions, the clinician has to rely on collateral history regarding family, peer group, and school functioning over time. Because a longitudinal perspective is shorter in this age group and adolescence can be a time of turmoil, it is especially important to rule out an Axis I disorder that can be masquerading as a personality disorder or as "adolescent turmoil." In the third section of this chapter, we have emphasized strategies to delineate this contribution of individual factors from situational or contextual factors.

Perugi and colleagues (2003) highlight the issue of bipolar versus personality disorder. They comment on how mood lability and interpersonal sensitivity traits appear to be related to a cyclothymic temperamental diathesis, which in turn appears to underline the complex pattern of anxiety, mood, and impulsive disorders, which atypical depressive patients with bipolar II disorder and/or borderline personality disorder display clinically. They conclude that the construct of borderline personality disorder is better covered by more conventional diagnostic entities.

Although this is a controversial position, it highlights the importance of ruling out the presence of bipolar disorder in patients who have a presentation that appears cross-sectionally to be characterized by behavioral disturbance and presumed personality disorder. It is important to obtain a longitudinal as well as family history from these patients. Early-onset depression, positive family histories for bipolar disorders, and/or antidepressant-induced hypomania should be considered regarding the possibility of a bipolar affective disorder. Akiskal and colleagues (2000) note mood lability with rapid shifts, often in a depressive polarity, was the hallmark of "unipolar" patients who switched to bipolar II. He added that, regrettably, such patients often get labeled "borderline."

Case Example

Ms. F was a 23-year-old woman who was well known to the inpatient psychiatric unit of a local hospital. She gave a long history that was characterized by affect instability, idealization, devaluation, and issues related to abandonment and identity disturbance going back to her early teens. She had required multiple admissions and was becoming too well known to the inpatient unit staff. The possibility of a bipolar affective disorder was overlooked given her stormy personality disorder on cross-sectional presentation. However, when a family history was obtained it was positive for bipolar illness. A closer history was elicited noting that the signs and symptoms of a hypomanic episode were present intermittently in this patient but that these episodes had been overlooked because of the more dramatic "characterological" presentation. She was started on a mood stabilizer and seen in follow-up. She went from one to three admissions per year from the age of 17–23 years to one to three admissions in the subsequent decade. The diagnosis that was more consistent with her history and her course was bipolar affective disorder with personality vulnerabilities. In this case, the mood stabilizer allowed the patient to have less behavioral fluctuations and affective instability but did not cause her to be seen only as having bipolar disorder with no Axis II vulnerabilities. When her bipolar disorder was diagnosed and treated, her functioning improved. She still had personality vulnerabilities, but these were no longer as florid or maladaptive.

The importance of ruling out substance abuse in adolescents with personality disorder and major depressive disorder is also very important. Grilo and colleagues (1997) showed that borderline personality disorder was diagnosed more frequently in patients with major depressive disorder and substance abuse disorder than in major depressive disorder or substance use disorder groups alone.

Careful attention to diagnosis and treatment helps avoid treatment nihilism and is especially important in treating adolescents. A medication approach that is acceptable and helpful to the patient and his or her parents is important. Strengthening the medication treatment alliance by exploring their experience and perception of medications is important. A review of the past history of medication trials is key to clarifying what medications have been used, what their mechanisms of action has been, and whether the medications have been helpful or unhelpful, causing a partial remission or stopped because of side effects or "poop out."

Currently, the additional challenge in medicating depressed adolescents is the controversy about antidepressants and suicide risk.

Gunnell and Ashby (2004) discuss the benefit/harm determination in adolescents. They note that the increase in prescribed antidepressants has coincided with a fall in suicide rates, causing some researchers to suggest a causal association. However, they note that a recent review of evidence from pediatric trials in Britain led to most selective serotonin reuptake inhibitors (SSRIs) being contraindicated in people age 18 years or younger. In their study, they review the evidence, find it inconclusive, and suggest clinical guidelines depending on the individual's underlying suicide risk. For patients with conditions that have a high suicide risk such as severe depression, they recommend using antidepressants but not in individuals with anxiety and/or mild depression. Furthermore, Isacsson and colleagues (1992) have indicated that adults who had completed suicide had a low rate of antidepressants that were prescribed often in a low dose.

March and colleagues (2004), in a randomized controlled trial of patients treated for adolescent depression, concluded that the combination of fluoxetine with cognitive-behavioral therapy offered the most favorable trade-off between benefit and risk for adolescents with major depressive disorder.

The Food and Drug Administration (FDA) statement on this issue indicated that the finding of an increased risk of suicidality in pediatric patients applied to all the drugs studied (Prozac, Zoloft, Remeron, Paxil, Effexor, Celexa, Wellbutrin, Levox, and Serzone) (U.S. Food and Drug Administration 2004). However, they concluded that these antidepressants should not be contraindicated because they felt that access to these substances was important for those who could benefit.

Some general clinical guidelines can be added to these observations. After establishing that there is an affective disorder present and that its severity warrants the use of antidepressants, clinicians should involve parents and patients in a discussion of the risks and benefits of using antidepressants. Clinicians should clearly document that this discussion has occurred. Patients and parents should be advised to call back and/or hold the antidepressant if the patient experiences any unusual restlessness or unusual thoughts such as self-harm ideation, especially if the patient has never experienced such thoughts before. Clinicians should monitor patients more closely when starting on an antidepressant and when increasing the dose, especially if there is a history of akathisia or hypomania. Although akathisia is much more common with neuroleptic individuals, it can occur as a rare side effect of SSRIs. The long-standing clinical teaching of monitoring patients more closely as they emerge from their depression and have increased energy while still dealing with the negative cognitions (hopelessness and despair) is especially apt in depressed teens with comorbid personality disorder characterized by affective liability and impulsivity.

While emphasizing the importance of not overlooking Axis I disorders in patients with Axis II diagnoses, we must also note that in a subgroup of patients the dilemma is the opposite in that patients receive an almost exclusive focus on their Axis I disorder without attending to Axis II issues.

Case Example

Ms. N was a 19-year-old woman with a lifelong history of chronic and intermittent depression and anxiety since age 6 years. After many years of medication trials throughout her teenage years for her Axis I disorders with only a partial and unsatisfactory response and with escalating behavioral disturbance (self cutting) and substance abuse, she was finally identified as having a borderline personality disorder in her late teens. She found this diagnosis to be comforting. She recounted that it helped her to know she did not "only" have depression. She was able to find therapy that focused on skills acquisition including identifying and anticipating triggers to her affective dysregulation, on how to overcome periods of what she termed disorganization, and on how she could learn to "distract myself sometimes and stay in the moment other times." Hearing about the diagnosis of borderline personality disorder "made sense" of her experience and gave her direction and made her feel like "less of a loser." It also enabled her mother but not her father to be more sympathetic to her struggles.

Kutcher and Kornblum (1992) have emphasized the need to use consistent longitudinal observation in the adolescent patient with possible personality disorder and comorbid Axis I disorder. The authors advocate documenting family, peer, and social behaviors over time. They emphasize that borderline personality disorder should not be diagnosed in the presence of an Axis I disorder, which can mimic similar symptoms. They suggest that clinicians need to be certain that the personality disorder symptoms profile is not a reflection of an underlying psychosis and also advocate the importance of ruling out substance abuse. They emphasize that all Axis I diagnoses must be carefully considered and that longitudinal observation and structured interviews be used. They also focus on helping the adolescent build up ego strengths using islands of functioning such as academic or athletic success as a starting point, and they emphasize cognitive approaches that help the adolescent to link cognitive distortion to maladaptive affect and behavior to decrease impulsivity and improve social skills.

Psychotherapeutically, it is important to teach the patient specific skills while focusing on "here and now" issues. The emphasis is on skill acquisition, attending to affect dysregulation and multiple crises. Also, optimizing the pharmacotherapy and stabilizing the Axis I disorder allows attention to be paid to the comorbid personality disorder, facilitating relapse prevention. In addition, adolescents challenge clinicians to involve family members, as family dysfunction (either contributing or secondary to the teen's distress) can drive, amplify, or exacerbate maladaptive behaviors (cutting, substance use) that complicate the clinical picture. Earlier in this chapter we commented on conceptual issues relating to how the family context may affect personality tendencies, characteristics, and expression. Collateral history from parents can reduce the impact of the patient's depressive thinking on the assessment by balancing the information gathered from the teen with information gathered from others. Family interventions from psychoeducation to psychotherapy can be especially important in this age group.

Conclusions

The relationship between personality factors and depressed mood is complex, especially so in adolescents. In this chapter, we have reviewed conceptual issues concerning the definition of personality and vulnerability, and how vulnerability factors may be related to depressed mood. Issues regarding tendencies versus characteristics, risk and vulnerability, interpersonal rejection, the context of the developmental framework, and how vulnerability relates to depressed mood have been highlighted. We have concluded the chapter by switching gears from conceptual issues to highlighting general clinical issues in the assessment and treatment of adolescents with comorbid affective and personality vulnerability.

References

Akiskal HS, Bourgeois ML, Angst J, et al: Re-evaluating the prevalence of and diagnostic composition within the broad clinical spectrum of bipolar disorders. J Affect Disord 59 (suppl 1):S5–S30, 2000

Alloy LB, Abramson LY: Depressive realism: four theoretical perspectives, in Cognitive Process in Depression. Edited by Alloy LB. New York, Guilford, 1988, pp 223–264

Alloy LB, Peterson C, Abramson LY, et al: Attributional style and the generality of learned helplessness. J Pers Soc Psychol 46:681–687, 1984

American Psychiatric Association: Diagnostic and Statistical Manual of Mental Disorders, 4th Edition, Text Revision. Washington, DC, American Psychiatric Association, 2000

Bandura A: Self-efficacy: toward a unifying theory of behavioral change. Psychol Rev 84:191–215, 1977

Barnett PA, Gotlib IH: Psychological functioning and depression: distinguishing among antecedents, concomitants, and consequences. Psychol Bull 104:97–126, 1988

Baron P, Peixoto N: Depressive symptoms in adolescents as a function of personality factors. J Youth Adolesc 20:493–500, 1991

Beck AT: Thinking and depression; I: idiosyncratic content and cognitive distortions. Arch Gen Psychiatry 9:324–333, 1963

Beck AT: Depression: Clinical, Experimental, and Theoretical Aspects. New York, Harper & Row, 1967

Beck AT, Epstein N, Harrison RP, et al: Development of the Sociotropy-Autonomy Scale: A Measure of Personality Factors in Depression. Philadelphia, PA, University of Pennsylvania, 1983

Becker D, Grilo C, Edell W, et al: Diagnostic efficiency of borderline personality disorder criteria in hospitalized adolescents: comparison with hospitalized adults. Am J Psychiatry 159:2042–2047, 2002

Blatt SJ: Levels of object representation in analytic and introjective depression. Psychoanal Study Child 29:107–157, 1974

Blatt SJ, Homann E: Parent-child interaction in the etiology of dependent and self-critical depression. Clin Psychol Rev 12:47–91, 1992

Blatt SJ, Shichman S: Two primary configurations of psychopathology. Psychoanalysis and Contemporary Thought 6:187–254, 1983

Blatt SJ, Zuroff DC: Interpersonal relatedness and self-definition: two prototypes for depression. Clin Psychol Rev 12:527–562, 1992

Blatt SJ, Schaffer CE, Bers SA, et al: Psychometric properties of the Depressive Experiences Questionnaire for Adolescents. J Pers Assess 59:82–98, 1992

Blatt SJ, Zuroff DC, Bondi CM: When and how perfectionism impedes the brief treatment of depression: further analyses of the National Institute of Mental Health Treatment of Depression Collaborative Research Program. J Consult Clin Psychol 66:423–428, 1998

Block J, Gjerde PF, Block JH: Personality antecedents of depressive tendencies in 18-year-olds: a prospective study. J Pers Soc Psychol 60:726–738, 1991

Boivin M, Shelly H, Bukowski WM: The roles of social withdrawal, peer rejection and victimization by peers predicting loneliness and depressed mood in childhood. Dev Psychopathol 7:765–785, 1995

Bond L, Carlin JB, Lyndal T, et al: Does bullying cause emotional problems? A prospective study of young teenagers. Br Med J 323:480–484, 2001

Bowlby J: Attachment and Loss, Vol 2: Separation: Anxiety and Anger. London, Hogarth Press, 1973

Bowlby J: Attachment and Loss, Vol 3: Loss: Sadness and Depression. London, Hogarth Press, 1980

Bretherton I, Munholland KA: Internal working models in attachment relationships: a construct revisited, in Handbook of Attachment: Theory, Research and Clinical Applications. Edited by Cassidy J, Shaver PR. New York, Guilford, 1999, pp 89–114

Brewin CR: Scientific status of recovered memories. Br J Psychiatry 169:131–134, 1996

Brewin CR, Andrews B, Gotlib IH: Psychopathology and early experience: a reappraisal of retrospective reports. Psychol Bull 113:82–98, 1993

Campbell RJ: Psychiatric Dictionary, 6th Edition. New York, Oxford University Press, 1989

Cantwell DP, Lewinsohn PM, Rohde P, et al: Correspondence between adolescent report and parent report of psychiatric diagnostic data. J Am Acad Child Adolesc Psychiatry 36:610–619, 1997

Christensen A, Phillips S, Glascow RE, et al: Parental characteristics and interactional dysfunction in families with child behavior problems: a preliminary investigation. J Abnorm Child Psychology 11:153–166, 1983

Cicchetti D, Rogosch FA: A developmental psychopathology perspective on adolescence. J Consult Clin Psychol 70:6–20, 2002

Cicchetti D, Toth S: Developmental psychopathology and disorders of affect, in Developmental Psychopathology, Vol 2: Risk, Disorder, and Adaptation. Edited by Cicchetti D, Cohen D. New York, Wiley, 1995, pp 369–420

Cicchetti D, Tucker D: Development and self-regulatory structures of the mind. Dev Psychopathol 6:533–549, 1994

Clark DA, Beck AT: Personality factors in dysphoria: a psychometric refinement of Beck's Sociotropy-Autonomy Scale. Journal of Psychopathology and Behavioral Assessment 13:369–388, 1991

Clark DA, Beck AT, Alford BA: Scientific Foundations of Cognitive Theory and Therapy of Depression. New York, Wiley, 1999

Clark LA, Watson D, Mineka S: Temperament, personality, and the mood and anxiety disorders. J Abnorm Psychol 103:103–116, 1994

Cohen LH, Towbes LC, Flocco R: Effects of induced mood on self-reported life events and perceived and received social support. J Pers Soc Psychol 55:669–674, 1988

Coyne JC: Toward an interactional description of depression. Psychiatry 39:28–40, 1976

Coyne JC, Gotlib IH: The role of cognition in depression: a critical appraisal. Psychol Bull 94:472–505, 1983

Dahl RE, Ryan ND: The psychobiology of adolescent depression, in Rochester Symposium on Developmental Psychopathology, Vol 7: Adolescence: Opportunities and Challenges. Edited by Cicchetti D, Toth SL. Rochester, NY, University of Rochester Press, 1996, pp 197–232

Digman JM: Personality structure: emergence of the five-factor model. Annu Rev Psychol 41:417–440, 1990

Fava M, Alpert JE, Borus JS, et al: Patterns of personality disorder comorbidity in early-onset versus late-onset major depression. Am J Psychiatry 153:1308–1312, 1996

Fichman L, Koestner R, Zuroff DC: Depressive styles in adolescence: assessment, relation to social functioning, and developmental trends. J Youth Adolesc 23:315–330, 1994

Flemming JE, Offord DR, Boyle MH: Prevalence of childhood and adolescent depression in the community: Ontario child health study. Br J Psychiatry 155:647–654, 1989

Folkman S, Lazarus RS: If it changes it must be a process: study of emotion and coping during three stages of a college examination. J Pers Soc Psychol 48:150–170, 1985

Forehand R, Wells KC, McMahon RS, et al: Maternal perception of maladjustment in clinic-referred children: an extension of earlier research. J Behav Assess 4:145–151, 1982

Giancola PR: Evidence for dorsolateral and orbital prefrontal cortical involvement in the expression of aggressive behavior. Aggress Behav 21:431–450, 1995

Giancola PR, Zeichner A: Neuropsychological performance on tests of frontal-lobe functioning and aggressive behavior in men. J Abnorm Psychol 103:832–835, 1994

Giancola PR, Zeichner A: Construct validity of a competitive reaction-time aggression paradigm. Aggress Behav 21:199–204, 1995

Gray JA: Anxiety and the brain: not by neurochemistry alone. Psychol Med 9:605–609, 1979

Gray JA: Precis of the neuropsychology of anxiety: an enquiry into the functions of the septohippocampal system. Behav Brain Sci 5:469–534, 1982

Grilo CM, Walker ML, Becker DF, et al: Personality Disorders in adolescents with major depression, substance use disorders, and coexisting major depression and substance use disorders. J Consult Clin Psychol 65:328–332, 1997

Grossmann KE, Grossmann K, Zimmermann P: A wider view of attachment and exploration: stability and change during the years of immaturity, in Handbook of Attachment: Theory, Research, and Clinical Applications. Edited by Cassidy J, Shaver PR. New York, Guilford, 1999, pp 760–786

Gunnell P, Ashby D: Antidepressants and suicide: what is the balance of benefit and harm. Br Med J 329:34–38, 2004

Hammen C: Generation of stress in the course of unipolar depression. J Abnorm Psychol 100:555–561, 1991

Hammen C, Burge D, Adrian C: Timing of mother and child depression in a longitudinal study of children at risk. J Consult Clin Psychol 59:341–345, 1991

Hankin BL, Abramson LY: Development of gender differences in depression: an elaborated cognitive vulnerability-transactional stress theory. Psychol Bull 127:773–796, 2001

Haynes SN: Models of Causality in Psychopathology. New York, MacMillan, 1992

Horwarth E, Johnson J, Klerman G, et al: Depressive symptoms as relative and attributable risk factors for first-onset major depression. Arch Gen Psychiatry 49:817–823, 1992

Ingram RE, Price JM: The role of vulnerability in understanding psychopathology, in Vulnerability to Psychopathology: Risk Across the Lifespan. Edited by Ingram RE, Price JM. New York, Guilford, 2001, pp 3–19

Isacsson G, Boethius G, Bergman U: Low level of antidepressant prescription for people who later commit suicide. Acta Psychiatr Scand 85:444–448, 1992

Johnson JG: Event-specific attributions and daily life events as predictors of depression symptom change. Journal of Psychopathology and Behavioral Assessment 17:39–49, 1995

Joiner TE: A test of the interpersonal theory of depression in youth psychiatric patients. J Abnorm Psychol 27:77–85, 1999

Joiner TE, Wagner KD: Attribution style and depression in children and adolescents: a meta-analytic review. Clin Psychol Rev 15:777–798, 1995

Joiner TE, Alfano MS, Metalsky GI: When depression breeds contempt: reassurance seeking, self-esteem, and rejection of depressed college students by their roommates. J Abnorm Psychol 101:165–173, 1992

Jorm AF, Christensen H, Henderson AS, et al: Predicting anxiety and depression from personality: Is there a synergistic effect of neuroticism and extraversion? J Abnorm Psychol 109:145–149, 2000

Kasen S, Cohen P, Skodol AE, et al: Childhood depression and adult personality disorder: alternate pathways of continuity. Arch Gen Psychiatry 58:231–236, 2001

Kendler KS, Kessler RC, Neale MC, et al: The prediction of major depression in women: toward an integrated etiologic model. Am J Psychiatry 150:1139–1148, 1993a

Kendler KS, Neale MC, Kessler RC, et al: A longitudinal twin study of 1-year prevalence of major depression in women. Arch Gen Psychiatry 50:843–852, 1993b

Kendler KS, Thornton LM, Gardner CO: Stressful life events and previous epi-
    sodes in the etiology of major depression in women: an evaluation of the
    "kindling" hypothesis. Am J Psychiatry 157:1243–1251, 2000
Kessler R: Childhood family violence and adult recurrent depression. J Health
    Soc Behav 35:13–27, 1994
Klein DN, Durbin CE, Shankman SA, et al: Depression and personality, in
    Handbook of Depression and Its Treatment. Edited by Gotlib IH, Hammen
    CL. New York, Guilford, 2002, pp 115–140
Klein MH, Wonderlich SA, Shea MT: Models of the relationship between per-
    sonality and depression: toward a framework for theory and research, in
    Personality and Depression: A Current View. Edited by Klein MH, Won-
    derlich S, Shea MT. New York, Guilford, 1993, pp 1–54
Kuperminc GP, Blatt SJ, Leadbeater J: Relatedness, self-definition, and early ad-
    olescent adjustment. Cognit Ther Res 21:301–320, 1997
Kutcher S, Kornblum M: Borderline personality disorder in adolescents: a criti-
    cal overview, novel speculations, and suggested future directions, in Hand-
    book of Borderline Disorders. Edited by Silver D, Rosenbluth M. Madison,
    CT, International Universities Press, 1992, pp 535–552
Lau MA, Pihl RO: Alcohol and the Taylor aggression paradigm: a repeated mea-
    sures study. J Stud Alcohol 55:701–706, 1994
Lewinsohn PM, Allen NB, Seeley JR, et al: First onset versus recurrence of de-
    pression: differential processes of psychosocial risk. J Abnorm Psychol
    108:483–489, 1999
Lewinsohn PM, Solomon A, Seeley JR, et al: Clinical implications of "subthresh-
    old" depressive symptoms. J Abnorm Psychol 109:345–351, 2000
Little S: Interpersonal and achievement orientations and specific stressors pre-
    dicting depressive and aggressive symptoms in children. Cognit Ther Res
    24:651–670, 2000
Luthar SS, Blatt SJ: Dependent and self-critical depressive experiences among
    inner-city adolescents. J Pers 61:365–386, 1993
Luthar SS, Blatt SJ: Differential vulnerability of dependency and self-criticism
    among disadvantaged teenagers. J Res Adolesc 5:431–449, 1995
Maddi SR: Myth and personality. Journal of Mind and Behavior 1:145–153, 1980
March J, Silva S, Petrycia S, et al: Fluoxetine, cognitive-behavior therapy, and
    their indication for adolescents with depression. JAMA 292:807–820, 2004
McCrae RR, Costa PT Jr, Terracciano A, et al: Personality trait development
    from age 12 to age 18: longitudinal, cross-sectional and cross-cultural anal-
    yses. J Pers Soc Psychol 83:1456–1468, 2002
Monroe SM, Simons AD: Diathesis-stress theories in the context of life stress re-
    search: implications for the depressive disorders. Psychol Bull 110:406–425,
    1991
Neufeld RWJ: Dynamic differentials of stress and coping. Psychol Rev 106:385–
    397, 1999
Nolen-Hoeksema S, Girgus JS, Seligman ME: Learned helplessness in children:
    a longitudinal study of depression, achievement, and explanatory style.
    J Pers Soc Psychol 51:435–442, 1986

Patterson GR, Capaldi DM: A mediational model for boys' depressed mood, in Risk and Protective Factors in the Development of Psychopathology. Edited by Rolf JE, Masten AS. New York, Cambridge University Press, 1990, pp 141–163

Perugi G, Toni C, Travierso MC, et al: The role of dysthymia in atypical depression: toward a database reconceptualization of the borderline–bipolar II connection. J Affect Disord 73:87–98, 2003

Petti TA, Vela RM: Borderline disorders of childhood: an overview. J Am Acad Child Adolesc Psychiatry 29:327–337, 1990

Post RM: Transduction of psychosocial stress into the neurobiology of recurrent affective disorder. Am J Psychiatry 149:999–1010, 1992

Poznanski EO, Mokros HB: Phenomenology and epidemiology of mood disorders in children and adolescents, in Handbook of Depression in Children and Adolescents. Edited by Reynolds WM, Johnston HF. New York, Plenum, 1994, pp 19–39

Rickard KM, Forehand R, Wells KC, et al: Factors in the referral of children for behavioral treatment: a comparison of mothers of clinic referred deviant, clinic-referred nondeviant, and non-clinic children. Behav Res Ther 19:201–205, 1981

Rothbart MK, Derryberry D: Temperament in children, in Psychology at the Turn of the Millennium. Edited by von Hofsten C, Bäckman L. Vol 2: Social, Developmental, and Clinical Perspectives. East Sussex, UK, Psychology Press, 2002, pp 17–35

Santor DA: Proximal effects of dependency and self-criticism: conceptual and methodological challenges for depressive vulnerability research. Cogn Behav Ther 32:49–67, 2003

Santor DA, Kusumakar V: Open trial of interpersonal therapy in adolescents with moderate to severe major depression: effectiveness of novice IPT therapists. J Am Acad Child Adolesc Psychiatry 40:236–240, 2001

Santor DA, Patterson RL: Frequency and duration of mood fluctuations: effects of dependency, self-criticism, and negative events. Pers Individ Dif 37:1667–1680, 2004

Santor DA, Zuroff DC: Interpersonal responses to threats to status and interpersonal relatedness: effects of dependency and self-criticism. Br J Clin Psychol 36:521–542, 1997

Santor DA, Zuroff DC: Controlling shared resources: effects of dependency, self-criticism, and threats to self-worth. Pers Individ Dif 24:237–252, 1998

Santor DA, Bagby RM, Joffe RT: Evaluating stability and change in personality and depression. J Pers Soc Psychol 73:1354–1362, 1997

Santor DA, Messervey D, Kusumakar V: Measuring peer pressure, popularity, and conformity in adolescent boys and girls: predicting school performance, sexual attitudes, and substance abuse. J Youth Adolesc 29:163–182, 2000

Santor DA, Pringle JD, Israeli AL: Enhancing and disrupting cooperative behavior in couples: effects of dependency and self-criticism following favorable and unfavorable performance feedback. Cognit Ther Res 24:379–399, 2001

Santor DA, Ingram AD, Kusumakar V: Influence of executive functioning difficulties on verbal aggression: moderating effects of winning and losing and increasing and decreasing levels of provocation. Aggress Behav 29:475–488, 2003

Schmitz N, Kugler J, Rollnik J: On the relation between neuroticism, self-esteem, and depression: results from the National Comorbidity Survey. Compr Psychiatry 44:169–176, 2003

Segal ZV, Ingram RE: Mood priming and construct activation in test of cognitive vulnerability to unipolar depression. Clin Psychol Rev 14:663–695, 1995

Solomon J, George C: The measurement of attachment security in infancy and childhood, in Handbook of Attachment: Theory, Research and Clinical Applications. Edited by Cassidy J, Shaver PR. New York, Guilford, 1999, pp 760–786

Spasojevic J, Alloy LB: Rumination as a common mechanism relating depressive risk factors to depression. Emotion 1:25–37, 2001

Spence SH, Sheffield J, Donovan C: Problem-solving orientation and attributional style: moderators of the impact of negative life events on the development of depressive symptoms in adolescence? J Clin Child Adolesc Psychol 31:219–229, 2002

Sund AM, Wichstrom L: Insecure attachment style as a risk factor for future depressive symptoms in early adolescence. J Am Acad Child Adolesc Psychiatry 41:1478–1485, 2002

Swann WB, Read SJ: Self-verification processes: how we sustain our self-conceptions. J Exp Soc Psychol 17:351–372, 1981

Swann WB, Wenzlaff RM, Krull DS, et al: Allure of negative feedback: self-verification strivings among depressed persons. J Abnorm Psychol 101:293–306, 1992

Teasdale JD: Negative thinking in depression: cause, effect, or reciprocal relationship? Advances in Behavior Research and Therapy 5:3–25, 1983

Teasdale JD: Cognitive vulnerability to persistent depression. Cognition and Emotion 2:247–274, 1988

Thase ME: The role of Axis II comorbidity in the management of patients with treatment-resistant depression. Psychiatr Clin North Am 19:287–309, 1996

Thomas A, Chess S, Birch HG, et al: Behavioral Individuality in Early Childhood. New York, New York University Press, 1963

Trull TJ, Widiger TA, Lynam DR, et al: Borderline personality disorder from the perspective of general personality functioning. J Abnorm Psychol 112:193–202, 2003

Trzesniewski KH, Donnellan MB, Robins RW: Stability of self-esteem across the lifespan. J Pers Soc Psychol 84:205–220, 2003

U.S. Food and Drug Administration: FDA statement on recommendation of psychopharmacologic drugs and pediatric advisory committees. September 16, 2004. Available at: www.fda.gov/bbs/topics/news/2004/NEW01116.html. Accessed February 5, 2005.

Veiel HOF: A preliminary profile of neuropsychological deficits associated with major depression. J Clin Exp Neuropsychol 19:587–603, 1997

Velting DM, Shaffer D, Gould MS, et al: Parent-victim agreement in adolescent suicide research. J Am Acad Child Adolesc Psychiatry 37:1161–1166, 1998

von Bertalanffy L: General Systems Theory. New York, Braziller, 1968

Webster-Straton C: Mothers' and fathers' perceptions of child deviance: roles of parent and child behaviors and parent adjustment. J Consult Clin Psychol 56:909–915, 1988

Westen D, Shedler J, Durrett C, et al: Personality diagnoses in adolescence: DSM-IV Axis II diagnoses and an empirically derived alternative. Am J Psychiatry 160:952–966, 2003

Windle M, Lerner RM: Reassessing the dimensions of temperamental individuality across the life span: the Revised Dimensions of Temperament Survey (DOTS–R). J Adolesc Res 1:213–229, 1986

Zimmerman P: Structure and functions of internal working models of attachment and their role for emotion regulation. Attach Hum Dev 1:291–306, 1999

Zimmerman P, Becker-Stoll F: Stability of attachment representations during adolescence: the influence of ego-identity status. J Adolesc 25:107–124, 2002

Zuroff DC: Depressive personality styles and the five-factor model of personality. J Pers Assess 63:453–472, 1994

Zuroff DC, Blatt SJ, Sotsky SM: Relation of therapeutic alliance and perfectionism to outcome in brief outpatient treatment of depression. J Consult Clin Psychol 68:114–124, 2000

CHAPTER 10

THE IMPACT OF PERSONALITY DISORDERS ON LATE-LIFE DEPRESSION

J. P. Cooper, M.D.

Alastair Flint, M.D.

There is a dearth of research on the impact of personality disorders on depression in late life compared with reports in younger age groups (Agronin and Maletta 2000). The definition of *elderly* varies among authors, but for the purposes of this chapter we refer primarily to those age 60 years and over. There is evidence that the presence of a personality disorder is associated with a chronic outcome of depression (less likelihood of recovery) and impaired social support in the elderly (Vine and Steingart 1994). This presence also affects the presentation, course, and treatment of depressive illness in younger groups (Andrews et al. 1990; Perry and Vaillant 1989).

In this chapter we examine the diagnostic issues related to personality disorders and dimensions in late-life depression; the impact on major depressive disorder, dysthymic disorder, and other types of depression (bipolar disorder, depression associated with medical conditions); and the relationship to suicide. We also examine the effects of personality disorders on the various forms of treatment for late-life depression, including pharmacotherapy, electroconvulsive therapy (ECT), and psychotherapy.

Diagnostic Issues

The prevalence of current or lifetime depressive illness among older persons with a personality disorder has not been adequately studied. The absence of a gold standard for diagnosis of personality disorders in late life results in contradictory prevalence rates (Agronin and Maletta 2000). Longitudinal data required for diagnosis in the elderly are often unavailable and unreliable. The lack of age-adjusted diagnostic instruments affects diagnosis. Also, changes in classification for both diagnostic entities have precluded retrospective study.

Personality disorder traits must be differentiated from DSM-IV-TR Axis I disorders (American Psychiatric Association 2000). These traits may reflect normal function, less severe personality dysfunction, or subthreshold depressive disorders, which remit with appropriate treatment. Individuals with maladaptive personality traits, including those who are suspicious, withdrawn, or who have difficult interpersonal relationships, often lack the insight to obtain treatment, which affects the study of this group.

Most investigators of late-life personality disorders and depression have focused on hospital in- and outpatients. This focus may relate to the methodological difficulties of accessing community samples of elderly depressed subjects with personality disorders because of stigma and their reluctance to participate in research. The bias in the diagnosis of a personality disorder in clinical populations may affect the outcome of studies. This group may have more severe symptoms and may be less responsive to treatment than those in the community who have not sought formal treatment. There is a need to determine if community samples differ from clinical populations in outcome measures, including prognosis and response to treatment modalities. Although there have been several community-based studies of depression in the elderly, these have not examined personality disorders (Cole and Dendukuri 2003; Cole et al. 1999; Sharma et al. 1998).

Any study of the impact of personality disorders on depressive illness must also differentiate between the type of depression, including major depressive disorder, dysthymic disorder, bipolar depression, recurrent brief depressive disorder, and depression associated with medical conditions, including dementia.

The elderly are often ashamed to describe intrapsychic and interpersonal difficulties (Wiener et al. 1997). They often are not aware of previous diagnoses, and clinicians may have not discussed these because of the negative connotations and diagnostic uncertainty. This lack of communication relates to concerns about the stigma of psychiatric diagnoses in earlier cohorts. The use of family and others to provide collateral history is essential. These informants have interacted with the patient over time and are less likely to deny difficult behaviors. They are able to recall details that the patient may not recall because of cognitive impairment. Interviews with family members of depressed older adults have been found to have higher reliability in the diagnosis of personality dimensions than interviews with the patients themselves (Molinari et al. 1998).

The time frame of a cross-sectional interview when personality is a longitudinal diagnosis often requires assessment over time to establish a diagnosis. A decade-by-decade review of patient behaviors may assist in determining whether current behavior is of long-standing origin or is related to other disorders such as chronic depression, organic brain changes, or age-related life events. Also, the cognitive effects of depression may affect recall of behavior patterns.

The major diagnostic approaches to personality psychopathology are dimensional and categorical. This approach may affect the results of studies depending on the focus of the scales being used (Mulder 2002). According to Cloninger's psychobiological (seven-factor) model of temperament and character, harm avoidance, novelty seeking, and reward dependence are independent dimensions that describe personality (Cloninger 1987; Cloninger et al. 1993). All of the studies based on this model use the Tridimensional Personality Questionnaire (TPQ) or, more recently, the Temperament and Character Inventory (TCI). Significant effects of age on personality dimensions have been reported; thus, it is necessary to have age-adjusted norms (Brandstrom et al. 2001). Although there has been limited research using these scales in older adults, there is evidence that the TCI is useful for research on personality in the elderly (Casey and Joyce 1999).

An alternative dimensional classification of personality is the five-factor model (Digman 1990), which uses the NEO (neuroticism, extraversion, openness) Personality Inventory (NEO-PI) and its revised version (NEO-PI-R) (Costa and McCrae 1985; Costa and McCrae 1992). There have been several studies of these dimensions in individuals ages 65–85 years old (Cappeliez and O'Rourke 2002; Costa et al. 1986; McCrae and Costa 1988; Roepke et al. 2001). There is very limited study in the "old-old" (those over 85 years), with small sample sizes and few cross-sectional approaches (Roepke et al. 2001).

Criteria for categorical diagnoses of personality disorder do not take into account age-related changes in social function, comorbid illness, cognitive impairment, and selective mortality of some personality disorders (Agronin and Maletta 2000). A focus on work and social behavior is often not relevant in the elderly. Avoidant or dependent personality disorders may be falsely diagnosed when physical illness and decreased mobility result in the elderly being more reliant on caregivers. It is often difficult to differentiate personality disorders from the features of depression, including dependency, helplessness, somatic preoccupation, and negative self-evaluation (Lazarus and Sadavoy 1996). There is also no established way to describe the severity of personality dysfunction, which is not controlled for in most studies.

The difficulty in making a diagnosis of personality disorder when one is experiencing an episode of depressive illness must be addressed because of the clinical and research implications. It is unclear whether the assessment methods tap into enduring characteristics or are manifestations of affective state. The clinical state of depression affects self-perception so that the assessment of personality disorders in those who are depressed may not accurately reflect enduring personality characteristics (Hirschfeld et al. 1983; Sadavoy and Fogel 1992). Personality disorders in late life are vulnerable to the exacerbation or reemergence of maladaptive traits or the development of secondary Axis I psychopathology secondary to an acute stressor or age related losses (Sadavoy 1987). In younger people, studies of personality dimensions rather than disorders have found personality scores to be relatively stable and not state dependent (McCrae et al. 2000; Santor et al. 1997). Further research is needed to clarify whether these findings apply to the older adult.

Major Depressive Disorder

Relatively little is known about the impact of personality disorder on the course of major and nonmajor late-life depression. Between 10% and 30% of those who experience late-life major depressive disorder or dysthymic disorder have a diagnosis of personality disorder (Devanand 2002). In one study of more than 500 elderly inpatients with major depression, 24% had a comorbid personality disorder (Kunik et al. 1994).

Abrams and colleagues (1987) noted that the elderly with a history of major depression had more lifetime personality dysfunction than those without this history, although no specific pattern was identified. Early-onset (less than age 60 years) major depressive disorder in the elderly was associated with increased personality dysfunction, particularly avoidant, dependent, and not otherwise specified diagnoses (Abrams et al. 1987, 1994). This finding may reflect postdepressive changes, predisposition, or a low-grade depressive subtype.

The presence of personality disorder in the elderly with major depressive disorder has been found to be associated with a history of recurrent depressive episodes, additional DSM-IV-TR Axis I diagnoses, and a history of suicide attempts. These results support the predictive validity of the presence of personality disorders being associated with a chronic outcome of late-life depression (Kunik et al. 1993; Vine and Steingart 1994).

Personality disorders in the elderly with major depressive disorder are more likely to belong to the Cluster C "anxious" category (avoidant, dependent, obsessive-compulsive, passive-aggressive) or the not otherwise specified category, with few meeting criteria for the Cluster B "dramatic" (antisocial, borderline, histrionic, narcissistic) diagnoses (Kunik et al. 1994). Perhaps Cluster A "odd or eccentric" (paranoid, schizoid, schizotypal) personality disorders are less vulnerable to old age depression, with more risk for paranoid states or late-onset schizophrenia.

Several authors have reported a decreased prevalence of Cluster B disorders in late-life depression compared with middle-life depression (Abrams et al. 1987; Kunik et al. 1994; Sadavoy 1987; Thompson et al. 1988; Weissman et al. 1988). The question raised is whether personality disorders in younger adults disappear with age. It is possible that dramatic behaviors decrease with age and are replaced with somatic complaints, depressive withdrawal, and aberrant family interactions (Sadavoy 1987). Death by suicide or other causes in patients with major depressive disorder may lower the proportion of those with personality disorder diagnoses present in old age. A cohort effect of older age subjects being less likely than young and middle-age subjects to meet criteria for personality disorders and major depression further explains this decreased prevalence (Devanand 2002). In contrast, a meta-analysis of personality disorder in older adults concluded that the rate of personality disorder in the elderly, including the depressed elderly, was as high as those under age 50 years (Abrams and Horowitz 1999; Morse and Lynch 2000).

It is unclear if personality disorders induce or trigger depression or whether depression of a chronic or recurrent type predisposes to a personality disorder. Shea and colleagues (1996) have described a "scar" hypothesis, which refers to lasting personality change beyond the recovery from a major depressive episode (reviewed by Shea and Yen in Chapter 3 of this book). The clinical implication is the need for aggressive treatment of personality disorders and depressive symptoms. Prospective study, particularly in the elderly, is required (Hirschfeld et al. 1983; Schrader 1994).

Elevated harm avoidance scores based on the Cloninger model of temperament and character have been reported in the general population with depression (Cloninger et al. 1993; Hansenne et al. 1999; Pelissolo and Corruble 2002). These elevated levels of harm avoidance persist in prospective studies of those whose depression has remitted, although harm avoidance scores are lower than before treatment. The role of harm avoidance and other dimensions of personality in late-life depression requires clarification.

Various authors have examined the impact of the dimension of neuroticism on depressive disorder. Oldehinkel and colleagues (2001) reported that older persons with low levels of both disability and neuroticism were less likely to develop depressive disorder. A high neuroticism score in younger study populations was associated with a worse long-term outcome in those with major depressive disorder with chronicity and resistance to treatment (Hirschfeld et al. 1986; Mulder 2002). Neuroticism has been suggested to be the most powerful predictor of depression, although the evidence of a true personality predisposition for depression is modest and not specific to the elderly (Enns and Cox 1997). Stressful life events, long-term difficulties such as an ill spouse or poverty, and high neuroticism are risk factors for depression in late life, particularly recurrent episodes of these (Ormel et al. 2001). High neuroticism and long-term difficulties increase the risk even without stressful life events, possibly because of the uncontrollable nature of stressful life events in later life.

Personality disorders in the elderly may be associated with disability and impaired social and interpersonal functioning after the acute depressive episode (Abrams et al. 1998). Elderly patients with persisting or recurrent depression who also had Cluster B personality symptoms after treatment of the acute episode reported that these diagnoses contributed to decreased global function and quality of life over 1 year (Abrams et al. 2001). This finding suggests that personality disorders act as a cofactor in exacerbating or amplifying the impact of residual depression on function and quality of life. The elderly who lack social supports have been found to have an increased vulnerability to depression, which is likely tied to personality factors (Krouse et al. 1990). This finding may have treatment implications for cases of geriatric depression that need to address characterological issues. Stek and colleagues (2002) found that personality disorder predicted a worse outcome of depression in elderly patients 6–8 years after clinical treatment.

Dysthymic Disorder

The rate of dysthymic disorder is lower in the elderly than younger groups (Bellino et al. 2000). The elderly with dysthymic disorder differ from younger adults who have more frequent comorbid Axis I and Axis II (personality disorder) diagnoses (Bellino et al. 2001). The onset of dysthymic disorder occurs later in the elderly, with onset at just over age 52 years in one study (Devanand et al. 1994). Elderly dysthymic individuals are generally not young dysthymic individuals who have grown old.

There are limited data on the impact of personality disorders on dysthymic disorder in the elderly. There are many similarities between chronic major depression and dysthymic disorder in the elderly (Devanand et al. 1994). Devanand and colleagues (2000) reported personality disorders in just over 30% of an elderly population with dysthymic disorder, with a distribution of personality disorders similar to early-onset major depressive disorder. Obsessive-compulsive, avoidant, and borderline personality disorders were the most frequent diagnoses. Personality disorders are associated with early age at onset of depressive illness, which is consistent with studies of major depression in late life (Abrams et al. 1987; Kunik et al. 1994).

Characterological depression is not described in DSM-IV-TR. It refers to a lifelong characteristic depressed mood perceived by the self and others. This condition may meet criteria for dysthymic disorder or major depressive disorder, with feelings of dejection, hopelessness, and discouragement between episodes (Chaisson-Stewart 1985; Scott 1988). It is closely related to "depressive personality traits" originally described by several of the pioneers of psychiatric nosology including Kraepelin, Kretschmer, and Schneider (Phillips et al. 1990). Some of these patients warrant a personality disorder diagnosis, with narcissistic, borderline, avoidant, and dependent personality disorders most likely to complicate a chronic depressive pattern. Little is known about the course and management of this diagnosis. Akiskal (1983) suggested that this diagnosis could be deemed an affective disorder with character pathology, or a personality disorder with secondary affective symptomatology, or subgroups of each depending on antidepressant response.

Chronic depressive disorder is often seen in the geriatric population and associated with personality psychopathology and referred to as "double depression." Post (1972) has referred to "depressive invalidism" to describe double depression in the elderly who also have severe recurrent depression and incomplete remissions. The relationship to dysthymic disorder and personality disorders in late life is unknown.

Other Types of Depression

Other types of depression include bipolar depression, recurrent brief depressive disorder and other atypical depressive disorders, depression associated with dementia, and other medical causes. There is little information on the impact of personality disorders on these types of mood disorders in the elderly. Most of the studies were based on research with younger adults. These studies included retrospective chart reviews and cross-sectional approaches. A methodological issue is the difficulty in the diagnosis of personality pathology in the presence of mood symptoms.

Bipolar Disorder

Personality disorders have been reported in 40%–50% of younger adults with bipolar disorder (Kay et al. 2002; Ucok et al. 1998). Bipolar patients with personality disorders have a lower rate of current employment, more prescribed psychotropics, increased alcohol consumption and substance use, and a more difficult course of bipolar illness (Kay et al. 2002). Obsessive-compulsive disorder and paranoid, histrionic, and borderline personality disorders have been reported as more prevalent in patients with bipolar disorder (Rossi et al. 2001; Ucok et al. 1998). One of the few studies of the prevalence and clinical features of bipolar depression in late life reported that bipolar II disorder and atypical depression were less common (Benazzi 2001). Unfortunately, this study excluded severe personality disorders. Research on the impact of personality disorders on bipolar depression in the elderly is lacking.

There are several personality dimensions associated with bipolar disorder in younger groups. Elevated harm avoidance has been associated with both bipolar disorder and unipolar depression. High novelty seeking has been associated with bipolar disorder (Young et al. 1995). Neuroticism, hostility, and social dysfunction were reported to have a negative prognostic value only for bipolar disorder and nonendogenous depression (Heerlein et al. 1998). Higher scores on the positive emotion facet (subscale) of extraversion have been reported in patients with euthymic bipolar disorder when compared with patients who have recovered from unipolar depression (Bagby et al. 1996).

Depression Associated With Medical Conditions

The implications of personality dimensions and disorders add a further level of complexity to the understanding of depression in various medical populations. Morris and Robinson (1995) found that neuroticism was higher in depressed patients after stroke. In those with supratentorial infarcts, the 1-year cumulative incidence of depression was just under 40%, and those with high neuroticism had an increased risk of poststroke depression regardless of lesion location (Aben et al. 2002).

The effects of premorbid personality disorders in the case of the demented patient with depression are unclear. Strauss and colleagues (1997) reported that a relationship between premorbid personality and depressive symptoms in Alzheimer's disease was found only if the informant for both personality and symptom assessment was the same person. Other studies had inconsistent results and suggested the need for prospective study of premorbid personality and its effects on the behavioral and psychological symptoms of dementia (Low et al. 2002). Increased neuroticism and rigidity predicted the occurrence of Alzheimer's disease, but the impact on depression in dementia was not examined (Meins and Dammast 2000).

Suicide

Suicide rates are higher in later life than any other age group (Conwell et al. 2002). Both depression and personality factors have been found to be important risk factors for suicide in older people (Harwood et al. 2001; Lawrence et al. 2000). These findings have been consistent with the results in younger groups in which several studies have found increased suicide risk in those with both depression and a personality disorder (Cheng et al. 1997; Isometsa et al. 1996; Van Gastel et al. 1997). A recent 10-year prospective study in younger persons found a similar pattern, with increased suicide rates in those with comorbid major depression and personality disorder (Hansen et al. 2003).

High novelty seeking has been associated with past suicide attempts in younger adults (Grucza et al. 2003). Low extraversion has been associated with lifetime history of attempted suicide, whereas high neuroticism has been associated with suicidal ideation in studies of depressed inpatients over age 50 years (Duberstein et al. 2000). In younger patients with bipolar depression, suicide attempts have been reported to be more frequent in those with a history of a personality disorder (Ucok et al. 1998). There is no information specific to suicide in patients with late-life bipolar depression.

The interaction between personality, mood, and the risk of suicide in the older adult needs clarification. Research in this area must differentiate between type of depression, suicide attempts, and completed suicide. Suicide is a serious and important outcome in late life depression and requires better prevention and treatment strategies.

Treatment Issues

Overview

Depression in late life is a significant public health problem that is often unrecognized or inadequately treated despite evidence of efficacious treatment being available (Lebowitz et al. 1997). The impact of personality disorder on early recognition, diagnosis, and treatment of late-life depression requires study to reduce suffering and permit optimal quality of life for older adults. Most of the literature concerning treatment has been based on studies in the general adult population. Earlier studies that were not specific to the elderly reported that those with neurotic, hypochondrical, or hysterical traits had poor response to amitriptyline or imipramine (Bielski and Friedel 1976; Paykel 1972). Also, high neuroticism scores predicted worse response to treatment in depressed inpatients and outpatients (Duggan et al. 1990; Faravelli et al. 1986; Shawcross and Tyrer 1985; Weissman et al. 1978; Zuckerman et al. 1980). These studies had significant methodological issues, including the emphasis on long-term outcome, and most were naturalistic.

Studies of dimensions of personality have found that neuroticism scores decrease with treatment of patients with depressive disorder, but the scores remain elevated relative to control subjects (Du et al. 2002; Mulder 2002; Pelissolo and Corruble 2002). Neuroticism predicts chronic poor outcome with psychotherapy and pharmacotherapy and may act as a predisposing factor for major depression, but it does not predict response when severity is controlled for (Bagby et al. 2002; Berlanga et al. 1999; Petersen et al. 2002). Harm avoidance scores are related to depression severity and decrease with treatment but remain elevated relative to control subjects (Agosti and McGrath 2002; Joyce et al. 1994; Mulder and Joyce 1994). Study is required regarding the role of neuroticism and harm avoidance as personality characteristics that affect response to treatment in those individuals with late-life depression.

Most of the evidence to support the finding that personality pathology predicts a worse outcome with treatment of depressed patients comes from the methodologically weakest studies or from those in which personality features overlap depressive features (Mulder 2002). More carefully designed studies (structured interviews and controlled for treatment) have found no difference in short-term outcome (Hirschfeld et al. 1998; Joyce et al. 1994; Krishnan 2003; Marijnissen et al. 2002; Mulder et al. 2003; Stuart et al. 1992). These studies were not specific to late-life depression. Research in the older adult is important to find the personality variables that may be clinically relevant in the prediction of treatment response.

Patients with depression and personality pathology are less likely to receive an adequate treatment course, and this may introduce a bias in research results. Charney and colleagues (1981) reported that ECT or psychotropic use in those with depression and personality disorders was much less frequent. Black and colleagues (1988) found that almost 30% of those with a personality disorder compared with almost 50% of those without a personality disorder received an adequate treatment with medication. These studies were not specific to late life but may be even more relevant in the elderly, in whom issues of ageism, concerns about adverse effects, and lack of accessibility to psychiatric treatment may decrease the likelihood of adequate treatment, particularly in those perceived by caregivers as "difficult." Just under 20% of those with recurrent, nonpsychotic geriatric depression are treatment resistant with a lack of response and relapse during the continuation and maintenance phases of treatment (Little et al. 1998). A question raised by this finding is the role of personality disorders in these resistant cases, and there is no information available from the research literature.

The approach to treatment of the depressed elderly with personality disorders includes obtaining relevant history and mental status examination; assessing physical health; providing feedback to the patient, family, and caregivers to assist in management and vigorous treatment using available biological and psychological treatments; and addressing social issues such as isolation, housing, and financial concerns (Table 10–1). Physical health must be assessed because chronic medical illness may affect the outcome of geriatric depression and the course of personality disorders. Medical disorders such as thyroid disorders and adverse reactions to medications may cause depression in the elderly and should be considered in the differential diagnosis. A physical examination including neurological examination is required to exclude structural brain changes that may be found in conditions such as vascular depression associated with late life (Blazer 2000). The patient's history should include information about alcohol consumption and a list of prescription and alternative medications. The mental status examination should include a formal assessment of cognition. A collaborative history from family members and caregivers is an important component of the assessment and assists in optimizing treatment for the older adult.

Personality disorders and dimensions and their impact on late-life depression must be communicated to patients, family, and caregivers in a practical manner that assists care, particularly in long-term care settings. Respect for privacy and confidential information and obtaining appropriate consent are essential. For example, depressed elderly in a long-term care setting with an external locus of control who are

TABLE 10–1. Approach to treatment of depressed elderly persons with personality disorders

History	• Onset of occurrence of affective, cognitive, somatic symptoms
	• Past psychiatric and alcohol history
	• Past medical history and role of physical illness and decreased mobility
	• Medications taken, including nonprescription and alternative medications
	• Collateral from family and caregivers
Mental status examination	• Affect and mood
	• Self-harm ideation
	• Cognition
	• Psychosis
	• Judgment and insight
	• Rapport
Rating scales	• Geriatric Depression Scale (Hamilton 1967)
	• Hamilton Depression Scale (Yesavage et al. 1983)
	• Mini-Mental State Examination (Folstein et al. 1975)
Treatment	• Work comprehensively and flexibly with other mental health professionals
	• Explore own feelings about aging
	• Formulate treatment plan and define goals
	• Accept limited treatment goals if applicable
	• Explain impact of personality dimensions and disorders on depression and care to patient, family, and other caregivers with appropriate consent
	• Treat adequately with therapeutic optimism
	• Use a biopsychosocial approach to treatment with pharmacotherapy, electroconvulsive therapy, and psychotherapy individually or in combination

demanding of caregiver attention may benefit from a more directive approach with reliable and consistent caregiver availability at specific times. Those with an internal locus of control may require more explanation, involvement in care decisions, and a flexible approach by caregivers (Beekman et al. 2001; Spar and LaRue 1997).

Age affects treatment, including drug interactions and pharmacokinetics, the dose and schedule of pharmacotherapy, and the format and pace of psychotherapy. A comprehensive and flexible approach that involves working closely with other health care professionals is needed. Treating the elderly requires the exploration of one's own feelings about aging, accepting limited treatment goals, and maintaining therapeutic optimism (Meador and Davis 1996; Spar and LaRue 1997).

Pharmacotherapy and Electroconvulsive Therapy

The role of pharmacotherapy and ECT in late-life depression associated with personality disorders has not been well studied. Kunik and colleagues (1993) reported that elderly inpatients with major depression benefited from pharmacotherapy with antidepressant medication or ECT regardless of whether there was a comorbid personality disorder. Studies in younger age groups have reported benefits of pharmacotherapy for depressive disorders with comorbid personality disorders (Mulder et al. 2003; Russell et al. 2003). Patients with major depressive disorder treated with selective serotonin reuptake inhibitors (SSRIs) were less likely to meet criteria for personality disorder diagnoses (Ekselius and von Knorring 1998; Fava et al. 1994, 2002). Others reported a worse outcome for medication or ECT in those with depression and characterological disorder (Peselow et al. 1992; Pfohl et al. 1984; Sato et al. 1993).

Factors to consider in the use of pharmacotherapy in this population include safety, efficacy, pharmacokinetics, and comorbid medical conditions (Montgomery 2002). Various agents have been used for the treatment of older adults with depressive disorders, including SSRIs, tricyclic antidepressants (TCAs), monoamine oxidase inhibitors, and other atypical antidepressants. Mittmann and colleagues (1997) found no difference between antidepressant classes in efficacy and tolerability. Others have suggested that SSRIs are the first choice in the depressed elderly (Montgomery 2002). A comparative review of SSRIs in patients with late-life depression concluded that there is no evidence to recommend any one agent, although less risk of drug interaction may be a reason to consider citalopram or sertraline (Solai et al 2001). The impact of personality disorders on the pharmacotherapy of patients with late-life depression requires careful study to permit an evidence-based approach to treatment.

There has been considerable interest in measures of personality dimensions and disorders at baseline and response to treatment of depressive illness (reviewed by Kennedy et al. in Chapter 5 of this book). Although there have been a number of studies of TCAs, SSRIs, and mood stabilizers in younger groups (see Chapter 5 of this book), it is unknown if these outcomes apply to late-life depression, dysthymic disorder, and bipolar depression. There is virtually no information on the impact of personality disorder on the treatment of late-life depression with ECT. A naturalistic study in younger patients reported that personality pathology affected short-term but not 12-month outcome (Casey et al. 1996). ECT was equally effective in depression with or without a personality disorder in four studies (Mulder 2002). Unfortunately, there were no studies of older adults. Also, the studies were not controlled and had small numbers who received the treatment. As a result there is the risk that the patients deemed suitable for ECT differed significantly in personality pathology from those receiving other treatments.

Psychotherapy

Older persons vary in their introspective ability and motivation to engage in psychotherapy. Age per se is not a contraindication to psychotherapy (Lazarus and Sadavoy 1996; Steuer 1982). The benefit and response to psychotherapy depends on the individual and the type of psychotherapy selected as most appropriate for that person. Cognitive-behavioral, interpersonal, life-review, and psychodynamic approaches have been described as useful when psychosocial factors contribute to personality disorders and depression or when somatic treatment is refused, ineffective, or poorly tolerated (Butler 1974; Lazarus and Sadavoy 1996; Yesavage and Karasu 1982). Unfortunately, the use of psychotherapy to modify the impact of personality disorders on late-life depression has not been adequately studied. This is not unlike the situation in other forms of treatment in this population. Research in this area requires better outcome and process measures and methods to determine the impact of choice of treatment on outcome (Arean et al. 2003).

It has been suggested that those with an externalizing style may do better with a directive therapy, whereas those with an internalizing style may respond more to an insight-oriented approach (Spar and LaRue 1997). Supportive psychotherapies are more appropriate for patients with cognitive impairment, psychosis, or increased somatic concerns. Goals and techniques must be flexible and individualized (Kennedy and Tanenbaum 2000). The approach used must address family conflicts, include advocacy, and use the psychotherapy as an adjunct to medication and to improve the social supports and environment (Lazarus 1989). Role transitions such as bereavement, career changes, and decreased social support and physical difficulties including pain and poor sleep require exploration (Spar and LaRue 1997).

Useful approaches include the clarification of pathological character patterns, tactful confrontation of the patient with these patterns, and interpretation as to whether the patient will react in a paranoid fashion, devalue and withdraw from treatment, or tolerate depression or loss of self-esteem (Grotjahn 1955; Yesavage and Karasu 1982). Psychodynamic approaches with behavioral techniques may be effective in the character-disordered patient in a long-term care setting (Sadavoy and Dorian 1983).

Psychotherapy with patients with personality disorder has been described as more difficult than psychotherapy with those who do not have one. Elderly patients with Cluster B personality disorders may be sensitive, labile, and impulsive and may frustrate the therapist with demands (Sadavoy 1987). Those with personality disorders are demanding of caregivers and family, and their behavior may affect the ability to engage in individual psychotherapy. The elderly, depressed, narcissistic patient is more able to accept an approach that acknowledges the realistic causes of depression (such as loss of self-esteem) and that provides hope for new emotional resources as a consequence of examining priorities (Grotjahn 1955). Dependent or avoidant elderly individuals may respond better to treatment because they are more likely to comply with treatment even though it is likely to be longer than for the older adult without personality disorder (Abrams and Horowitz 1999).

One of the few studies in the elderly with major depression and personality disorders treated with psychotherapy reported decreased response to psychotherapy (Thompson et al. 1988). Elderly outpatients with major depression treated with brief (16–20 sessions) cognitive, behavioral, or psychodynamic psychotherapies resulted in a 70% overall response rate for these modalities (Thompson et al. 1987). The presence of a personality disorder increased the risk of treatment failure by four times. Cognitive and behavioral approaches maintained improvement more than psychodynamic approaches. Those with more severe personality disorder had a more protracted course, although one-half of the patients where there was a low expectation of improvement responded to cognitive and behavioral therapy. Gallagher and Thompson (1983) reported that over 50% of depressed elderly treated with these brief psychotherapies had not relapsed at 1 year.

In younger age groups, there is limited evidence in favor of structured psychotherapeutic interventions such as cognitive-behavioral therapy in those with major depression and personality pathology (Mulder 2002). Dialectical behavior therapy (DBT) and interpersonal therapy may be useful in the treatment of older adults with personality disorders (DeLeo et al. 1999). DBT is a cognitive-behavioral therapy developed to treat suicidal and borderline personality disorders that has been applied to many clinical populations (Rizvi and Linehan 2001). It involves skills training, coaching, and behavior analysis. This therapy has resulted in reduced suicidal behavior, hospitalization, anger, and withdrawal from treatment (Swenson et al. 2001). Interpersonal therapy is a brief psychotherapy that addresses interpersonal problems linked to depression. There is no information about the use of these approaches in the depressed elderly with personality disorders. There is also no data about the psychotherapy of late-life dysthymic disorder (Bellino et al. 2000).

In addition to individual psychotherapies, group and family therapies are often useful in the care of the depressed elderly with personality disorders (Pearlman 1993). Family members are often required to provide history, to assist in patient management and enhance treatment compliance, to provide transportation, and to address family conflicts (Lazarus and Sadavoy 1996; Spar and LaRue 1997). Group therapies include cognitive-behavioral and psychodynamic approaches. Klausner and colleagues (1998) described a goal-focused, time-limited group psychotherapy approach with psychoeducation and skills training to achieve individual goals compared with a reminiscence group therapy that involved a life review to facilitate decisions in a group of older adults who failed to attain complete remission of late-life depression. Most of the subjects in this study were receiving antidepressants, and both group approaches improved depressed mood and degree of disability. The goal-focused group psychotherapy resulted in a greater change in depressive symptoms, improved hope, reduced anxiety, and enhanced social function.

Lynch and colleagues (2003) added group dialectical behavior therapy to antidepressant medication and clinical management in chronically depressed older adults (over age 60 years). Over 70% of those who received the DBT remitted after treatment compared with 47% of those who only received the medication and clinical management. During 6 months of follow-up, 75% of the DBT group were in remission compared with 30% of those who did not receive this group psychotherapy. Dependency and adaptive coping, which may create a vulnerability to depression, also improved in the DBT group. These findings suggest the potential for a useful intervention, but research is required to examine the impact of personality disorders on the use of this modality for the treatment of late-life depression.

Case Example

Ms. L, a 72-year-old married woman, presented with a 3-month history of depressed mood, vegetative symptoms, hopelessness, and passive suicidal ideation following her father's death and her husband's retirement. She had a history of recurrent episodes of depressed mood since age 35 years that had been treated with antidepressants and anxiolytics. Her mood symptoms were in remission over the past 15 years, with no psychotropics or other psychiatric treatment. Her past medical history was unremarkable. Ms. L described a lifelong pattern of seeking attention, approval, and reassurance from others and preoccupation with her appearance. A thorough history, mental status examination including cognitive assessment, and interview with her husband were obtained. Her husband described her as "shallow and self-absorbed." Ms. L presented in a rather dramatic manner, wearing a large, colorful hat and dark sunglasses. Her speech and gestures created the impression that she was focused on capturing the attention of the interviewer with her choice of words, often for effect. The diagnoses included a major depressive disorder and histrionic personality disorder traits. She was started on antidepressant and cognitive-behavioral psychotherapy that explored her depressed mood, coping skills, and losses. She did not respond to full trials at therapeutic doses of two SSRIs. Ms. L became more dramatic in her behavior, seeking the therapist's approval and reassurance during sessions and calling between sessions. She also demanded attention from her husband and on one occasion threw herself down the stairs at home when she felt ignored. Venlafaxine was started at full therapeutic doses, with a partial improvement in depressive symptoms. Lithium carbonate was added as an adjuvant, with remission of the major depressive disorder within 2 weeks at therapeutic doses. Also, the patient was seen in individual psychotherapy, and couple sessions were held to address marital tensions and provide support for her husband. Unexpectedly, the histrionic personality traits were significantly reduced with resolution of the depressive symptoms. Although still enjoying the attention of others, Ms. L was less focused on herself and demonstrated insight into her difficulties. She was able to direct her desire to be the center of attention to appropriate settings such as performing with a charity musical review.

This case highlights some of the issues related to the effect of personality disorder traits on the management of late-life depression. A biopsychosocial approach was most useful. Collateral history from family members assisted in diagnosis. The need for aggressive treatment despite the significant character pathology was demonstrated by the excellent response to a combination of pharmacotherapy, individual psychotherapy, and couple therapy. In this case, the presence of personality disorder traits did not adversely affect outcome. Also, on an individual basis, a personality disorder diagnosis should not deter vigorous treatment of late-life depression.

Conclusions

The impact of personality disorders on late-life depression remains unclear. Depression may affect the manifestation of symptoms that lead to a personality disorder diagnosis, especially in those with early-onset chronic depression. Whether personality disorders induce depression or whether depression affects personality disorders is tautological.

The assessment of personality in the elderly has been difficult because of the absence of reliable standardized rating instruments. Differences in the measures of personality as dimensions versus categorical diagnoses further complicate assessment. There has been a paucity of research, particularly randomized trials, in the elderly. There is also a dearth of literature that differentiates between types of depression (major depressive disorder, dysthymic disorder, or bipolar depression).

Several studies in the elderly have found that the presence of a personality disorder is associated with worse long-term outcome. The limited data on the impact of personality on treatment in late-life depression prevent clear conclusions, with one study finding biological treatments equally benefited those with or without a personality disorder, whereas another study of psychotherapy concluded decreased likelihood of treatment response. Research on personality pathology and treatment outcome in major depression has produced conflicting results in younger adults. High neuroticism scores generally were found to be associated with a worse outcome over the long-term. Study design affected the rate of personality pathology, depending on how it was measured. Depressed patients with personality pathology were less likely to receive adequate treatment. Studies did not control for severity and chronicity of depression and other characteristics.

The best-designed studies suggested that personality pathology had the least effect on depression outcome in younger age groups. Until there is evidence to the contrary, the presence of personality disorder in the depressed elderly should not affect therapeutic optimism.

References

Aben I, Denollet J, Lousberg R, et al: Personality and vulnerability to depression in stroke patients: a one-year prospective follow-up study. Stroke 33:2391–2395, 2002

Abrams RC, Horowitz SV: Personality disorders after age 50: a meta-analytic review of the literature, in Personality Disorders in Older Adults: Emerging Issues in Diagnosis and Treatment. Edited by Rosowsky E, Abrams RC, Zweig RA. Mahwah, NJ, Lawrence Erlbaum, 1999, pp 55–68

Abrams RC, Alexopoulos GS, Young RC: Geriatric depression and DSM-III-R personality disorder criteria. J Am Geriatr Soc 35:383–386, 1987

Abrams RC, Rosendahl E, Card C, et al: Personality disorder correlates of late and early onset depression. J Am Geriatr Soc 42:727–731, 1994

Abrams RC, Spielman LA, Alexopoulos GS, et al: Personality disorder symptoms and functioning in elderly depressed patients. Am J Geriatr Psychiatry 6:24–30, 1998

Abrams RC, Alexopoulos GS, Spielman LA, et al: Personality disorder symptoms predict declines in global functioning and quality of life in elderly depressed patients. Am J Geriatr Psychiatry 9:67–71, 2001

Agosti V, McGrath PJ: Comparison of the effects of fluoxetine, imipramine, and placebo on personality in atypical depression. J Affect Disord 71:113–120, 2002

Agronin ME, Maletta G: Personality disorders in late life: understanding and overcoming the gap in research. Am J Geriatr Psychiatry 8:4–18, 2000

Akiskal HS: Dysthymic disorder: psychopathology of proposed chronic depressive subtypes. Am J Psychiatry 140:11–20, 1983

American Psychiatric Association: Diagnostic and Statistical Manual of Mental Disorders, 4th Edition, Text Revision. Washington, DC, American Psychiatric Association, 2000

Andrews G, Neilson M, Hunt C, et al: Diagnosis, personality and the long-term outcome of depression. Br J Psychiatry 157:13–18, 1990

Arean PA, Cook BL, Gallagher-Thompson D, et al: Guidelines for conducting geropsychotherapy research. Am J Geriatr Psychiatry 11:9–16, 2003

Bagby RM, Young LT, Schuller DR, et al: Bipolar disorder, unipolar depression and the five-factor model of personality. J Affect Disord 41:25–32, 1996

Bagby RM, Ryder AG, Cristi C: Psychosocial and clinical predictors of response to pharmacotherapy for depression. J Psychiatry Neurosci 27:250–257, 2002

Beekman AT, Deeg DJ, Geerlings SW, et al: Emergence and persistence of late life depression: a 3-year follow-up of the Longitudinal Aging Study Amsterdam. J Affect Disord 65:131–138, 2001

Bellino S, Bogetto F, Vaschetto P, et al: Recognition and treatment of dysthymia in elderly patients. Drugs Aging 16:107–121, 2000

Bellino S, Patria L, Ziero S, et al: Clinical features of dysthymia and age: a clinical investigation. Psychiatry Res 103:219–228, 2001

Benazzi F: Bipolar depression in late life: prevalence and clinical features in 525 depressed outpatients. J Affect Disord 66:13–18, 2001

Berlanga C, Heinze G, Torres M, et al: Personality and clinical predictors of recurrence of depression. Psychiatr Serv 50:376–380, 1999

Bielski RJ, Friedel RO: Prediction of tricyclic antidepressant response: a critical review. Arch Gen Psychiatry 33:1479–1489, 1976

Black DW, Bell S, Hulbert J, et al: The importance of axis II in patients with major depression: a controlled study. J Affect Disord 14:115–122, 1988

Blazer D: Depression, in Merck Manual of Geriatrics, 3rd Edition. Edited by Abrams WB, Beers MH, Berkow R. Philadelphia, PA, Merck, 2000, pp 310–322

Brandstrom S, Richter J, Przybeck T: Distributions by age and sex of the dimensions of temperament and character inventory in a cross-cultural perspective among Sweden, Germany, and the USA. Psychol Rep 89:747–758, 2001

Butler RN: Successful aging and the role of the life review. J Am Geriatr Soc 22:529–535, 1974

Cappeliez P, O'Rourke N: Profiles of reminiscence among older adults: perceived stress, life attitudes, and personality variables. Int J Aging Hum Dev 54:255–266, 2002

Casey JE, Joyce PR: Personality disorder and the temperament and character inventory in the elderly. Acta Psychiatr Scand 100:302–308, 1999

Casey P, Meagher D, Butler E: Personality, functioning, and recovery from major depression. J Nerv Ment Dis 184:240–245, 1996

Chaisson-Stewart GM: An integrated theory of depression, in Depression in the Elderly. Edited by Chaisson-Stewart GM. New York, Wiley, 1985, pp 56–104

Charney DS, Nelson JC, Quinlan DM: Personality traits and disorder in depression. Am J Psychiatry 138:1601–1604, 1981

Cheng AT, Mann AH, Chan KA: Personality disorder and suicide: a case control study. Br J Psychiatry 170:441–446, 1997

Cloninger CR: A systematic method for clinical description and classification of personality variants: a proposal. Arch Gen Psychiatry 44:573–588, 1987

Cloninger CR, Svrakic DM, Przybeck TR: A psychobiological model of temperament and character. Arch Gen Psychiatry 50:975–990, 1993

Cole MG, Dendukuri N: Risk factors for depression among elderly community subjects: a systematic review and meta-analysis. Am J Psychiatry 160:1147–1156, 2003

Cole MG, Bellavance F, Mansour A: Prognosis of depression in elderly community and primary care populations: a systematic review and meta-analysis. Am J Psychiatry 156:1182–1189, 1999

Conwell Y, Duberstein PR, Caine ED: Risk factors for suicide in later life. Biol Psychiatry 52:193–204, 2002

Costa PT Jr, McCrae RR: Manual for the NEO Personality Inventory. Odessa, FL, Psychological Assessment Resources, 1985

Costa PT Jr, McCrae RR: Revised NEO Personality Inventory (NEO-PI-R) and NEO Five-Factor Inventory (NEO-FFI): Professional Manual. Odessa, FL, Psychological Assessment Resources, 1992

Costa PT Jr, McCrae RR, Zonderman AB: Cross-sectional studies of personality in a national sample, 2: stability in neuroticism, extraversion, and openness. Psychol Aging 1:144–149, 1986

DeLeo D, Scocco P, Meneghel G: Pharmacological and psychotherapeutic treatment of personality disorders in the elderly. Int Psychogeriatr 11:191–206, 1999

Devanand DP: Comorbid psychiatric disorders in late life depression. Biol Psychiatry 52:236–242, 2002

Devanand DP, Nobler MS, Singer T, et al: Is dysthymia a different disorder in the elderly? Am J Psychiatry 151:1592–1599, 1994

Devanand DP, Turret N, Moody BJ, et al: Personality disorders in elderly patients with dysthymic disorder. Am J Geriatr Psychiatry 8:188–195, 2000

Digman JM: Personality structure: emergence of the five-factor model. Annu Rev Psychol 41:417–440, 1990

Du L, Bakish D, Ravindran AV, et al: Does fluoxetine influence major depression by modifying five-factor personality traits? J Affect Disord 71:235–241, 2002

Duberstein PR, Conwell Y, Seidlitz L, et al: Personality traits and suicidal behavior and ideation in depressed inpatients 50 years of age and older. J Gerontol B Psychol Sci Soc Sci 55:P18–P26, 2000

Duggan CF, Lee AS, Murray RM: Does personality predict long-term outcome in depression? Br J Psychiatry 157:19–24, 1990

Ekselius L, von Knorring L: Personality disorder comorbidity with major depression and response to treatment with sertraline or citalopram. Int Clin Psychopharmacol 13:205–211, 1998

Enns MW, Cox BJ: Personality dimensions and depression: review and commentary. Can J Psychiatry 42:274–284, 1997

Faravelli C, Ambonetti A, Pallanti S, et al: Depressive relapses and incomplete recovery from index episode. Am J Psychiatry 143:888–891, 1986

Fava M, Bouffides E, Pava JA, et al: Personality disorder comorbidity with major depression and response to fluoxetine treatment. Psychother Psychosom 62:160–167, 1994

Fava M, Farabaugh AH, Sickinger AH, et al: Personality disorders and depression. Psychol Med 32:1049–1057, 2002

Folstein MF, Folstein SE, McHugh PR: "Mini-Mental State": a practical method for grading the cognitive state of patients for the clinician. J Psychiatr Res 12:189–198, 1975

Gallagher DE, Thompson LW: Effectiveness of psychotherapy for both endogenous and nonendogenous depression in older adult outpatients. J Gerontol 38:707–712, 1983

Grotjahn M: Analytic psychotherapy with the elderly. Psychoanal Rev 42:419–427, 1955

Grucza RA, Przybeck TR, Spitznagel EL, et al: Personality and depressive symptoms: a multidimensional analysis. J Affect Disord 74:123–130, 2003

Hamilton M: Development of a rating scale for primary depressive illness. Br J Soc Clin Psychol 6:278–296, 1967

Hansen PE, Wang AG, Stage KB, et al: Comorbid personality disorder predicts suicide after major depression: a 10 year follow-up. Acta Psychiatr Scand 107:436–440, 2003

Hansenne M, Reggers J, Pinto E, et al: Temperament and character inventory (TCI) and depression. J Psychiatr Res 33:31–36, 1999

Harwood D, Hawton K, Hope T, et al: Psychiatric disorder and personality factors associated with suicide in older people: a descriptive and case control study. Int J Geriatr Psychiatry 16:155–165, 2001

Heerlein A, Richter P, Gonzalez M, et al: Personality patterns and outcome in depressive and bipolar disorders. Psychopathology 31:15–22, 1998

Hirschfeld RM, Klerman GL, Clayton PJ, et al: Assessing personality: effects of the depressive state on trait measurement. Am J Psychiatry 140:695–699, 1983

Hirschfeld RM, Klerman GL, Andreasen NC, et al: Psychosocial predictors of chronicity in depressed patients. Br J Psychiatry 148:648–654, 1986

Hirschfeld RM, Russell JM, Delgado PL, et al: Predictors of response to acute treatment of chronic and double depression with sertraline and imipramine. J Clin Psychiatry 59:669–675, 1998

Isometsa ET, Henriksson MM, Heikkinen ME, et al: Suicide among subjects with personality disorders. Am J Psychiatry 153:667–673, 1996

Joyce PR, Mulder RT, Cloninger CR: Temperament predicts clomipramine and desipramine response in major depression. J Affect Disord 30:35–46, 1994

Kay JH, Altshuler LL, Ventura J, et al: Impact of axis II comorbidity on the course of bipolar illness in men: a retrospective chart review. Bipolar Disord 4:237–242, 2002

Kennedy GJ, Tanenbaum S: Psychotherapy with older adults. Am J Psychotherapy 54:386–407, 2000

Klausner EJ, Clarkin JF, Spielman L, et al: Late-life depression and functional disability: the role of goal-focused group psychotherapy. Int J Geriatr Psychiatry 13:707–716, 1998

Krishnan KR: Comorbidity and depression treatment. Biol Psychiatry 53:701–706, 2003

Krouse N, Liang J, Keith V: Personality, social support and psychological distress in later life. Psychol Aging 5:315–326, 1990

Kunik ME, Mulsant BH, Rifai AH, et al: Personality disorders in elderly inpatients with major depression. Am J Geriatr Psychiatry 1:38–45, 1993

Kunik ME, Mulsant BH, Rifai AH, et al: A study of personality disorder in elderly psychiatric inpatients (abstract). Am J Psychiatry 151:603–605, 1994

Lawrence D, Almeida OP, Hulse GK, et al: Suicide and attempted suicide among older adults in Western Australia. Psychol Med 30:813–821, 2000

Lazarus L: Psychotherapy in the ambulatory care setting, in Geriatric Psychiatry. Edited by Busse E, Blazer D. Washington, DC, American Psychiatric Press, 1989, pp 567–576

Lazarus LW, Sadavoy J: Individual psychotherapy, in Comprehensive Review of Geriatric Psychiatry, 2nd Edition. Edited by Sadavoy J, Lazarus LW, Jarvik LF, et al. Washington, DC, American Psychiatric Press, 1996, pp 819–850

Lebowitz BD, Pearson JL, Schneider LS, et al: Diagnosis and treatment of depression in late life: consensus statement update. JAMA 278:1186–1190, 1997

Little JT, Reynolds CF, Dew MA, et al: How common is resistance to treatment in recurrent, nonpsychotic geriatric depression? Am J Psychiatry 155:1035–1038, 1998

Low LF, Brodaty H, Draper B: A study of premorbid personality and behavioral and psychological symptoms of dementia in nursing home residents. Int J Geriatr Psychiatry 17:779–783, 2002

Lynch TR, Morse JQ, Mendelson T, et al: Dialectical behavior therapy for depressed older adults: a randomized pilot study. Am J Geriatr Psychiatry 11:33–45, 2003

Marijnissen G, Tuinier S, Sijben AE, et al: The temperament and character inventory in major depression. J Affect Disord 70:219–223, 2002

McCrae RR, Costa PT Jr: Age, personality, and the spontaneous self-concept. J Gerontol 43:S177–S185, 1988

McCrae RR, Costa PT Jr, Ostendorf F, et al: Nature over nurture: temperament, personality, and life span development. J Pers Soc Psychol 78:173–186, 2000

Meador KG, Davis CD: Psychotherapy, in The American Psychiatric Press Textbook of Geriatric Psychiatry, 2nd Edition. Edited by Busse EW, Blazer DG. Washington, DC, American Psychiatric Press, 1996, pp 395–412

Meins W, Dammast J: Do personality traits predict the occurrence of Alzheimer's disease? Int J Geriatr Psychiatry 15:120–124, 2000

Mittmann N, Herrmann N, Einarson TR, et al: The efficacy, safety and tolerability of antidepressants in late life depression. J Affect Disord 46:191–217, 1997

Molinari V, Kunik ME, Mulsant B, et al: The relationship between patient, informant, social worker, and consensus diagnoses of personality disorder in elderly depressed inpatients. Am J Geriatr Psychiatry 6:136–144, 1998

Montgomery SA: Late-life depression: rationalizing pharmacologic treatment options. Gerontology 48:392–400, 2002

Morris PL, Robinson RG: Personality, neuroticism, and depression after stroke. Int J Psychiatry Med 25:93–102, 1995

Morse JQ, Lynch TR: Personality disorders in late life. Curr Psychiatry Rep 2:24–31, 2000

Mulder RT: Personality pathology and treatment outcome in major depression: a review. Am J Psychiatry 159:359–371, 2002

Mulder RT, Joyce PR: Relationships of the Tridimensional Personality Questionnaire to mood and personality measures for depressed patients. Psychol Rep 75:1315–1325, 1994

Mulder RT, Joyce PR, Luty SE: The relationship of personality disorders to treatment outcome in depressed outpatients. J Clin Psychiatry 64:259–264, 2003

Oldehinkel AJ, Bouhuys AL, Brilman EI, et al: Functional disability and neuroticism as predictors of late life depression. Am J Geriatr Psychiatry 9:241–248, 2001

Ormel J, Oldehinkel AJ, Brilman EI: The interplay and etiological continuity of neuroticism, difficulties, and life events in the etiology of major and subsyndromal first and recurrent depressive episodes in later life. Am J Psychiatry 158:885–891, 2001

Paykel ES: Depressive typologies and response to amitriptyline. Br J Psychiatry 120:147–156, 1972

Pearlman IR: Group psychotherapy and the elderly. J Psychosoc Nurs Ment Health Serv 31:7–10, 1993

Pelissolo A, Corruble E: Personality factors in depressive disorders: contribution of the psychobiologic model developed by Cloninger. Encephale 28:363–373, 2002

Perry JC, Vaillant GE: Personality disorder, in Comprehensive Textbook of Psychiatry, 5th Edition. Edited by Kaplan HI, Saddock BJ. Baltimore, MD, Williams & Wilkins, 1989, pp 13–52

Peselow ED, Fieve RR, DiFiglia C: Personality traits and response to desipramine. J Affect Disord 24:209–216, 1992

Petersen T, Papakostas GI, Bottonari K, et al: NEO-FFI factor scores as predictors of clinical response to fluoxetine in depressed outpatients. Psychiatry Res 109:9–16, 2002

Pfohl B, Stangl D, Zimmerman M: The implications of DSM-III personality disorders for patients with major depression. J Affect Disord 7:309–318, 1984

Phillips KA, Gunderson JG, Hirschfeld RMA, et al: A review of the depressive personality. Am J Psychiatry 147:830–837, 1990

Post F: The management and nature of depressive illnesses in late life: a follow-through study. Br J Psychiatry 121:393–404, 1972

Rizvi SL, Linehan MM: Dialectical behavior therapy for personality disorders. Curr Psychiatry Rep 3:64–69, 2001

Roepke S, McAdams LA, Lindamer LA, et al: Personality profiles among normal aged individuals as measured by the NEO-PI-R. Aging Ment Health 5:159–164, 2001

Rossi A, Marinangeli MG, Butti G, et al: Personality disorders in bipolar and depressive disorders. J Affect Disord 65:3–8, 2001

Russell JM, Kornstein SG, Shea MT, et al: Chronic depression and comorbid personality disorders: response to sertraline versus imipramine. J Clin Psychiatry 64:554–561, 2003

Sadavoy J: Character disorders in the elderly: an overview, in Treating the Elderly With Psychotherapy: The Scope for Change in Later Life. Edited by Sadavoy J, Leszcz M. Madison, CT, International Universities Press, 1987, pp 175–229

Sadavoy J, Dorian B: Treatment of the elderly characterologically disturbed patient in the chronic care institution. J Geriatr Psychiatry 16:223–240, 1983

Sadavoy J, Fogel B: Personality disorders in old age, in Handbook of Mental Health and Aging, 2nd Edition. Edited by Birren J, Slane RB, Cohen GD. San Diego, CA, Academic Press, 1992, pp 433–462

Santor DA, Bagby RM, Joffe RT: Evaluating stability and change in personality and depression. J Pers Soc Psychol 73:1353–1362, 1997

Sato T, Sakado K, Sato S: Is there any specific personality disorder or personality disorder cluster that worsens the short-term treatment outcome of major depression? Acta Psychiatr Scand 88:342–349, 1993

Schrader G: Chronic depression: state or trait? J Nerv Ment Dis 182:552–555, 1994

Scott J: Chronic depression. Br J Psychiatry 153:287–297, 1988

Sharma VK, Copeland JR, Dewey ME, et al: Outcome of the depressed elderly living in the community in Liverpool: a 5 year follow-up. Psychol Med 28:1329–1337, 1998

Shawcross CR, Tyrer P: Influence of personality on response to monoamine oxidase inhibitors and tricyclic antidepressants. J Psychiatr Res 19:557–562, 1985

Shea MT, Leon AC, Mueller TI, et al: Does major depression result in lasting personality change? Am J Psychiatry 153:1404–1410, 1996

Solai LK, Mulsant BH, Pollock BG: Selective serotonin reuptake inhibitors for late-life depression: a comparative review. Drugs Aging 18:355–368, 2001

Spar JE, LaRue A: Concise Guide to Geriatric Psychiatry, 2nd Edition. Washington, DC, American Psychiatric Press, 1997, pp 34–49, 97–101

Stek ML, Van Exel E, Van Tilburg W, et al: The prognosis of depression in old age: outcome six to eight years after clinical treatment. Aging Ment Health 6:282–285, 2002

Steuer J: Psychotherapy with the elderly. Psychiatr Clin North Am 5:199–213, 1982

Strauss ME, Lee MM, DiFilippo JM: Premorbid personality and behavioral symptoms in Alzheimer disease: some cautions. Arch Neurol 54:257–259, 1997

Stuart S, Simons AD, Thase ME, et al: Are personality assessments valid in acute major depression? J Affect Disord 24:281–289, 1992

Swenson CR, Sanderson C, Dulit RA: The application of dialectical behavior therapy for patients with borderline personality disorder on inpatient units. Psychiatry Q 72:307–324, 2001

Thompson LW, Gallagher D, Breckenridge JS: Comparative effectiveness of psychotherapies for depressed elders. J Consult Clin Psychol 55:385–390, 1987

Thompson LW, Gallagher D, Czirr R: Personality disorder and outcome in the treatment of late life depression. J Geriatr Psychiatry 21:133–146, 1988

Ucok A, Karaveli D, Kundakci T, et al: Comorbidity of personality disorders with bipolar mood disorders. Compr Psychiatry 39:72–74, 1998

Van Gastel A, Schotte C, Maes M: The prediction of suicidal intent in depressed patients. Acta Psychiatr Scand 96:254–259, 1997

Vine RG, Steingart AB: Personality disorder in the elderly depressed. Can J Psychiatry 39:392–398, 1994

Weissman MM, Prusoff BA, Klerman GL: Personality and the prediction of long-term outcome of depression. Am J Psychiatry 135:797–800, 1978

Weissman MM, Leaf PJ, Bruce ML, et al: The epidemiology of dysthymia in five communities-rates, risks, comorbidity, and treatment. Am J Psychiatry 145:815–819, 1988

Wiener P, Alexopoulos GS, Kakuma T, et al: The limits of history taking in geriatric depression. Am J Geriatr Psychiatry 5:116–125, 1997

Yesavage JA, Karasu TB: Psychotherapy with the elderly. Am J Psychother 36:41–55, 1982

Yesavage JA, Brink TL, Rose TL, et al: Development and validation of a geriatric depression screening scale: a preliminary report. J Psychiatr Res 17:37–49, 1983

Young LT, Bagby RM, Cooke RG, et al: A comparison of Tridimensional Personality Questionnaire dimensions in bipolar disorder and unipolar depression. Psychiatry Res 58:139–143, 1995

Zuckerman DM, Prusoff BA, Weissman MM, et al: Personality as a predictor of psychotherapy and pharmacotherapy outcome for depressed outpatients. J Consult Clin Psychol 48:730–735, 1980

INDEX

*Page numbers printed in **boldface** type refer to tables or figures.*

Acetylcholine, and borderline
personality disorder, **25**
Adolescence and adolescents
depression and risk of personality
disorders in, 58–59
hypomanic traits in unipolar
depression and, 199
personality factors and
depression in, 229–258
treatment of bipolar disorder in,
215
Adrenocorticotropic hormone
(ACTH), and borderline
personality disorder, 21–22
Affect dysregulation, and treatment
of depression complicated by
personality disorders, 136
Affective instability, and personality
disorders, 20–24, 207–208
Age at onset
of depression in adolescents,
253
of depression comorbid with
personality disorders, 58–59,
97, 124
of dysthymic disorder in elderly,
273
Aggression, and dimensions of
personality, 25–27, 244
Agreeableness, as dimension of
personality. *See also* Dimensional
models

compliance with treatment and,
107
in conduct disorder and antisocial
personality disorder, 60
definition of, 7, **77**
depressive personality disorder
and, 75, 79
Akiskal, H.S., **67,** 194, 198, 199, 216,
273
Alcohol abuse. *See also* Substance
abuse
bipolar disorder comorbid with
personality disorders and,
190–191
social anxiety and, 32
Alzheimer's disease, 275
Amisulpride, 24
Amitriptyline, 22
Amoxapine, 169
Amphetamines
borderline personality disorder
and, 21, **25**
schizotypal personality disorder
and, 34
Anaclitic depression, 47
Anhedonia, and depressive
personality disorder, 78, 82
Animal models
of impulsivity and aggression,
25
personality types and, 14
psychoanalytic theory and, 6–7

Anticonvulsant drugs. *See also*
  Pharmacotherapy
  borderline personality disorder
    and, 23, 29
  refractory depression and, 168,
    170
Antidepressants. *See also*
  Pharmacotherapy; Selective
  serotonin reuptake inhibitors;
  Tricyclic antidepressants
  decrease of personality pathology
    in depressed patients and,
    160–161
  major depressive disorder and,
    104, **105,** 108–112, 141
  personality factors and response
    to, 108–112, 141, 161–165
  suicide risk in adolescents and,
    255–256
Antipsychotic drugs, and chronic
  depression comorbid with
  personality disorders, 169. *See
  also* Atypical antipsychotics
Antisocial behavior, and genetics, 24
Antisocial personality disorder
  conscientiousness and
    agreeableness dimensions
    and, 60
  neuroimaging studies of
    aggression and, 28
  role of serotonin in impulsivity
    and, 27
Anxiety
  negative affectivity/negative
    emotionality/neuroticism
    (NA/N) dimension and, 51,
    53
  psychobiology of personality
    disorders and, 30–32
Anxiety disorders
  borderline personality disorder
    and, 205
  cognitive-behavioral therapy for
    personality disorders and,
    170

incidence of comorbidity with
    Cluster C personality
    disorders, 31
Arabs, and history of concepts of
    personality, 4
Asian cultures, comparison to
    European in eighteenth century,
    14
Assessment. *See also* Diagnosis
  of chronic depression comorbid
    with personality disorders,
    165–166
  of depressive vulnerability factors
    in adolescents, 241–246
  of depressive personality
    disorder, 79–85
  of major depressive disorder
    complicated by personality
    disorders, 123–125
Asthenic personality disorder, **67**
Attachment, and vulnerability to
    depression in adolescents, **242,**
    244–245
Attention, and depression in
    adolescents, 243–244
Attributional style, and depression
    in adolescents, 241–242
Atypical antipsychotics. *See also*
    Antipsychotic drugs
  borderline personality disorder
    and, 30
  major depression complicated by
    personality disorders and,
    143
  refractory depression with
    comorbid personality
    disorders and, 168, 169, **170**
Autonomy/self-criticism (AUT-SC)
    personality dimension, 47–49,
    52, 54, 61
Avoidant personality disorder
  comorbidity of with social
    phobia, 30
  depressive personality disorder
    and, 81

Beard, Charles, 5
Beck, A.T., 47, 48
Beck, J., 130, 243
Beck Anxiety Inventory (BAI), 130
Beck Depression Inventory II (BDI-II), 129
Beck Hopelessness Inventory, 130
Behavior. *See* Aggression; Antisocial behavior; Behavior facilitation system; Behaviorism; Help-seeking behavior; Therapy-interfering behaviors
Behavioral therapy, for depression in elderly, 281. *See also* Cognitive-behavioral therapy; Dialectical Behavior Therapy
Behavior facilitation system, and negative affectivity/negative emotionality/neuroticism (NA/N) dimension, 51
Behaviorism, and concept of temperament, 9
Benefit/harm determination, and antidepressants for adolescents, 255–256
Benzodiazepines, and social anxiety, 32
Biopsychosocial approach, to treatment of depression in elderly, 283
Biosocial model, of treatment for depression complicated by personality disorders, 136
Bipolar disorder
    borderline personality disorder spectrum and, 202–209, 254
    elderly patients with personality disorders and, 274
    personality and continuum from disposition to disorder of, 194, 198–202
    personality disorders and comorbidity with, 188–194, **195–197,** 217–222

personality factors in treatment of, 213–217, **218**
    pharmacotherapy for chronic depression and, 167–168
    temperament and trait markers of, 209–213
Bipolar personality or bipolar temperament, 194, 198, 200–201, 206
Bipolar spectrum disorder, 125, 201–202
Borderline personality disorder
    adolescents and, 252–253, 255
    bipolar disorder and, 191, 193, 202–209, 214
    depressive personality disorder and, 81–82
    dialectical behavior therapy and, 172
    major depressive disorder comorbid with, 125
    pharmacotherapy for chronic depression and, 167–168
    psychobiology of affective instability and, 20–30
    research findings on depression and, 56–57
    substance abuse and, 255
Boundaries, and treatment of depression complicated by personality disorders, 150
Bupropion, 168
Buspirone, 167

Carbamazepine, and borderline personality disorder, 23, 29–30
Case examples
    of bipolar disorder comorbid with personality disorders, 202–204, 220–222
    of compliance with medication, 107
    of depression in adolescents, 247–252, 254–255, 256–257
    of depression in elderly, 282–283

Case examples *(continued)*
of depressive personality
disorder, 80
of major depressive disorder, 105,
107
of mixed personality disorder and
major depression, 122–123,
124–125, 127–129, 130–140
Case formulation, and major
depression complicated by
personality disorders, 130–135
Categorical approach, to depression
and personality disorders, 66–
73, 269–270
Center for Epidemiologic Studies
Depression Scale (CES-D), 103
Central nervous system (CNS), and
role of serotonin in aggression,
27
Characteristics, and definition of
personality, 230
Character spectrum dysphoria, **55,**
56
Cheever, John, 8
Chess, Stella, 9–10
Childhood abuse, and borderline
personality disorder, 21–22
China, definition of personality in
ancient, 3
Cholinergic system, and affective
instability, 20–21
Chronic depression. *See* Major
depressive disorder;
Refractory depression
Citalopram
depression in elderly and,
279
impulsive-aggressive behavior in
personality disorders and, 29
Clinical typologies, and personality-
depression relationship, 54–60
Clomipramine
chronic depression comorbid
with personality disorders
and, 167

major depressive disorder and,
109, 110
Clonazepam, 31
Clonidine, 31
Cloninger, C.R., 47, 101. *See also*
Dimensional models
Clozapine, 30
Cluster A personality disorders
DSM-IV-TR categorization of, 19,
158
pharmacotherapy for chronic
depression comorbid with,
168–169
psychobiology of,
32–34
Cluster B personality disorders
DSM-IV-TR categorization of, 19,
158
pharmacotherapy for aggression
in, 29–30
pharmacotherapy for refractory
depression comorbid with,
167–168
psychotherapy for depression in
elderly and, 281
Cluster C personality disorders
anxiety-related traits and, 30,
31
DSM-IV-TR categorization of, 19,
158
major depressive disorder in
elderly and, 271
pharmacotherapy for chronic
depression comorbid with,
167
Cognitive Behavioral Analysis
System of Psychotherapy
(CBASP), 86, 127, 136, 174,
175
Cognitive-behavioral therapy (CBT).
See also Behavioral therapy;
Cognitive therapy;
Psychotherapy
for adolescents with depression,
255

for chronic or refractory
depression comorbid with
personality disorders, 162,
169–172
for depression in elderly, 281
for depressive personality
disorder, 86–87
for major depressive disorder
complicated with personality
disorders, 126, 144–151
Cognitive conceptualization
diagram, 130, **132**
Cognitive function. *See also*
Cognitive personality factors;
Cognitive theory;
Neurocognitive factors
diagnosis of depression in elderly
and, 269
schizotypal personality disorder
and, 33, 34
Cognitive model, of depression, 130–
135, 243
Cognitive personality factors, and
depression in adolescents, 241–
243
Cognitive theory, of depression, 47
Cognitive therapy, for relapse
prevention in bipolar disorder,
216. *See also* Cognitive-
behavioral therapy
Collateral sources
diagnosis and treatment of
depression in elderly and,
269, 277, 283
of information on depression in
adolescents, 251
Combination treatment
of chronic or refractory
depression comorbid with
personality disorders, 174–
175
of depression in elderly, 283
Common-cause models, of
personality-depression
relationship, 45, 238

Communication, and split treatment,
142
Comorbidity, of psychiatric
disorders
of anxiety disorders and Cluster
C personality disorders, 31
of bipolar disorder and borderline
personality disorder,
202–209
of bipolar disorder with
personality disorders, 188–
194, 217–222
depressive personality disorder
and, 70–71
treatment of major depressive
disorder complicated by
personality disorders and,
121–151
Compensatory strategies, and
depression complicated by
personality disorders, **132,** 134
Compliance, with treatment. *See also*
Resistance
major depressive disorder with
comorbid personality
disorder and, 104–107, 113,
139–140
personality factors in bipolar
disorder and, 214
psychotherapy for treatment-
refractory depression and,
171
Complication (scar) models, of
personality-depression
relationship, **45,** 46, 57, 217, 238
Conditional assumptions, and major
depression complicated by
personality disorders, **131**
Conduct disorder, and
conscientiousness or
agreeableness dimensions, 60
Confidentiality, and treatment of
depression in elderly, 277
Congruency model, of vulnerability,
232, 238

Conscientiousness, as dimension of personality. *See also* Dimensional models
  bipolar disorder and, 211
  in conduct disorder and antisocial personality disorder, 60
  definition of, 7, **77**
  depressive personality disorder and, 75, 79
Constraint, temperamental, 11–12
Contextual factors, and depression in adolescents, 249–250
Continuity, of personality over time, 231
Coolidge Axis II Inventory (CATI), 84
Cooperativeness, and major depressive disorder, 101–102
Core beliefs, and major depression complicated by personality disorders, **131**, 133, 149
Cost, and pharmacotherapy for major depression complicated by personality disorders, 141–142
Countertransference, and major depression complicated by personality disorders, 140
Creativity, and bipolar disorder, 212
Criminal offenders, and role of serotonin in impulsive aggression, 26, 27
Cross-sectional interviews, for diagnosis of depression in elderly, 269
Culture and cultural factors
  major depressive disorder and, 98
  personality types and, 13–14
  self-report evidence and, 15–17
Cyclothymia, and borderline personality disorder, 206
Cyclothymic personality disorder, 67
Cyclothymic temperament, and bipolar disorder, 199

Defense mechanisms, and major depression complicated by personality disorders, 134–135
Dementia, and depression in elderly, 275
Dependency. *See also* Dimensional models; Interpersonal dependency
  bipolar disorder and, 212
  cognitive theory of depression and, 47
  personality in adolescents and, 235, 241
  treatment of depression in adolescents and, 249
Dependent personality disorder
  bipolar disorder and, 193
  depressive personality disorder and, 81
Depression. *See also* Depressive personality disorder; Double depression; Major depressive disorder; Refractory depression
  borderline personality disorder and comorbid, 21–22
  clinical typologies and relationship of to personality, 54–60
  impulsivity and risk of suicidal behavior in, 28
  models of relation to personality, 44–54
  personality disorders and assessment or treatment of chronic and refractory, 157–176
  personality disorders in elderly and, 267–284
  personality factors in adolescents and, 229–258
Depression spectrum disease, 55
Depressive invalidism, 273
Depressive neurosis, **67**

Depressive personality disorder
(DPD)
affective instability and, 23–24
assessment of, 79–85
categorical approach to, 66–73
clinical description of, 80
construct validity of, 65–66
dimensional approach to, 73–79
DSM-IV-TR and, 23, 65
treatment of, 72–73, 85–88
Depressive Personality Disorder
Inventory (DPDI), 85
Depressive reaction, **67**
Depressive realism, 249
Depressive temperament (DT), 216
Desipramine, 109, 110
Developmental framework, for
vulnerability factors in
adolescence, 235–238, **242**
Diagnosis. *See* Assessment;
Diagnostic validity; Differential
diagnosis
of depressive personality
disorder, 69
misdiagnosis of borderline
personality disorder and, 209
of personality disorders and
depression in elderly, 268–
270
Diagnostic Interview for Depressive
Personality (DIDP), 84–85
Diagnostic Interview for DSM-IV
Personality Disorders (DIPD),
83
Diagnostic Interview for Genetic
Studies, 216
Diagnostic validity, of depressive
personality disorder, 69–70
Dialectical Behavior Therapy (DBT).
See also Behavioral therapy
chronic or refractory depression
comorbid with personality
disorders and, 172
depression in elderly and, 281,
282

major depression complicated by
personality disorders and,
136, 144, 146
Diathesis model, of vulnerability, **232**
Diathesis-stress model, of
personality-depression
relationship, 46, 49, **232**
Differential diagnosis. *See also*
Diagnosis
of depression in elderly, 277
of depressive personality
disorder, 79–83
Dimensional models, of personality.
See also Agreeableness;
Conscientiousness;
Dependency; Extraversion;
Five-factor model; Harm
avoidance; Neuroticism;
Novelty seeking; Openness;
Seven-factor model
comorbidity of bipolar disorder
and borderline personality
disorder, 208
depressive personality disorder
and, 73–79
development of, 7–8
major depressive disorder and,
99–102, 109–112
personality-depression
relationship and, 47–54
Directive therapy, and depression in
elderly, 280
Disciplined personal involvement
concept, and treatment of
depression complicated by
personality disorders, 150
Distal effects, of vulnerability, 239–241
Divalproex sodium, and borderline
personality disorder, 23, 29
Dominant goal personalities, 48
Dopamine and dopaminergic system
affective instability in borderline
personality disorder and, **25**
schizophrenia and, 32
social anxiety and, 31

Double depression
  chronic depression in elderly and,
    273
  comorbid personality disorders
    and treatment outcome in,
    163, 175
Draper, George, 4
DSM-III
  depressive personality disorder
    and, 68
  separate axis for personality
    disorders in, 43
DSM-III-R, and depressive
    personality disorder, 67
DSM-IV, and depressive personality
    disorder, 67, 68, **69**, 82
DSM-IV-TR
  categorization of personality
    disorders in, 19, 158
  definition of personality
    disorders in, 246
  depressive personality disorder
    and, 23, 65, 67
  major depressive disorder and, 98
  mixed personality disorder
    comorbid with unipolar
    affective illness in, 125
  personality disorders in
    adolescence and, 252
Dynamic model, of vulnerability, 239
Dysfunctional attitudes, and acute
    depression, 159
Dysfunctional Attitudes Scale (DAS),
    130
Dysregulation. *See* Regulation
Dysthymic disorder
  bipolar disorder and, 198
  comorbid personality disorders
    and, 124, 163
  depressive personality disorder
    and, 24, 67–68, 70–71, 80, 82
  elderly patients and, 272–273
  subaffective form of, **55**, 56

Education. *See* Psychoeducation

Elderly
  definition of, 267
  diagnostic issues in, 268–270
  dysthymic disorder in,
    272–273
  longitudinal review of affective
    disorder and personality
    disorder in, 253
  major depressive disorder in,
    270–272
  suicide and, 275
  treatment issues for, 276–283
Electroconvulsive therapy (ECT)
  chronic depression comorbid
    with personality disorders
    and, 169
  depression in elderly and, 279–
    280
Emotional dysregulation, in
    depressed patients with
    personality disorders,
    172
Emotional strength, and bipolar
    disorder, 212
Environment
  concepts of temperament and, 10,
    12
  genetics and development of
    personality, 159
Epidemiologic Catchment Area
    study, 102
Epidemiology, of depressive
    personality disorder, 71. *See also*
    Prevalence
Equifinality, and development of
    personality in adolescence,
    236–237
Europe, comparison to Asian
    cultures of eighteenth century,
    14
European Depression
    Epidemiological Survey
    (DEPRES), 102
Evolution, and personality
    disorders, 100

Exacerbation model, of personality-depression relationship, 238

Executive functioning, and depression in adolescents, 243–244

Explanatory style, and depression in adolescents, 241–242

Extraversion, as dimension of personality. *See also* Dimensional models; Introversion
  bipolar disorder and, 211, 212
  compliance with treatment and, 107
  definition of, 7, **76**
  depressive personality disorder and, 75, 79
  major depressive disorder and, 100–101, 102, 110–112

Eysenck, H. J., 100

Eysenck Personality Inventory, 101, 103, 105, 109–110, 214

Factor analysis
  of depressive personality disorder, 75
  of mania subtypes in bipolar disorder, 199–200
  of temperamental dimensions associated with depression, 49–53

Family. *See also* Collateral sources; Family studies; Family therapy; Parents
  depression in adolescents and dysfunction of, 257
  diagnosis and treatment of depression in elderly and, 269, 277
  psychotherapy for refractory depression and, **171**

Family studies. *See also* Genetics
  of bipolar disorder, 199, 201, 254
  of borderline personality disorder, 20

of depressive personality disorder, 72, **73**

Family therapy, for depression in elderly, 282

Feedback, and treatment of patients with chronic or refractory depression, **167, 171**

Fenfluramine, 31

Five-factor model (FFM), of personality dimensions. *See also* Dimensional models
  bipolar disorder and, 210, 211–212
  depressive personality disorder and, 74–79
  integrative model and, 59–60
  major depressive disorder and, 102
  stability of personality in adolescents and, 234

Fluoxetine
  borderline personality disorder and, 22, 29
  depression in adolescents and, 255
  major depressive disorder and, 109, 110, 111, 124, 143
  refractory depression comorbid with personality disorders and, 168

Fluvoxamine, 22

Food and Drug Administration, U.S. (FDA), 256

Freud, Sigmund, 5–7, 13

Galen, 3, 4, 8, 13, 17, 231

Gall, Franz, 4

Gender
  help-seeking behavior in major depressive disorder and, 103, 113
  prevalence of major depressive disorder and, 97

Genetics. *See also* Family studies; Twin studies
  antisocial behavior and, 24

Genetics *(continued)*
contribution of to personality and
temperament, 13
environment and development of
personality, 159
serotonergic system and
aggression, 27
stress responsiveness and, 165
Geriatric patients. *See* Elderly
Greece, definition of personality in
ancient, 3, 4. *See also* Galen
Group therapy
for depression in elderly, 282
for major depression complicated
by personality disorders,
150
Growth hormone, and borderline
personality disorder, 21, **25**
Guidelines
for antidepressant use in
adolescents, 256
for pharmacotherapy with
treatment-refractory
depression, **170**
for psychotherapy with
treatment-refractory
depression, **171**
for treatment of major depression
complicated by personality
disorders, 126–140

Haloperidol
borderline personality disorder
and, 30
schizotypal personality disorder
and, 34
Hamilton Rating Scale for
Depression (Ham-D), 109, 112,
129
Harm avoidance. *See also*
Dimensional models
bipolar disorder and, 211, 212
depression in elderly and, 276
depressive personality disorder
and, 79

major depressive disorder and,
101–102, 103, **104,** 113, 271–
272
Help-seeking behavior, and major
depressive disorder, 102–103,
113
Hippocrates, 4
Histrionic personality disorder
bipolar disorder and, 190, 191,
193, 214
schizophrenia and, 189
Homework assignments, and
treatment of depression
comorbid with personality
disorders, 170–171
Hooton, Ernst, 9
Hopelessness, and depressive
personality disorder, 68,
71
Human Genome Project, 13
Human immunodeficiency virus
(HIV), and bipolar disorder,
199
Hyperthymic temperament (HT),
216
Hypomania, and bipolar disorder,
198, 199, 206
Hypothalamic-pituitary-adrenal
(HPA) axis, and borderline
personality disorder associated
with depression, 21–22

Ibn Ridwan, 4
Imipramine
major depressive disorder and,
108
social anxiety and, 31
Impaired functioning, and treatment
of depressive personality
disorder, 72–73
Impulsivity
bipolar disorder and, 199, 207–
208, 212
borderline personality disorder
and, 24–30, 207–208

Independence model, of personality-depression relationship, 44, **45,** 60

Inhibition
definition of personality and, 3
mood disorders and control of, 244

Insight-oriented approach, to psychotherapy for depression in elderly, 280

Integrative models, of personality traits and disorders, 59–60

Integrative treatment, of chronic depression and comorbid personality disorders, 165–175

Intermittent explosive disorder (IED), 28

International Personality Disorder Examination (IPDE), 83–84

Interpersonal dependency, and cognitive theory of depression, 47. *See also* Dependency

Interpersonal Dependency Inventory, 214

Interpersonal models, of depression, 244–245

Interpersonal psychotherapy (IPT)
for chronic or refractory depression comorbid with personality disorders, 162, 172–173
for depression in elderly, 281–282

Interpersonal rejection. *See also* Relationships
bipolar disorder and sensitivity to, 212
personality in adolescents and, 235

Introjective depression, 48

Introversion, sources of data and meaning of, 15. *See also* Extraversion

Inventory of Interpersonal Problems, 106

Ipsapirone, 27

James, Alice, 8

Kant, Immanuel, 4
Karolinska Scales of Personality, 106
Kraepelin, Emil, 66, **67,** 194
Kretschemer, Ernst, 4, 194
Kuhn, Thomas, 16

Lamotrigine
major depression complicated by personality disorders and, 143
refractory depression in bipolar patients and, 168

Lenin, V.I., 5

Levodopa, 31

Life-charting approach, to treatment of bipolar disorder, 215

Life events. *See also* Stress
association of depression and personality disorders with, 160, 165
depression in adolescents and, 241–242, 249–250
depressive episodes in borderline personality disorder and, 57
treatment outcome in chronic depression and, 163

Life history, and major depression complicated by personality disorders, **131**

Life review, and depression in elderly, 282

Limited reparenting, and treatment of major depression complicated by personality disorders, 150

Lithium
bipolar and borderline personality disorders and, 168
chronic or refractory depression comorbid with personality disorders and, **170**
major depressive disorder and, 108

Locus of control, and depression in elderly, 277–278

Lombroso, Cesare, 4

Longitudinal review, of depression in adolescents, 253, 257

Major depressive disorder (MDD). *See also* Depression
borderline personality disorder comorbid with, 205
comorbid personality disorders and treatment of, 121–151
dimensional models of personality and, 99–102
in elderly patients, 270–272
maladaptive personality functioning as risk factor for, 112
personality disorder and development of, 98–99
personality and response to antidepressants in, 108–112
personality and treatment of, 102–107
prevalence of, 97
vulnerabilities to, 97–98

Mania, and personality disorders comorbid with bipolar disorder, 191–192, 198

Maprotiline, 110

Mayr, Ernst, 13

Medical illness, and depression in elderly, 270, 274–275, 277

Medication Event Monitoring System (MEMS), 106–107

Mental status examination, and depression in elderly, 277, **278**

Millon Clinical Multiaxial Inventory—III (MCMI-III), 84

Mind Over Mood: Change How You Feel By Changing the Way You Think (Greenberger and Padesky 1995), 145

Minnesota Multiphasic Personality Inventory (MMPI-2), 106

Mirtazapine, 167

Moclobemide, 105

Monoamine oxidase inhibitors (MAOIs). *See also* Pharmacotherapy
borderline personality disorder and, 22–23
chronic depression comorbid with personality disorders and, 167
social anxiety and, 32

Mood cycling, and bipolar disorder, 198–199

Mood stabilizers. *See also* Pharmacotherapy
bipolar disorder and, 200, 206, 217
borderline personality disorder and, 23, 29, 206
major depression complicated by personality disorders and, 143

Multifinality, and development of personality in adolescence, 236–237

Multimodal approach, to treatment of major depression complicated by personality disorders, 126–127

Narcissistic personality disorder, 191, 192

National Comorbidity Survey, 102

National Institute of Mental Health Treatment of Depression Collaborative Research Program, 248

Nefazodone
chronic depression comorbid with personality disorders and, 167, 175
major depressive disorder and, 110

Negative affectivity/negative emotionality/neuroticism (NA/N) dimension, 49–53

NEO (neuroticism, extraversion, openness) Personality Inventory (NEO-PI), 269
NEO short version (NEO-FFI), 114
Neurasthenic neurosis, **67**
Neurochemistry, and concepts of temperament, 11
Neurocognitive factors, and vulnerability to depression in adolescents, **242**
Neuroimaging studies
    of impulsivity and aggression in personality disorders, 27–28
    of schizotypal personality disorder, 33
Neuroleptics. *See also* Pharmacotherapy
    borderline personality disorder and, 30
    schizotypal personality disorder and, 33
Neurological examination, and depression in elderly, 277
Neuropsychological studies
    of prefrontal cortex and aggression, 28
    of schizotypal personality disorder, 33
Neurotic depression, 54, **55**
Neuroticism, as dimension of personality. *See also* Dimensional models
    bipolar disorder and, 211, 212
    definition of, 7, **76**, 159
    depressive personality disorder and, 75, 79
    major depressive disorder and, 100–101, 102, 110–112, 113–114, 272
    risk for personality disorders and depression and, 60–61
    suicidal ideation and depression in elderly patients and, 275
    theoretical and referential meanings of, 15

treatment of depression in elderly and, 276
Norepinephrine and noradrenergic system, and borderline personality disorder, 21, **25**
Normal variation, and depressive personality disorder, 82–83
Nortriptyline
    borderline personality disorder and, 22
    major depressive disorder and, 109
Novelty seeking. *See also* Dimensional models
    bipolar disorder and, 211, 212
    compliance with medication and, 107
    definition of, 101
    major depressive disorder and, 103, **104**, 113

Obsessive-compulsive personality disorder
    bipolar disorder and, 190, 191, 193
    depressive personality disorder and, 81
Olanzapine, 143, 168
Ontario Health Survey, 102
Openness, as dimension of personality. *See also* Dimensional models
    bipolar disorder and, 211
    compliance with treatment and, 107
    definition of, 7, **76**
    depressive personality disorder and, 78
Others, interchange with, and cognitive models of depression, 242–243

Parents, and treatment of depression in adolescents, 251, 256, 257. *See also* Family; Limited reparenting
Parkinson's disease, 31

Paroxetine, 111
Passive-aggressive personality disorder, 108
Pathoplasty models, of personality-depression relationship, 44–45, 52, 53, 57–58, 217, 238
Patient history, and depression in elderly, 277, **278**
Pavlov, I.P., 5
Peer pressure, and vulnerability factors in adolescents, 235, 244
Perfectionism
    bipolar disorder and, 212
    treatment of depression in adolescents and, 248, 252
Persistence
    definition of, 101
    major depressive disorder and, **104**
Personality. *See also* Dimensional models; Personality disorders; Personality traits; Personality types; Temperament
    bipolar disorder and continuum of, 194, 198–202
    concepts of temperament and, 12–13
    definition of, 3–4, 230–231
    depression in adolescents and, 229–258
    depressive personality disorder and, 87–88
    Freud and psychoanalytic theory on, 5–7
    major depressive disorder and maladaptive functioning of, 112
    models of relationship of depression to, 44–54
    theoretical and referential meanings of, 15–17
    treatment of bipolar disorder and, 213–217, **218**

treatment of major depressive disorder and, 102–107
Personality Diagnostic Questionnaire-4+ (PDQ-4+), 84
Personality Diagnostic Questionnaire—Revised (PDQ-R), 108, 189–190, 214, 215
Personality dimensions. *See* Dimensional models; Five-factor model; Personality traits; Seven-factor model
Personality disorders. *See also* Cluster A personality disorders; Cluster B personality disorders; Cluster C personality disorders; *specific disorders*
    antidepressant response in chronic depression and, 161–165
    assessment and treatment of refractory and chronic depression and, 157–176
    bipolar disorder and comorbidity with, 188–202, 217–222
    clinical typologies and relationship of depression to, 54–60
    definition of in DSM-IV-TR, 246
    depression in elderly and, 267–284
    major depressive disorder and, 98–99, 121–151
    psychobiology of, 19–35
Personality traits, and classification of personality, 158–161. *See also* Dimensional models; Five-factor model; Seven-factor model
Personality types, and cultural influences, 13–14

Pharmacotherapy. *See also*
Anticonvulsant drugs;
Antidepressants; Antipsychotic
drugs; Compliance; Monoamine
oxidase inhibitors; Mood
stabilizers; Neuroleptics;
Selective serotonin reuptake
inhibitors; Side effects;
Treatment
affective instability in borderline
personality disorder and, 22–
23
aggression in Cluster B
personality disorders and,
29–30
chronic or refractory depression
comorbid with personality
disorders and, 166–169, **170**
depression in adolescents and,
255–256, 257
depression in elderly and, 278,
279
depressive personality disorder
and, 85–86
major depressive disorder
comorbid with personality
disorders and, 113, 140–143
schizotypal personality disorder
and, 33–34
social anxiety disorder and, 31–32
Phenelzine
affective instability in borderline
patients and, 23
chronic depression comorbid
with personality disorders
and, 167
social anxiety and, 32
Phenytoin, 30
Physical examination, and diagnosis
of depression in elderly, 277
Physostigmine, and affective
instability, 20
Positive affectivity/positive
emotionality/extraversion (PA/
E) dimension, 49–53, 60

Poststroke depression, 275
Predisposition models. *See*
Vulnerability models
Prevalence. *See also* Epidemiology
of alcohol use disorder comorbid
with personality disorders,
191
of depressive personality
disorder, 71
of major depressive disorder, 97,
270, 271
of mood disorders in adolescents,
238
of personality disorders in bipolar
patients, 188–189, 190, 191–
192, 193, **195–197**, 274
of personality disorders in
chronic depression patients,
162
of personality disorders and
depression in elderly
patients, 268
Privacy, and treatment of depression
in elderly, 277
Procaine, and affective instability,
20–21
Prolactin response, and borderline
personality disorder, 21, **25,** 26–
27
Proximal effects, of vulnerability,
239–241
Psychoanalytic theory, and concepts
of personality and
temperament, 5–7
Psychobiology, of personality
disorders
anxiety-related traits and,
30–32
bipolar disorder and, 210–211
borderline personality disorder
and, 20–30
DSM-IV-TR categorization system
and, 19
major depressive disorder and,
100–101

Psychobiology, of personality
  disorders *(continued)*
  schizotypy and Cluster A
    personality disorders,
    32–34
Psychodynamic psychotherapy. *See
  also* Psychotherapy
  for depression in elderly,
    281
  for major depressive disorder
    comorbid with personality
    disorders, 126,
    144–151
Psychoeducation
  major depression complicated by
    personality disorders and,
    149
  treatment of depression in
    adolescents and,
    257
  treatment of depression in elderly
    and, 282
Psychometric instruments. *See*
  Rating instruments
Psychosis and psychotic symptoms.
  See also Psychotic depression;
  Psychoticism
  pharmacotherapy for chronic or
    refractory depression and
    Cluster A
    personality disorders, 168–
    169
  psychobiology of Cluster A
    personality disorders and,
    32
Psychosocial factors
  proximal and distal effects of
    vulnerability and,
    239–240
  in treatment of bipolar disorder,
    214–215
Psychosocial therapy, for treatment
  of refractory depression
  comorbid with personality
  disorders, 169, 173

Psychotherapy. *See also* Cognitive-
  behavioral therapy; Dialectical
  Behavior Therapy; Family
  therapy; Group therapy;
  Interpersonal psychotherapy;
  Psychodynamic psychotherapy;
  Treatment
  for depression in adolescents,
    257
  for depression in elderly, 280–283
  for depressive personality
    disorder, 86–87
  for major depressive disorder
    complicated by personality
    disorders, 126, 143–151
  for refractory or chronic
    depression comorbid with
    personality disorders, 169–
    174
Psychotic depression, 169
Psychoticism, and major depressive
  disorder, 100–101. *See also*
  Psychosis and psychotic
  symptoms
Public health, and depression in late
  life, 276

Quality of life, and depression in
  elderly, 272
Questionnaire data, and personality
  dimensions, 8

Rating instruments
  assessment of depression in
    adolescents and, 246
  depressive personality disorder
    and, 83–85
  treatment of depression in elderly
    and, **278**
  treatment of major depression
    complicated by personality
    disorders and, 129–130
Reactivity, and concepts of
  temperament, 10–11, 11–12,
    244

Reassurance seeking, and depression in adolescents, 244–245

Refractory depression. *See also* Depression; Major depressive disorder
pharmacotherapy for, 167–169
psychotherapy for, 169–174
relationship between personality and, 164–165

Regulation, and concepts of temperament, 10–11. *See also* Affect dysregulation; Emotional dysregulation; Self-regulation

Reinventing Your Life: How to Break Free From Negative Life Patterns and Feel Good Again (Young and Klosko 1994), 145

Relapse prevention
cognitive therapy for bipolar disorder and, 216
depression in adolescents and, 257
major depression complicated by personality disorders and, 149–151

Relationships. *See also* Interpersonal rejection; Peer pressure; Social support
depressive personality disorder and, 81
vulnerability factors in adolescence and, 235

Reliability, and diagnosis of depressive personality disorder, 69

Reminiscence group therapy, 282

Resistance, and treatment of major depression complicated by personality disorders, 139–140. *See also* Compliance

Response Style Questionnaire (RSQ), 112

Revised NEO Personality Inventory (NEO-PI-R), 85, 102, 106, 107, 111, 112

Reward dependence
definition of, 101
major depressive disorder and, 103, **104**

Risk and risk taking
bipolar disorder and, 199
definition of vulnerability and, 231–233

Risperidone, 30

Rothbart, Mary, 10–11

Scar hypothesis, and major depressive episodes in elderly, 271

Scar models. *See* Complication models

Schema-based therapy, for depressive personality disorder, 86–87

Schemas, and major depression complicated by personality disorders, 130, 133, 134

Schizoid personality disorder, and bipolar disorder, 193

Schizophrenia
bipolar disorder and, 189
dopamine hypothesis for, 32
schizotypal personality disorder and, 32

Schizotaxia, 34

Schizotypal personality disorder
bipolar disorder and, 193
psychobiology of, 32–34

Schneider, Kurt, 66–67

Seasonal affective disorder, 211

Selective serotonin reuptake inhibitors (SSRIs). *See also* Antidepressants; Pharmacotherapy
affective instability in borderline personality disorder and, 22
chronic or refractory depression comorbid with personality disorders and, 167, **170**

Selective serotonin reuptake
inhibitors (SSRIs) *(continued)*
depression in adolescents and,
255, 256
depression in elderly and, 279
major depressive disorder and,
109
social anxiety and, 31
Self, and cognitive models of
depression, 242–243
Self-consciousness, and depressive
personality disorder, 79
Self-criticism, and depression in
adolescents, 233, 241, 249. *See
also* Autonomy/self-criticism
personality dimension
Self-directedness, and major
depressive disorder, 101–102
Self-esteem
bipolar disorder and, 216
depressive personality disorder
and, 68, 71
Self-Esteem and Stigma
Questionnaire, 216
Self-help cognitive-behavioral
therapy manuals, 145
Self-regulation, and concepts of
temperament, 10–11, 244. *See
also* Regulation
Self-report evidence
assessment of major depression
complicated by personality
disorders and, 127–129
cultural influences on, 15
diagnosis of personality disorders
and, 189–190
Self-transcendence, and major
depressive disorder, 101
Serotonin and serotonergic system
affective instability in borderline
personality disorder and,
21
impulsivity and aggression in
Cluster B personality
disorders and, 25–27, 29

refractory depression and, 164–
165
social anxiety and, 31
Sertraline
depression in elderly and, 279
impulsive-aggressive behavior in
personality disorder and, 29
major depressive disorder and,
108
social anxiety and, 31
Seven-factor model, of personality
dimensions. *See also*
Dimensional models
depression in elderly and, 269
major depressive disorder and,
101–102, 109–110
Severity, of vulnerability to
depression in adolescents, 245–
246
Side effects, of medication and
compliance issues, 105
Skills training, and treatment of
depression in adolescents,
257
Social network. *See* Social support
Social phobia
comorbidity of with avoidant
personality disorder, 30
pharmacotherapy for, 31–32
psychobiology of, 31
Social skills training (SST), and
chronic or refractory depression
comorbid with personality
disorders, 173
Social support. *See also* Relationships
chronic depression with
comorbid personality
disorders and, 163, 164, 165
depression in adolescents and,
244–245
depressive personality disorder
and, 81
Socialization, and major depression
complicated by personality
disorders, 135–140

Sociotropy/dependency (SOC-DEP) personality dimension, 47–49, 52, 54, 61

Spectrum models, of personality-depression relationship, 45–46, 53, 57, 217, 219. *See also* Bipolar spectrum disorder

Split treatment, for major depression complicated by personality disorders, 142

Spontaneous mania, and bipolar disorder, 206

Spurzheim, Johann Gaspar, 4

Stability
diagnosis of depressive personality disorder and, 69
of personality over time, 231
of personality in young adults, 234–235

Staged therapy, for major depression with personality disorders, 127

Stanley Foundation Bipolar Network, 215, 219

State dependence model, of personality-depression relationship, 238

Strategic approach, to treatment of major depression with personality disorders, 126–127

Stress. *See also* Life events
genetics and response to, 165
relationship between depression and personality disorders and, 160, 165

Stroke, and depression, 274–275

Structured Clinical Interview for DSM-III Personality Disorders (SCID), 108, 191

Structured Clinical Interview for DSM-IV Axis II Personality Disorders (SCID-II), 83, 192, 213, 214, 215, 253

Structured Interview for DSM Personality (SIDP), 188–189

Structured Interview for DSM-IV Personality (SIDP-IV), 83–84

Structured Interview for the Five Factor Model (SIFFM), 85

Subclinical model. *See* Spectrum models

Substance abuse. *See also* Alcohol abuse
in adolescents with personality disorder and depression, 255
borderline personality disorder and, 205

Suicide and suicidal ideation
antidepressant use in adolescents and, 255–256
bipolar disorder and, 168, 215
elderly patients and, 275
impulsivity in depression and risk of, 28
major depressive disorder with comorbid personality disorder and, 103, 137–138, 271

Supportive psychotherapy, for depression in elderly, 280

Symptom presentation, and personality factors in major depressive disorder, 103, **104**

Systematic Treatment Enhancement Program for Bipolar Disorder (STEP-BD), 219

Temperament. *See also* Personality
bipolar disorder and, 209–213
classification of personality and, 158–161
definition and concepts of, 3–4, 8–13
depression in adolescents and, 243–244
seven-factor model of, 101–102
theoretical and referential meanings of, 15–17

Temperament and Character
Inventory (TCI), 101–102, 103,
109, 269
Tendencies, and definition of
personality, 230
Therapeutic alliance, and major
depression complicated by
personality disorders, 139, 147
Therapy-interfering behaviors, and
major depression complicated
by personality disorders, 135–
140
Thiothixene
borderline personality disorder
and, 30
schizotypal personality disorder
and, 34
Thomas, Alexander, 9–10
Trait markers, of bipolar disorder,
209–213. *See also* Personality
traits
Tranylcypromine, 22
Treatment. *See also* Combination
treatment; Compliance;
Countertransference;
Electroconvulsive therapy;
Integrative treatment;
Pharmacotherapy;
Psychotherapy; Relapse
prevention; Split treatment;
Therapeutic alliance
chronic depression comorbid
with personality disorders
and integrative, 165–175
of depression in adolescents, 247–
257
of depression in elderly,
276–283
of depressive personality
disorder, 72–73, 85–88
of major depressive disorder with
comorbid personality
disorder, 102–107, 121–151
personality factors in bipolar
disorder and, 213–217, **218**

Tricylic antidepressants (TCAs). *See
also* Antidepressants
chronic depression comorbid
with personality disorders
and, 167
major depressive disorder and,
108, 109
psychobiology of affective
instability and, 21,
22
Tridimensional Personality
Questionnaire (TPQ), 101, 106,
109, 110, 210–211, 269
Tripartite model, of personality-
depression relationship,
49–53
Tryptophan hydroxylase (TPH), and
aggression, 27
Twin studies. *See also* Genetics;
Family studies
of borderline personality
disorder, 24
of personality and major
depression in women,
53

Venlafaxine, 167
von Zerssen, D., 194, 201
Vulnerabilities, to psychiatric
disorders
assessment of depression in
adolescents and, 241–246,
248–252
definition of personality and,
230–234
major depressive disorder and,
97–98
personality in adolescents and,
234–241
Vulnerability models, of personality-
depression relationship, 46, 47–
49, 57, 58, 217

Wisconsin Card Sorting Test
(WCST), 33, 34